MYSTERIOUSLY MISSING
COLLEGE COURSES

MYSTERIOUSLY MISSING COLLEGE COURSES

—— **IMPORTANT** ——
Information That Is Nearly
—— **NEVER** ——
Covered in a University or College Course

JOHN M. MEMORY, Ph.D., J.D.

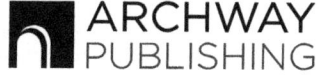
ARCHWAY
PUBLISHING

Scriptures taken from the Holy Bible, New International Version®, NIV®. Copyright © 1973, 1978, 1984, 2011 by Biblica, Inc.™ Used by permission of Zondervan. All rights reserved worldwide. www.zondervan.com The "NIV" and "New International Version" are trademarks registered in the United States Patent and Trademark Office by Biblica, Inc.™

Archway Publishing books may be ordered through booksellers or by contacting:

Archway Publishing
1663 Liberty Drive
Bloomington, IN 47403
www.archwaypublishing.com
1 (888) 242-5904

Because of the dynamic nature of the Internet, any web addresses or links contained in this book may have changed since publication and may no longer be valid. The views expressed in this work are solely those of the author and do not necessarily reflect the views of the publisher, and the publisher hereby disclaims any responsibility for them.

Any people depicted in stock imagery provided by Getty Images are models, and such images are being used for illustrative purposes only. Certain stock imagery © Getty Images.

ISBN: 978-1-4808-6565-5 (sc)
ISBN: 978-1-4808-6564-8 (hc)
ISBN: 978-1-4808-6566-2 (e)

Library of Congress Control Number: 2018909644

Print information available on the last page.

Archway Publishing rev. date: 11/09/2018

ACKNOWLEDGMENTS

The most fortunate aspect of the early decades of my life was having Odessa Arnette Memory (1908–1989) as my mother. As people who knew her well realized, she was a very intelligent, capable woman who greatly enjoyed living. One of the important things I inherited or learned from her was strong enjoyment of living.

My son, Alexander Clinton Memory, was born in 1978. Having him as my son has been the most fortunate thing I have experienced in the later decades of my life. His example of strong scholarship and learning in his education and working career has encouraged me to continue to acquire, even after retirement, important and interesting information.

My father died tragically in 1949. I have had the great good fortune that six fine and accomplished men (and other men and women) I have enjoyed and respected have shown special interest in me. All of these men had successful marriages. They were Jasper L. Memory, my uncle, Dan Smith, my neighbor and cousin, William Watkins, my uncle, Winfield Blackwell, the husband of a cousin, Howard Boozer, an acquaintance in a Unitarian-Universalist fellowship, and Dick Perry, duplicate bridge player and director. I learned important things about life from these men. Also, their continuing interest in me bolstered my self-esteem.

CONTENTS

FOREWORD

How can I live a long, healthy, happy, and bountiful life? How can I spend my time and money in productive ways? How can I cope with failure? How can I be a good parent? How can I translate my values into moral behavior in the civic and political arena? How can I stay well informed and improve my decision-making?

These questions emerge in adolescence and continue to engage us throughout adulthood. John Memory's book takes a novel approach to addressing them through scholarly findings and a lifetime of experiential wisdom: 36 chapters and 5 essays, each focused on "Important Information that Is Nearly Never Covered in a University or College Course." Dr. Memory encourages readers to improve heart and brain health and "discover elusive truth" in the face of daunting discouraging factors: psychological conditions, social & cultural pressures, and "incomplete or incorrect information" promulgated by experts and industries, and even professors.

Dr. Memory's training as a social scientist, criminologist, and lawyer give him a breadth of intellectual curiosity and analytic skills that have led to this compendium of information. His life experiences in the university, the prosecutor's office, the U.S. Army Judge Advocate General Corps, and in consulting give him contextual awareness of the role of research and the synthesis of multi-disciplinary findings necessary for an encompassing view of multi-faceted personal and social problems. His family life, especially parenting a son, has motivated him to share his views so that others can consider alternatives to established medical advice and choose healthy life habits.

Dr. Memory's early chapters on health would be of value to readers of all ages. Healthy choices made in youth and early adulthood have the greatest potential outcomes for brain and heart health, but adults in their 50s through 70s can make significant changes to prolong life and mitigate illness. Older and health-compromised adults will be interested in new approaches to reversing heart and brain damage.

I am pleased to say that I am the mother of his son – divorced and with arms-length contact over the years. As such I am honored to be able to write this Foreword. As my life's work has been music therapy (itself an interdisciplinary subject and health-care profession) I am especially interested in Dr. Memory's chapters on mental health and the importance of recreation in a healthy life. He includes not only sports and music but also bridge (the card game) – all areas in which he has observed and experienced the value of creative and expressive activities in which the participant becomes totally involved, both individually and as partners and team players.

There is controversial information in many chapters. To defy a physician's prescription to take statin drugs, to take multiple nutritional supplements, to draw conclusions about race relations, to use statistics as a basis for personal choices – these positions will cause debate. Dr. Memory's sharing of both his personal risk factors for heart and brain disease and his experiences with coping with various challenges in life demonstrate his authenticity, integrity and qualifications to spur all of us to making choices for healthy, happy, and productive lives.

Contributed by Barbara Cobb Memory, Ph.D., Music Therapist (Ret.)
Associate Professor of Music Therapy, Emeritus,
East Carolina University (1986 – 2013)

PREFACE

The main reason I decided to write this book was that, in spite of my very serious heart and brain disease risk factors, my performance of a **statin-free** supplement-and-exercise routine I developed in 1982 has resulted in my having, at 74, excellent cardiovascular health and brain health and function. **I do not believe this is a trivial or small achievement. Since 1987, all of my primary physicians and cardiologists (except a lipids expert at Duke) have strongly recommended that I take a statin drug.** If I had followed their strong recommendation in the 1980s, the extremely enjoyable part of my life would have ended several decades ago as a result of adverse side effects of the statin drug. I believe that I have a duty to make this information available to many people.

The five health problems Americans fear the most are 5-type 2 diabetes, 4-stroke, 3-heart disease and heart attack, 2-Alzheimer's, 1-cancer. I feel extremely fortunate that I am and have been dealing very successfully with very serious risks of developing disease number five (diabetes) through 2 (heart disease and heart attack). In nearly all cases, my approach has been non-conventional, holistic. Fortunately, I learned in 2018 that three homeopathic anti-cancer measures have stopped the advance of my aggressive prostate cancer. Of course, the table of contents will help you to find my discussion of each of these subjects except stroke, which is in chapter 6.

On November 13, 2017, the guidelines for hypertension (high blood pressure) were changed to include as hypertension readings of 130 and above for the top (systolic) number and 80 and above for the bottom (diastolic) number. I am glad that chapter 7 of this book is precisely about dealing with somewhat elevated blood pressure without medication.

The information in this book about heart and brain health involves,

to a large extent, prevention of disease through life style and non-medical approaches. **Nothing in this book about heart and brain health is intended for use by a person who has had a heart attack, has serious heart disease, is subject to severe heart attack risk, is subject to severe stroke risk, is subject to severe sudden cardiac death risk, has congestive heart failure, or has other severe heart disease risks.**

Early in 2017, I decided to try to determine whether I have or am aware of "clusters of information" that are nearly never covered in university and college undergraduate courses. I listed 36 clusters of information. I have not requested or gotten from others suggestions of information to include. So, this is genuinely the product of one person's thinking and work. Later, I read a semester list of undergraduate course descriptions of a respected university in the U.S. Southeast and found no evidence that any of the subjects of those clusters were covered extensively in one or more of the university's courses during that semester. Of course, there may be coverage in courses of other universities and colleges.

I want to acknowledge that some of the information in this book's 17 chapters relating to health are covered in the relatively very small number of U.S. college and university programs about alternative, holistic, homeopathic, naturopathic health methods.

I failed in attempts to find one or more qualified professors who would cooperate in a survey study about this. So, I decided to convert the project into writing this book.

In addition to attempting to provide a wide variety of worthwhile and interesting information, I am trying to shed some light on an important subject—the adequacy of undergraduate course content in the U.S. Greg Ludianoff and Jonathan Haidt in 2018 had published an important book, *The Coddling of the American Mind* (2018), which includes extensive discussion of strong resistance of college and university students to being exposed to ideas and even words the students believe are offensive. That phenomenon may partially explain the absence of some material in this book from college and university curricula.

Though I certainly have not done a literature review concerning graduates' satisfaction with their higher education, I found an interesting quote in a 2014 article, "Chapter 2: Public views on the value of education," on the Pew Research Center website. The education referred to undergraduate higher education.

"[S]ome 41% of Millenials ages 25 to 32, 45% of Gen Xers and 47% of Baby Boomers say their schooling was 'very useful' in getting them ready to enter the labor force."

I am surprised that the percentages answering "very useful" were as low as they were and that the percentage giving that answer declined from the oldest group to the youngest.

Additional motivation for writing this book was my strong desire for this book to help many young adults to be healthy, happy, and successful. I hope, also, that many older Americans will benefit especially from the 17 chapters about health.

Since writing this type of book must be an intellectually daunting task, you may justifiably wonder whether my background and skills qualify me to do the work. I hold a JD degree (Wake Forest University, 1968) and PhD in criminology (FSU, 1981), wrote a lead law review article (Memory, 1967), and was an associate editor of the WF law review. Seven articles on various subjects by me have been published in scholarly journals, some of which were refereed. I developed and directed a very significant grant-funded study of disciplinary infractions of inmates in North Carolina prisons. A resulting article (Memory et al, 1999), of which I was the lead author, was published in a refereed journal and, I hope, made a significant contribution to the fields of criminology and criminal justice. I developed and was the senior editor and the major contributor to a 500-page reader (Memory & Aragon, 2001) about patrol policing. Chapter 35 provides additional information about my writing.

Though **I am not a health expert**, I am a "health nut." Like many other "health nuts," I have been subjected to "good-natured ribbing" concerning my health-related practices. When it started to become obvious during my 60s that I was getting substantial benefits from working very hard for decades on my health, that ridicule inexplicably ended.

I have had scholarly and professional experiences that have helped me to be able to write responsibly on health subjects. First, my doctoral dissertation in criminology at Florida State University (Memory, 1981) was on work-related stress of judges. The body's physiological stress reaction is importantly related to health outcomes. Second, I am a PhD research social scientist. The research capabilities of a criminologist are very similar to those of an epidemiologist. Third, I had an article (Memory, 1989) published in a refereed health journal. Fourth, I was a consulting editor of a refereed health journal for two years. Fifth, in recent years a book (Memory & Evatt, 2012) about heart health approaches for women written by me and a co-author was released by digital publishing at Wake Forest University.

Though I put my strident criticism of the 2017 Republican tax cut into chapter 29, chapters 26 through 29 mainly concern conflict, sometimes violent conflict, between White and Black Americans. Some of my statements in chapters 26 through 29 seriously violate political correctness. I think it is appropriate to provide here some information about my background. As I mention several times in this book, I am a life-long Democrat, have never voted for a Republican, and worked especially hard in support of Barack Obama in 2008 and Hillary Clinton in 2016.

I grew up in Riverton, which is an unincorporated family resort and retirement community in south-central North Carolina. While I lived there from 1949 to 1961, when I left for college, there were eight Black families living in Riverton in what were or had been tenant-farmer houses. I liked and enjoyed Black people. After having nearly no contact with African Americans at WFC and WFU law school, my positive interactions with African Americans continued when I was in the Army from 1969–74.

During my working career relating mainly to Criminal Justice, my interactions with African Americans were uniformly positive. In 2006, I would have readily said that three of my all-time favorite people were Black, and I continue to think they are very fine people. I care deeply about the welfare of all ethnic groups in the U.S., including African Americans.

I am related to many intelligent, moral, caring, well educated, capable, and accomplished people, many of whom are now deceased, who made improving the circumstances of Black people in the U.S. an important part of their lives. Those people have included an important historian-author and a member of the North Carolina Supreme Court. While I have not achieved the prominence or influence of those men, I have always supported, sometimes to my own detriment, improvement of the circumstances of Black people in the U.S. and meaningful implementation of liberal/progressive values.

If you read this entire book, you will realize that something I have written will annoy members of many groups—conservatives and liberals, Democrats and Republicans, Christians and agnostics/atheists, doctors, professors,

African Americans, and others. I don't write or say things because of my ideology or values. I write and say things because I believe there is strong evidence that they are true.

In this book, there is repetition of some information. Repetition helps me to learn important information. Also, I've wanted to make sure that readers will be able to acquire especially important information. Headings will help you to determine whether you have already read particular information.

Two friends have suggested that I put all information about "author's relevant expertise and experiences" in the preface and not put any of that information in individual chapters. There are several reasons for my decision not to follow that advice.

(1) I have had a long and complex life and have had significant, illuminating experiences relating to the subjects of many of this book's chapters. A friend who is a retired PhD physicist once said to me, "I'm sort of amazed by the information you have on many diverse subjects." Putting all of my "expertise and experiences" information into the preface would produce an extremely long preface. You can read in the "About the Author" section near the end of the book information about extraordinary challenges I have encountered and about outcomes that were made possible by my decades-long pro-health efforts. I hope that reading that information will encourage readers to "keep up the good fight" for excellent health.

(2) My relevant expertise and experiences have produced very important content of about 30 of the chapters. For example, my determined work preventing my development of heart disease has produced valuable information included in about 12 chapters that readers would probably not be able to obtain through ordinary Internet searches. I don't know of another highly qualified PhD social scientist who writes and disseminates information similar to my thinking found in chapters 26 through 29 about potential for conflict, including violent conflict, between Black and White Americans

(3) This book is more like a collection of essays than a conventional book with an over-arching subject. Because some readers probably will select a modest number of chapters to read, I want the content of each chapter to be to a large extent sufficient without reference to other chapters.

(4) I hope that learning some about my lifelong determined efforts to discover elusive truth will encourage some readers to do that in their own lives. Remember: Sometimes, the "information" that experts, an industry, and/or professors make available to people is not the "whole truth" and may not genuinely be true at all.

REFERENCES

Lukianoff, Greg & Haidt, Jonathan (2018). *The coddling of the American mind: how good intentions and bad ideas are setting up a generation for failure.* NY, NY: Penuin Press.

Memory, John M. (1997). *Some relationships.* (self-published)

Memory, John M. (1989). Juvenile suicide in secure detention facilities: correction of published rates. *Death Studies,* Vol. 13, pp. 455–63.

Memory, John M. (1981). *Work-related stress of criminal trial court judges.* Unpublished doctoral dissertation, Florida State University, Tallahassee, FL.

Memory, John M. (1967). N.C.G.S. 15-4.1: "Due process of law" under *Gideon v. Wainwright? Wake Forest Law Review,* Vol. 3, pp. 1–32.

Memory, John M. & Aragon, R. (Eds.). (2001). *Patrol officer problem solving and solutions.* Durham, NC: Carolina Academic Press.

Memory, John M., Guo, G., Parker, K., & Sutton, T. (1999). Comparing disciplinary infraction rates of North Carolina Fair Sentencing and Structured Sentencing inmates. *The Prison Journal,* Vol. 79, pp. 45–71.

Memory, John M. & Evatt, Lynn (2012). *Vascular cleansing routines: safe and effective heart health programs for women (and men).* Released by Wakexpress (Digital publishing at Wake Forest University), Winston-Salem, NC.

INTRODUCTION

Many non-fiction books tell one long and complex story that may be helpful. This book tells 36 stories, any number of which may be helpful. Nearly every chapter provides information concerning one or more professional or vocational fields.

Some "ivory-tower intellectuals" might say that much of the content of this book is "light weight" intellectually. My answer is, "Information does not have to be hard to understand and learn for it to be important and interesting." Also, please remember that it is impossible for me to include in one book definitive treatments of 36 important, challenging, and, in some cases, broad subjects. I have tried to put early in each chapter important information that is not widely known. I have used headings, underlining, and bold font to help readers to find information they would like to acquire.

As the table of contents indicates, the chapters are extremely varied in content. I do not now and never have had expertise concerning a significant number of these subjects. Though I have worked very hard on producing well written chapters that contain genuinely important and interesting information, it has not been feasible for me to carry out a full literature review concerning the topics of 36 widely diverse chapters. I am confident that experts will be able to point out ways that many of the chapters can be improved. There are a few situations in which I have failed to provide a cite to a relevant article or book. For example, in chapter one I don't provide a reference concerning individuals' resistance to urging by others relating to health. In that case, I have misplaced the reference information. The point is that I would not include a statement if I did not know that there is substantial support for the statement. Except for chapters 27 and 33, contributing to scholarly literature is not a goal I have for this book.

Though I have previously written several documents that are included in this book, I have not previously developed strong knowledge of the subjects of some chapters. My approach in the latter chapters is mainly to provide references to websites, articles, and books which include potentially helpful information. While I believe that about 26 of the chapters could provide some important content for future undergraduate courses on their subjects, I assume that developers of courses on the other ten subjects (e.g., parenting, sociobiology, geography/history) would have fully sufficient generally available information to develop good courses.

I included 17 chapters about health partly because I believe that, unfortunately, physicians and other health professionals and even professors with health-related specialties do not want anyone to give away high quality health information that will reduce the need for people to have paid medical appointments and care.

All or nearly all of the ideas and information in the chapters about health are supported by ideas and information of holistic and integrative medical doctors (MDs) and osteopathic physicians (DOs) and naturopathic doctors (NDs). All of those practitioners are licensed health practitioners. Virtually all of the methods they utilize are supported by research. Additional indication that the types of approaches in this book's chapters relating to health can be legitimately addressed in responsible discussion about health is found in the fact that the National Institutes of Health (NIH) has a National Center for Complementary and Alternative Medicine.

I have an obligation to state that, though I have tried to provide fully current information in the 17 chapters on health subjects, there undoubtably have been some recent developments. Instead of being information about the safety of measures I have recommended, I believe the information is more likely to concern a recently developed alternative, holistic health measure. Of course, I believe I have been well informed and prudent about actions I have recommended.

Here's an important thing to remember while reading the chapters about health: Anything that helps heart health nearly certainly helps brain health, and vice versa, and good approaches concerning heart and brain health help greatly in cancer prevention. Working intelligently and diligently on anti-aging approaches will help greatly with heart and brain health and cancer prevention. These approaches, which overlap greatly, tend to help significantly with prevention of Parkinson's disease.

A high percentage of readers of the chapters on health subjects probably, like me, have personal health challenges relating to the subjects of several chapters. I suggest that readers select the chapter which addresses the highest percentage of their health challenges. Then, using ideas in that chapter as a starting point, they can develop a fairly comprehensive health plan by adding supplements and other measures from other chapters. For some late middle-age readers, starting with ideas in chapter 13 on anti-aging approaches may make sense.

There are four chapters which relate to conflict, sometimes violent conflict, between White persons and Black persons in the U.S. I have provided information about my background and life experiences relating to this in the preface. Some of my statements in those chapters seriously violate political correctness. Now, as I discuss in those chapters, we are experiencing in the U.S. a rapid deterioration of race relations and an increase of interracial violence. **Political correctness has not prevented these very negative things from happening.** I believe that acknowledging important reality in the U.S. may be an important step in reversing these trends and solving some of our intractable problems.

You will notice that there are five "essays." Though most cover a subject found in a nearby chapter, each essay can be read separately.

— SECTION 1 —
Basics of Healthful Living

— CHAPTER 1 —
Ways to Bolster Your Health Motivation

Elaboration. This chapter is intended to help people with health motivation problems. Health motivation is the subject of the first chapter of this book because, as documented in the 17 chapters about health, many types of meaningful action relating to health cannot occur if the person is not sufficiently motivated. Information in chapters about incidence of various types of health problems (e.g., obesity, heart disease, depression, stress-related disorders, Alzheimer's, and self-destructive behavior) shows that deficiency of health motivation is extremely common.

It is intended, also, to encourage adults to teach healthy lifestyle to children. I started teaching that to my son Alex when he was 2½.

You may think it would be good to learn about improving health motivation from a person with great health-related genes, great health-related habits, and no problems relating to health motivation. That does not describe me. I have serious risk factors regarding many adverse health conditions, and I have to work determinedly protecting my health. As I detail later, I have several major personality problems relating to health motivation. I hope that my struggle since 1969 trying to protect and improve my health will inspire some readers to stay with that effort in their own lives. It has paid off for me more than you can imagine.

Achievability of healthful, bountiful living. The most important statement in this book is that **it doesn't take much time, energy, and**

money to gain benefits from exercise (not necessarily strenuous or long exercise) and nutrition (diet and supplements that don't take much time or money) that can greatly improve nearly every aspect of your life and wellbeing. That has occurred for me.

Several experts argue that, if your exercise is moderate in intensity, you need 150 minutes of exercise per week. I've become convinced that 17 to 20 minutes of very brisk walking can provide meaningful exercise. In chapter 4, I give detailed information about how buying 15 very important supplements can cost less than $1 per day.

Finding several ideas that work for you. I realize that this chapter includes many ideas that can possibly be overwhelming. If you find several ideas about health motivation that you think will work for you, I encourage you to implement those ideas in your life. Emphasizing the unbelievably great benefits of exercise worked for me.

Benefits of exercise. Because the benefits of exercise constitute especially good and important knowledge that can help us with health motivation, that information is given here, very early in chapter 1. (A qualified university professor, Len Kravitz, PhD, has on the Internet an excellent article about exercise motivation, "Exercise motivation: what starts and keeps people exercising.")

In some cases, I have been able to provide the citation of a research article. Based on extensive reading since 1982, I have a high level of confidence that this is accurate information. So, I'll now list the astonishingly numerous and wonderful benefits of physical exercise I have become aware of:

> **Deterrence of cardiovascular disease and related conditions, including hypertension, type 2 diabetes, obesity, and problems with endothelial function (function of blood vessels)** (Taka-aki Okabe et al, 2006)
> **Strengthening of the heart**
> **Improvement of blood circulation** (Thompson et al, 2003)
> **Most effective way to build brain power** (Ratey, 2008)

Combined with Mediterranean diet, reduces Alzheimer's risk by 60% (Scarmeas et al, 2009)

For older persons with serious depression, as effective as taking an anti-depressant drug in depression control (Blumenthal et al, 1999)

Reverses detrimental effects of the physiological stress reaction (Salmon,2001).

Helps with troublesome anxiety

Moderate exercise produces growth of new brain cells in the hippocampus.

Improvement of brain function

Promotion of production of DHEA

Improvement of sex life

Help with achieving healthful sleep

Promotion of production of human growth hormone (HGH)

Promotion of production of glutathione after taking alpha-lipoic acid

Help with delivery of nutrients and oxygen to body tissues

Promotion of production of serotonin and dopamine

Release of endorphins

Reduction of risk of coronary artery disease, type 2 diabetes, osteoporosis, obesity, depression, and cancer of breast and colon (Thompson et al, 2003)

Reducing the most important part of this chapter to a short question. **What type of moderate exercise are you willing to do for at least 150 minutes per week?** If you will, for example, walk briskly for 20 minutes during four of your lunch hours every week, you "have it in your grasp" to protect and improve your health. You don't know yet that I will want you to take several carefully selected supplements 30 minutes before your walking. In addition to probably providing many health benefits, the supplements and exercise will help you to feel better, think better, and function better for the rest of the day.

Benefits of diet and supplements you need to be very aware of. Chapter 3 tells about achieving great lifestyle and health through excellent diet and exercise, and probably only a few supplements. Chapter 4 provides detailed information about the benefits of many nutritional supplements relating primarily to heart and brain health. Just as the information about benefits of exercise above is, I think, astonishingly great, you can remember the encouraging information in chapters 3 and 4 when you are making decisions about lifestyle (such as whether to rise off of the couch and take a 25-minute brisk walk).

Benefits of exercise and supplements resulting in improvement of sexual enjoyment and performance. There is no doubt whatsoever that exercise and carefully chosen supplements can substantially improve sexual enjoyment and performance. A chart in chapter four indicates supplements that have this benefit. If you want to improve your sexual enjoyment and performance, I recommend that you (1) take carefully selected supplements, (2) wait 30 minutes, and then (3) get 30 to 45 minutes of exercise that is at the top of the moderate range in strenuousness. Especially for people past middle age, I recommend performing this routine earlier in the day of all sexual activity. Add several heart- and brain-healthy supplements (Fortunately, they tend to help sexual enjoyment and performance.) to this routine, and you will be well down the road toward healthful living.

Three very important "sets" of information.

(1) Satisfactory health motivation helps a person to eat a healthful diet, learn about and take needed supplements, exercise regularly, have a physician and regular health tests and checkups, have a generally healthy lifestyle (which doesn't include smoking or drinking alcoholic beverages "too much"), and avoid troublesome weight gain (such as gain that could trigger development of type 2 diabetes).

(2) Recently, I heard a friend, who is a physician, say, "You can't beat genetics." I believe that is incorrect. It is possible for a person with "great health genes" to, through very bad lifestyle, squander those assets and suffer serious health problems. (I later tell about a friend who did that.) It is also sometimes possible for a person with "bad health genes" to, through excellent lifestyle, overcome those disadvantages and enjoy excellent health.

(3) Some people, including me and my son, are most effectively motivated regarding health by learning about the astonishingly great benefits of healthful lifestyle. Other people are most effectively motivated by learning about the often catastrophic results of very bad lifestyle.

Three health motivation posters. After this page, you will find my **Dr. WALSH** health motivation poster. In 1982, I wanted to over-learn and be constantly aware of the wonderful benefits of excellent nutrition and exercise. So, I dreamed up the Dr. WALSH poster. I had that poster on my bathroom mirror for more than 10 years. Dr. WALSH also helped my son! On the following page is my **WELLNESS+** poster, which presents the same information. On the next page is a poster I recently developed for people who respond well to learning the horrible consequences of bad lifestyle. Feel free to copy and share any of these posters.

I'm Dr. WALSH. You'll develop better exercise and diet habits if you read or look over this poster daily and remember that regular moderate exercise and a healthful, moderate diet, along with some supplements, will help you to achieve or improve many wonderful things, including:

W

Weight control
Waist you're proud of
Work productivity
Wardrobe that looks good & keeps fitting

A

Attractiveness
Aging s l o w l y
Anxiety & depression control
Arthritis prevention
Avoidance or control of diabetes
Agility & flexibility
Athletic performance
Alzheim. prevention
Avoidance of taking a statin drug

L

Longer life
Liveliness, energy & endurance
Limitation of weight fluctuation
Lower burnout risk
Less fat, more muscle

S

Sex appeal & sex life
Stress coping
Self-confidence & self-esteem
Sounder sleep
Sounder thinking
Strength
Stronger bones
Savings on medical care and wardrobe

H

Happiness
Health in general
Headache prevention
Heart & cardiovascular health
Hypertension prevention or control

The person in the picture is actually John M. Memory, PhD, age 74. He developed and wrote the first version of this poster in 1982 to help himself to over-learn and always remember the wonderful benefits of excellent nutrition, from food and supplements, and exercise. That has happened!

DIET AND EXERCISE MOTIVATOR POSTER

REGULAR MODERATE EXERCISE, HEALTHFUL DIET, AND CAREFULLY SELECTED SUPPLEMENTS HELP ME TO ACHIEVE OR IMPROVE <u>MANY WONDERFUL THINGS</u>, INCLUDING

W
WEIGHT CONTROL & PREVENTION OF HAZARDOUS WEIGHT FLUCTUATION
WAISTLINE THAT LOOKS GOOD & IS HEALTHFUL
WORK PRODUCTIVITY
WARDROBE THAT LOOKS GOOD & KEEPS FITTING

E
ENJOYMENT OF LIFE
ENJOYMENT OF SEX & PERFORMANCE IN SEX
ENHANCEMENT OF HEALTH
ENHANCEMENT OF AGILITY& FLEXIBILITY

L
LONGER LIFE
LIFESTYLE IMPROVEMENT
LARGER MUSCLE MASS (if desired)

L
LOWER-BACK HEALTH
LOWER "BAD" CHOLESTEROL (LDL) & TRIGLYCERIDES
LUNG CAPACITY

N
NATURAL PREVENTION OR CONTROL OF
    HEART & CARDIOVASCULAR DISEASE
    HYPERTENSION (HIGH BLOOD PRESSURE)
    TYPE 2 DIABETES
    CANCER (SEVERAL TYPES)
    ARTHRITIS (HIPS & BELOW)

E
EMOTIONAL HEALTH
DEPRESSION CONTROL
    ANXIETY CONTROL
    BURNOUT PREVENTION
ENERGY & ENDURANCE

S
SELF-ESTEEM & SELF-CONFIDENCE
SEX APPEAL & ATTRACTIVENESS
SENILITY & ALZHEIMER'S PREVENTION
SLOWER AGING
SOUND SLEEP

S
SOUND THINKING
SPORTS PERFORMANCE
STRENGTH
STRESS COPI NG
STRONGER BONES (OSTEOPOROSIS PREVENTION)
"SUCCESS" IMAGE

+
I'll develop better exercise and diet habits if I read this motivator daily and remember these WELLNESS+ benefits when I make a decision about diet or exercise.

HEADING DOWN TO HEART-DISEASE HELL

Weight gain V V	Results from bad diet, eating too much, and sedentary life style (little or no exercise).
Artery occlusion (atherosclerosis) V	Unhealthy diet, smoking and excess alcoholic beverages increase this risk.
Elevated blood pressure (hypertension) V	Uncontrolled hypertension in mid-life increases risk of heart attack and Alzheimer's/dementia.
Metabolic syndrome V V V	Involves symptoms including hypertension, excess waist measurement and belly fat, insulin resistance, bad "lipids profile" and blood sugar.
Type 2 diabetes V V	Early noticeable symptoms can be foot and lower leg pain and elevated blood sugar.
Alzheimer's V	or other dementia
Heart attack V	Risk starts much earlier.
Heart failure	Things such as heart attack and heart damage due to deficiency of coenzyme Q10 resulting from taking a statin drug can cause congestive heart failure, which can be fatal.

It's not hard to prevent this sequence, especially if you start early in your life.

Motivation assists. Many people have more trouble with exercise motivation than any other aspect of health motivation. Here is some information about things you can do to support your exercise motivation.

Recruit friends to exercise with.

Set exercise goals for yourself. For example, you can set goals for yourself of walking briskly or jogging two miles three times each week. I know from experience that, at some point, setting higher goals is not a good idea. Don't cause yourself to dread exercise.

An article by a PhD including ten motivational tips. On the WebMD website, you can find an article by Debra Fulghum Bruce, PhD, with the title "10 motivational tips to keep you healthy." The article seems to be more concerned with health motivation of females than males.

Dealing with cravings. Being able to deal healthfully with food and drink cravings is an important part of health motivation. Here are ten suggestions about dealing with cravings.

"Top 10 tips to curb your cravings." This list is found in a short book (2013), *The Daniel plan: 40 days to a healthier life*, by Rick Warren and "the Daniel Plan Team." As the title suggests, this book provides a coherent strategy for achieving a healthier life.

1. **Avoid your triggers**. Triggers of cravings can involve memories of indulging in cravings.

2. **Balance your blood sugar**. Low blood sugar can be associated with low blood flow to the brain.

3. **Eliminate sugar, artificial sweeteners, and refined carbs.**

4. **Eat SLOW carb, not LOW carbs.** High fiber carbs keep you fuller longer.

5. **Drink more water.**

6. **Make protein 25 percent of your diet.**

7. **Manage your stress.**

8. **Follow the 90/10 Rule.** Make excellent food choices 90% of the time, and allow yourself to "break the rules" some.

9. **Get moving.** Get physical exercise regularly.

10. **Get seven to eight hours of sleep a night.**

If I have super tasty snacks and desserts (e.g., Rocky Road ice cream, dark chocolate-covered almonds) in my house, I will not have sufficient will power to avoid eating the goodies. So, I am very careful not to buy and take home goodies I can't handle.

The importance of motivation relating to weight control. Since many people achieve major weight loss, that doesn't appear to be very difficult or remarkable. Tragically, nearly all of us regain that weight. It is very important to have enough motivation to **prevent undesirable weight gain**. In the summer of 2015 I reached 222 lbs., which may have moved me into type 2 diabetes. So, I lost to 205, which stopped my diabetes symptoms. In June 2018, I weighed 205. In life, you must do what you have to do.

Important information about the overweight and obesity problem in the U.S. is on the website of the NIH National Institute of Diabetes and Digestive and Kidney Diseases. The data are from the National Health and Nutrition Examination Survey, 2013–2014. It was found that:

More than one in three adults are overweight.

More than one in three adults are obese.

One in six adults have extreme obesity.

One in six children from 2 to 19 years old have obesity.

Of non-Hispanic Black persons, 48.4% are obese.

Obesity in the U.S. started increasing rapidly in the 1976–1980 period.

During the fall of 2017, President Trump designated the epidemic of opioid addiction and overdoses as a health emergency. I believe that the problems of extreme obesity, obesity, and overweight among Americans constitute, together, a health emergency.

A type of exercise that can fit into even a tight schedule. As mentioned earlier, a crucial aspect of achieving adequate health motivation is discovering meaningful exercise that you are willing to do regularly.

I have discovered that taking very carefully selected supplements, waiting 30 minutes, and then walking as briskly as I can for 17 to 20 minutes has great benefits for me. I can do that walking without needing to dress for exercise or shower after walking. Recently, I decided to, as needed, do meaningful brisk walking for 20 to 30 minutes as I am pushing a shopping cart and shopping at Walmart. As part of my efforts against prostate cancer, I have decided to do exercise with oxygen therapy (EWOT) nearly every day for the rest of my life.

Importance of this subject. Protecting and improving your health requires motivation sufficient to carry out concerted effort consistently. Also, for some people, sufficient motivation is necessary to avoid falling prey to self-destructive behaviors, such as smoking or overeating.

Unfortunately, there undoubtedly are tens of millions of Americans, many of them young adults, who do not have enough health motivation and, consequently, don't do the things needed to protect and improve their health.

Relevance for young adults. There is currently an epidemic of cardiovascular disease among young adults in the U.S. (Lee, 2008). It is important for a person to develop good health habits at an early age.

Author's relevant experience. My earliest health motivation was rooted in my morbid fear of death that arose soon after my father's tragic death when I was five. Fortunately, that fear prompted me to make good early decisions relating to health and eventually morphed into strong enjoyment of living.

As I discuss in more detail in chapter 6, I learned in 1982 that I have very severe heart- and brain-disease risk factors. Unfortunately, my health motivation has not been strong enough for me to exercise exclusively for health benefits. **I have had to bolster my motivation**. So, I have walked about 22,000 miles playing golf, since 1982 have exercised before about 3600 duplicate bridge games, and have always mowed my yard. Since 1982, I have taken carefully selected supplements, waited 30 minutes, and then exercised more than 8000 times. Because this routine has done a great job of keeping my arteries free from occlusion, I call it a "vascular cleansing routine" or VCR. Since I, at 74 years of age, have very good health, it appears that I am managing to win my health-motivation fight.

I have two other health motivation problems–difficulty limiting consumption of tasty treats and unwillingness to expend the money, effort, and time needed to prepare excellent meals "from scratch."

Of course, many people my age have exercised much more than I have. Many people have overcome much more serious health challenges than mine. My point is that I have managed, in spite of very severe heart and brain disease risk factors and motivation problems, to do what has been needed to achieve excellent heart and brain health outcomes.

The importance of hope concerning the future. I believe that a person needs to have hope concerning the future to be able and willing to do the difficult things needed to have excellent or, at least, good health.

The importance of enjoyment of life. Two exceptional and important people in the early decades of my life were my mother, Odessa Memory, and my uncle Jasper Memory, who was a much loved professor at Wake Forest College/University. Each of them greatly enjoyed many aspects of life and living. Mother especially enjoyed her grandchildren and playing bridge, and Jasper enjoyed several types of recreation, students, and friends. This enjoyment of life supported hope for the future for each of them.

If you don't genuinely enjoy living, it will be difficult for you to have enough health motivation. For example, a woman in an unhappy marriage works in her job and then at home works on parenting and housework until late every night. It may be difficult for her to have motivation, time, and energy to do the things needed to have a healthful lifestyle.

A wonderful example of health motivation. My friend Sarah does not have heart disease risk factors that are nearly as serious as mine. During early adulthood she smoked, very seldom exercised, became obese, became a diabetic, had a heart attack, and actually died in a hospital operating room. Fortunately, the doctors revived her. In later years, when her many prescribed drugs were not helping her enough, she very carefully studied non-traditional health approaches. Over years, she used that information in returning to normal weight, reversing and eliminating her diabetes, improving enough to need none of her medications, and returning to very good health. This is one of the most inspiring health stories I know of. She had to have great knowledge, motivation, and courage.

A chapter from an uncompleted book by me about health motivation. It includes information and ideas that I hope will help people with significant problems relating to health motivation.

The inherent difficulty of this subject. Even though the rest of this chapter concerns an extremely serious, intractable problem for many people, I hope that reading it can be encouraging for you. Though I am a PhD criminologist and not a psychologist, I have tried to develop potentially helpful ideas for people with this problem. Let me remind you: **I have this problem, which makes me unable to do physical exercise just for the health benefits, creates "cravings" problems for me, and keeps me from preparing excellent, healthful meals.**

WAYS TO INCREASE YOUR HEALTH MOTIVATION

It seems to me that there is a regrettable lack of discussion by health experts, people on TV, and the public of the importance of motivation in preventing and overcoming health problems. In this chapter, I share a variety of ideas which may help people to improve their health motivation.

The Importance of Self-Control (Will Power)

For every individual, how much self-control (will power) the individual has will strongly influence how much health motivation the individual has. I very recently found an extremely important article about this in which the author (Weir, 2012) interviews a top research scientist on the subject (Florida State University psychology professor Dr. Roy F. Baumeister). In his research on this subject, Dr. Baumeister reached several conclusions that he and other experts would not have expected. I encourage you to read this fairly short article, which you can access easily on the Internet.

Human Nature's Effect on Diet and Exercise Motivation

It is unlikely that our very distant ancestors engaged in vigorous physical activity for the fun of it or for health benefits. Because life then could be physically difficult and sometimes exhausting, they probably tried to conserve energy for the times when it was needed. This point of view may make the exercise-motivation problems of many humans more understandable. I deal with this difficulty by making my exercise have some purpose other than making me healthy (e.g., winning at bridge or golf or getting my lawn mowed). Maybe doing something similar to that will work for you. (At nearly 75 and with cancer, I am now willing to do EWOT (exercise with oxygen therapy) just for many great health benefits.)

Before development of agriculture, our distant ancestors probably did not have to be careful to limit their eating in order to avoid gaining weight. So, humans probably don't have tendencies built into human nature to do physical exercise or limit our eating. If this is true, we need to develop strategies for limiting how much we eat.

A main idea of this book is that, in spite of human nature that may not dovetail well with a healthful lifestyle, **it is clearly possible for people to overcome these factors, develop strong health motivation, adopt a healthful lifestyle, and reap giant health and quality of life benefits.**

Ideas from the Scholarly Literature on Motivation

For decades, I have continued to assume that health experts would once and for all solve the diet- and exercise-motivation riddle and help Americans to improve significantly regarding weight control and health. **That obviously hasn't happened**. Starting between 1976 and 1980, obesity has exploded as a disastrous health problem in the U.S. Nearly everyone who loses a lot of weight gains all of it back within five years.

Experts on exercise, diet, and health motivation have obviously done such a poor job of helping Americans to do the right things for their health that **I do not believe that it is crucial for me to provide a full review of the "scholarly literature" on exercise, diet, and health motivation**. Below are some selected ideas which may help you.

Several studies have indicated that a majority of subjects report that it is very important to make dietary changes to feel better and to control an existing medical problem, but extremely few were motivated by pressure from others (cf., Seltzer, 2012). In fact, in one study, greater social pressure from others concerning diet was associated with **higher fat intake** by the persons being pressured. These findings support this book's emphasis on **helping individuals to build their own motivation**, as opposed to helping people to build the health motivation of other people.

According to Hill and Stone in *Success through a Positive Mental Attitude* (2007), there are **ten sources of human motivation: desire for self-preservation, love, fear, sex, desire for life after death, desire for freedom of body and mind, anger, hate, desire for recognition and self-expression, and desire for material gain.**

Hill and Stone believe also that **hope is the magic ingredient that makes motivation to action possible.** So, hope helps you to have motivation; motivation helps you to do important things to improve your health and life; and improving your health and life helps you to have more hope concerning various aspects of your life. **If you think this is circular, you're right.** As I discuss later, this type of circular development can help your life to **spiral upward** in wonderful ways.

Based partly on ideas from Hill and Stone, here are things which can tend to increase your diet, exercise, and health motivation:

Fear of death, disability, disease, and illness

Knowledge of the benefits of good diet, supplements, and exercise

Knowledge of the bad effects of bad diet and inadequate exercise

Confidence in your ability to do difficult things

Role models who exhibit or have exhibited good diet and exercise lifestyle

Desire to be a good health role model for important others

Love of life and enjoyable life activities, including sex and activities with friends

Enjoyment of aspects and activities of the good-health-practices lifestyle

Competitive dynamics (e.g., desire to do better on wellness than another person)

External motivating factors and forces (e.g., need to avoid gaining weight to retain a job)

Realizing it when you have achieved some benefits of good diet and exercise

Feedback and encouragement from important others

Obviously, the more of the factors above that apply to you, the greater your health motivation will tend to be.

Self-Control

Here's a fascinating quote from an article by two University of Miami psychologists:

> "[W]e found four studies that supported . . . and only one that refuted . . . the proposition that religion's ability to promote self-control or self-regulation can explain some of religion's associations with health, well-being, and social behavior." (McCullough & Willoughby, 2009)

McCullough and Willoughby concluded that self-control does not result from an adult becoming religious but rather from growing up with religious parents. Since religious affiliation is declining in the U.S. (Pew Research Center, 2015), it is reasonable to predict an increase in "self-control problems" of young people in the U.S. This is one of the reasons I think parents should enjoy teaching their children, even quite young children, about healthful lifestyle.

Working to Improve Your Health

To succeed in many sectors of life, one must be willing to work and, probably, work hard. Here are some points to remember. (1) You may need to work hard to maintain or achieve good health; (2) working intelligently on your health can have giant payoffs; and (3) working hard and intelligently on your health can be very enjoyable (e.g., walking briskly with a loved one or friend for 45 minutes on a seashore during a beautiful sunset).

Taking Charge of Your Own Health

Many in the medical and the prescribed-drug establishment want us to think that, if we have a health problem, we can go to a doctor and get a solution that won't require any or much effort on our part. Partly because of this, many people simply don't know the giant health benefits they can get from substantial effort on their part. Maybe partly because of what operates as brainwashing by the medical/drug establishment, many people seem lazy and complacent about their own health and about the health of their children.

While I, of course, am not suggesting that you abandon doctors and all of your medication, the research clearly shows that getting involved in determining what needs to be done to protect or improve your health tends to improve your health prospects.

My Hope for You

I hope that this book will give you a glimmer of hope that you can have the motivation needed to do the things required to meet your health challenges. As time goes by, I hope the following things will gradually reinforce and strengthen each other in your life:

Hope for the future
Knowledge of achievable benefits
Belief that you can achieve benefits

Confidence in your ability to do what you need to do

Motivation sufficient to get good exercise and consume a good diet

Awareness that you are receiving benefits

Once you start getting benefits, such as lowering your blood pressure, through diet, exercise, and supplements, a new and stronger cycle of reinforcement can occur. Over time, your **HOPE, KNOWLEDGE, BELIEF, CONFIDENCE, MOTIVATION, AND AWARENESS** can get **stronger and stronger as you get healthier and healthier.** That is how it has worked for me over 36 years.

Inhibition of Health Motivation by Stress, Depression, Irrationality, Self-Destructiveness, and Addictions

Understanding why some people do have health motivation is only part of the story. Unfortunately, **health motivation can be inhibited by stress, depression, irrationality, self-destructiveness, addictions, bad diet, and loss of hope.** You may benefit from doing some "detective work" to figure out why you have the amount of health motivation that you have. I did and discovered that my low oxygen, low thyroid function, and tendency to become depressed were limiting my ability to do the right things for my health.

Stress. Many people who feel over-stressed feel that they can't find the time or energy to have a healthful diet and healthful exercise. Of course, if a person becomes "burnt-out" from long-term, cumulative stress, these problems can become even worse. Chapter 14 is about dealing healthfully with problems regarding stress and anxiety.

Wayne Froggatt is a counselor and very successful writer on subjects relating to psychology and psychotherapy who lives in New Zealand. He is the author of a book, *Taking Control* (2006), which is primarily intended to help people with problems concerning stress management.

Depression. Depression often involves incorrectly thinking that you have no hope for the future. Of course, this can undercut health motivation. Also, depression can cause one to feel lethargic, which can inhibit health motivation. Chapter 15 is about dealing healthfully with a tendency to become depressed.

Irrationality. The benefits of healthful diet and exercise are so great that it seems obvious that **anyone who knows a good bit about these benefits but still fails to have healthful lifestyle relating to diet and exercise is failing to act rationally.**

A question arises: How is depression connected with stress and irrationality? There are many possibilities. If the quality of your life is reduced by severe problems with stress, your ability to perform important life roles well enough can be diminished. This can be depressing. Of course, depression can reduce your effectiveness in stress management and coping. If you fail in important ways to be realistic and rational, your effectiveness in performance in important roles and in stress management/coping can be compromised. A connection that may not be obvious to a person who has not experienced serious depression is that **depression has the ability to cause the depressed person to think irrationally about important things.** For example, many people who are depressed believe that they can't have real hope for the future, while the truth is that many of them have very important resources that could be used to fashion a successful and enjoyable life.

I believe that making progress in these areas—stress, depression, and rationality—can help one to have more health motivation, which, of course, can lead to improvements in health and enjoyment and quality of life. As discussed later in this chapter, this can lead to a spiraling upward of one's life and health.

Self-destructiveness. There is an epidemic of self-destructive behavior in the U.S. (Chapter 16 is about this.). Becoming obese tends to destroy one's health and life. Completely failing to exercise, especially along with bad diet, can cause a young adult to have the blood vessels of a much older person. Driving without using your seat belt, riding a motorcycle without a helmet, smoking, subjecting yourself to dangerous people and situations, and drinking alcohol to excess qualify as self-destructive behaviors. All of these behaviors can interfere with ability to have good health motivation.

Addictions. Of course, addiction to smoking, alcohol, prescribed or illicit drugs, sex, hoarding, spending, or possibly other things can interfere with exhibiting good health motivation.

Bad diet. Eating a bad diet can make you feel bad and sluggish. This can undercut your health motivation.

The point here is that, if you see yourself as fitting into one or more of these categories, you may gain some self-knowledge that can help you to muster enough motivation to do the right things for your health.

The Dilemma of Over-Extended People

Research and our life experiences indicate that there are many people who have so many life activities and obligations that, realistically, they are over-extended and, possibly, over-stressed. As mentioned earlier, many women get up very early on every week day, prepare breakfast for family members, help kids to prepare for and get off to school, and dress for and drive to work. After a full work day, they drive toward home, with a stop to shop for food. Home again, they cook supper, eat supper on a tray in front of a TV, do house cleaning and laundry, help kids with homework, and get kids to bed. More tired and later than they would like, they get to bed, maybe with a husband. Of course, some men are in similar situations. Many of these people are headed toward some combination of burnout, stress-related health problems, and depression. **Of course, many feel/think that they can't possibly get healthful exercise or prepare really healthful meals for themselves and family members.**

Motivation Problems Resulting from Poor Brain Function

Dr. Daniel Amen, who is a very important expert on brain function, has concluded that lack of motivation can result from problems in function of the brain's deep limbic system (2015). Ways to improve the functioning of that part of the brain include strenuous aerobic exercise and working to overcome negative thoughts. As with all aspects of brain function, a healthful, balanced diet is important. Supplements which may help include DL-phenylalanine, SAMe, and L-tyrosine. Dr. Amen recommends that you take only one of the supplements at a time.

Connection of Health Motivation to Will Power and Related Concepts

The January 2009 issue of *Prevention Magazine* (p. 109) includes helpful suggestions from Kathleen D. Vohs, PhD, concerning "using your willpower wisely." She recommends that you use your limited amount of willpower sparingly; that you eat to avoid dips in your blood sugar (which can lead to strong food cravings); that you not try to maintain a diet that is too strict for you; and that you make sure that you get enough sleep.

Below are some adjectives and nouns and their opposites which relate to health motivation. If nearly all of the terms and phrases on the left apply to you, you don't need to read this chapter. **If several of the terms and phrases on the right apply to you to some degree (which is the case for most people), I think this chapter can probably help you.**

SELF-CONTROLLED	v.	LACKING SELF-CONTROL
SELF-DISCIPLINED	v.	LACKING SELF-DISCIPLINE
MUCH WILL POWER	v.	LITTLE WILL POWER
INDUSTRIOUS	v.	LAZY
ENERGETIC	v.	LETHARGIC
FIGHTER	v.	QUITTER
PERSISTENT	v.	NOT PERSISTENT
DRIVEN	v	HAVING LITTLE DRIVE
FOCUSED	v.	NOT ABLE TO FOCUS WELL
INGENIOUS IN PROBLEM SOLVING	v.	NOT INGENIOUS IN PROBLEM SOLVING
HOPEFUL	v.	NOT HOPEFUL
SELF-CONFIDENT	v.	LACKING SELF-CONFIDENCE
NOT "BURNT OUT"	v.	"BURNT OUT" OR OVER-STRESSED
NOT DEPRESSED	v.	DEPRESSED
FULLY RATIONAL	v.	SOMETIMES NOT FULLY RATIONAL

Most of us are described by some of the words on the left and also some of the words on the right. Maybe you can use the descriptors above to develop a little more self-knowledge. Then, maybe you can become somewhat better in capitalizing on your strengths and minimizing your weaknesses.

This book doesn't emphasize being harsh with yourself in order to build your will power and self-discipline. I don't recommend that you go through exercises involving entirely depriving yourself of things you want. *The Biggest Loser* show on TV shows personal trainers dealing harshly with overweight people who experience extreme discomfort and pain. While those approaches may help some people, they are not found in this book.

To help you to "stick with it," I suggest that you **not** condemn yourself. Condemnations can damage your self-esteem and actually hurt your ability to improve your health life style. Try to be gentle and encouraging with yourself. (I understand that being tough with themselves works for some people.)

Overcoming Inertia and Getting Started

Just getting started can be difficult. Since you are reading this chapter, something has gotten you started. Shock concerning my "bad lipids profile" overcame my inertia in 1981.

Several Internet sites allow you to get an estimation of your life expectancy. The results may help you to overcome inertia and get motivated. The results may include suggestion of specific ways that you can move toward a healthier lifestyle and improve your life expectancy.

Ways to Probably Get Payoffs Surprisingly Quickly from Exercise and Supplements

Nearly all of chapters 6 through 15 include a recommended routine (which I call a vascular cleansing routine (VCR)) that involves taking carefully selected supplements, waiting 30 minutes, and then getting at least 20 minutes (preferably 30 minutes) of at least moderate exercise. Unless you feel exhausted, my guess is that you'll feel better, healthier, and sharper mentally after doing a VCR. Exercise and good nutrition tend to improve sex life and enjoyment of sex. Later in this book I tell you about the dramatic positive outcomes doing my VCR for 36 years has given me. Do a VCR before a poker game. You will probably play better than usual.

The Power of Belief and Optimism

Being optimistic and believing in your health-related actions don't just increase your motivation: The medical literature and the non-medical measures literature both emphasize that **believing in the effectiveness of a treatment can increase its effectiveness**. This is the famous "placebo effect." That is why I encourage readers to call a supplement-and-exercise routine a vascular cleansing routine (VCR).

I encourage you to identify ways that you can know nearly immediately whether your exercise, diet, and supplements are helping you. **In 2007, when my friend Sarah weighed 266 lbs., she went on the Michael Thurman diet and started walking regularly. Within three weeks, her blood pressure and blood sugar had lowered to healthy levels.** So, she quickly got indication that what she was doing was working. I think that a high percentage of readers of this chapter can pretty quickly start getting benefits from healthful diet and exercise and supplements appropriate for their health challenges.

Sticking with It

We all know about the many millions of Americans who have a New Year's resolution to exercise and/or eat a more healthful diet. A high percentage have given up on that effort in a few weeks or months. I don't want that to include you. I hope that, earlier in this chapter, you acquired knowledge of the **giant benefits of good diet, supplements, and exercise**. If so, you should have better prospects for "sticking with" your health-improvement efforts. It will help to avoid making your exercise and/or diet too severe for you.

Spiraling Down and Spiraling Up

If a person "lets his health go," with bad diet, no exercise, no helpful supplements, and no attention to early signs of health problems, his health, enjoyment of life, and performance in important roles can gradually or even suddenly collapse. There can be a spiraling down as various types of health and life problems emerge.

We want you to know and remember that the opposite—having your life and health spiral upward—can happen also. I think that my last 39 years (during which I have had a wonderful son) have involved slow **spiraling upward**, with some fairly brief setbacks along the way.

Some Support from the Bible

I grew up in a small-town Southern Baptist church and had a very good experience with the surprisingly progressive Sunday school. So, it wasn't hard for me to think of ways that Christian doctrine supports doing even difficult things that will be good for your health.

Corinthians lists "faith, hope, and charity" as crucial for humans. While faith undoubtedly has a religious connotation, hope has a more generic meaning. As we've discussed earlier, hope is crucial to getting enough motivation and possibly even to the success of medical treatment. The Bible teaches to "Love your neighbor as yourself." The point is often made in sermons and Sunday school lessons that this inferentially teaches that you should love yourself. When you work seriously and determinedly on your own health, you are expressing love for yourself. Gluttony, including a pattern of overeating, is one of the "seven deadly sins." Sloth, including laziness, is also. Many people who won't work on their health when they know they need to are being lazy.

Overcoming Internal Resistance to Improvement of Motivation

If none of these approaches succeed in motivating you to get healthful diet and exercise, you may want to consider taking your resistance up with a good psychologist or counselor. While I'm not a psychologist, I'll share a little thinking about possible sources of this resistance.

1. **A life script that includes you being unhealthy.** "Script analysis" is a very interesting approach to psychological therapy. It argues that all of us have a life script that we probably learned early in life. If a man smokes and drinks like his father, maybe he has subconsciously accepted that as his life script. Sometimes, patients are able to get rid of an unhealthy script and accept a healthier script.

2. **A "martyr complex."** Some people, many of them parents, get a type of psychological payoff from feeling that they are being martyrs for the benefit

of others. The truth is that, usually, taking care of your own health is the right thing to do in relation to other family members.

3. Depression. It is nearly impossible to be fully motivated when you are depressed.

4. Fear of sexual pressure if you become more healthy and attractive. Improved diet, supplements, and selected supplements definitely tend to improve one's enjoyment of sex.

5. **Low self-esteem**. You may feel that you aren't important or lovable enough for you to really work to have good health.

6. **Anger for important others**. It is said that suicide can be motivated partly by anger for important persons in the suicide's life. Bad health lifestyle can be slow suicide.

Working with a competent psychologist or counselor can help a person to overcome problems like these.

REFERENCES

Amen, Daniel (2015). *Change your brain, change your life* (revised and expanded). NY, NY: Harmony Books.

Blumenthal, J. A. et al (1999). Effects of exercise training on older patients with major depression. *Archives of Internal Medicine*, Vol. 159, No. 19, pp. 2349–2356.

Froggatt, W. (2006). *Taking control.* Auckland, NZ: Harper Collins.

Hill, Napoleon & Stone, Clement W. (2007). *Success through positive mental attitude.* NY, NY: Pocket Books.

Lee, Joyce (2008). Why young adults hold the key to assessing the obesity epidemic of children. *Archives of Pediatric and Adolescent Medicine*, Vol. 162, No. 7, pp. 682–7.

McCullough, M. & Willoughby, B. (2009). Religion, self-regulation, and self-control: associations, explanations, and implications. *Psychological Bulletin*, Vol. 135, No. 1, pp. 69–93.

Pew Research Center (2015). America's changing religious landscape. *Pew Research Center Religion and Public Life* website (May 12, 2015).

Ratey, John J. with Hagerman, Eric (2008). *Spark: the revolutionary new science of exercise and the brain*. NY, NY: Little, Brown and Company.

Salmon, Peter (2001). Effects of physical exercise on anxiety, depression, and sensitivity to stress: a unifying theory. *Clinical Psychology Review*, Vol. 21, Issue 1, pp. 33–61.

Scarmeas, Nikolaos et al (2009). Physical activity, diet, and risk of Alzheimer's disease. *Journal of the American Medical Association*, Vol. 302, No. 6, pp. 627–637.

Seltzer, Leon (2012). Rebuffed? 4 reasons someone might reject your help. Psychology Today website. October 3, 2012.

Taka-aki Okabe, B.M. et al (2006). Effects of exercise on the development of atherosclerosis in apolipoprotein E-deficient mice. *Experimental Clinical Cardiology*, Vol. 11, No. 4, pp. 276–279.

Thompson, Paul D. et al (2003). American Heart Association scientific statement: exercise and physical activity in the prevention and treatment of atherosclerotic cardiovascular disease. *Arteriosclerosis, Thrombosis, and Vascular Biology*, Vol. 23, e42–49.

Weir, Kirsten (2012). The power of self-control. *Psychology Today*, Vol. 43, No. 1, p.36.

CHAPTER 2
Healthful Living

Importance of this subject. It's very clear that your lifestyle (the way you live) influences your health in many important ways. Therefore, this subject is terrifically important.

I believe that probably the most important health-related truth for a person to come to understand and believe is: **If you start genuinely healthful living early enough and stay with it, you probably will have substantially more benefits and payoffs than you could have imagined when you started**. That is what has happened to me, in spite of very numerous and significant health challenges. In the About the Author section at the end of this book, I tell about extraordinary problems, mainly health challenges, I have encountered and, fortunately, have overcome.

If a person fails to achieve and continue healthful living early in life, one of the many adverse effects will be that she or he will be much more vulnerable to depression during old age which is prompted by health problems that might have been prevented.

Two of this book's chapters (32 and 33) concern in very important ways the lifestyle of hunter-gatherer bands of humans in Africa between 200,000 bp (before present) and 70,000 bp. I believe that, in most important ways, those people achieved healthful living. So, one can argue (contrary to some of my discussion in chapter 1) that it is normal and natural for humans to live healthfully.

Several of the other chapters of this book include a description of a supplement-and-exercise routine (which I call a vascular cleansing routine, VCR, because it provides that benefit for me). Each of these chapters contains description of types of health problems which should prompt a person to implement and continue to perform a VCR. I recommend that persons who don't seem to have problems and symptoms described in those chapters go to chapters 4 and read the discussion about intended benefits of particular supplements, and select supplements to take before moderate exercise. Supplements I've taken for 35+ years have benefits regarding heart and blood vessel strength which have made it possible for my heart to beat at 180 beats per minute for literally hours during tachycardia. For many people, that would be life threatening.

Professional review of this chapter. This chapter was favorably reviewed by an experienced nurse-practitioner, who did not suggest any changes.

Author's relevant experience. Earlier in this book, you have learned some about my life experiences relating to health. Since my late 30s, I have been a serious "health nut." In my late 30's, I took a magazine test of knowledge relating to health and made 100%. So, I strongly encourage you to use this book to build your knowledge about health and then to continue to build and update your knowledge.

"Healthful living" was my uncle Jasper Memory's favorite course at Wake Forest College in the late 1910s. During his 90 years of living, he had remarkably good health. I and, no doubt, many others learned a great deal about healthful living from him. Many people can learn about healthful living from a relative.

Unfortunately, some MDs lack very important information about use of supplements and exercise in prevention of disease and illness. I recently saw an MD for the first time. Though I was nearly 74 years old, had been doing my own non-statins heart health routine since 1982, and have excellent cardiovascular health in spite of extremely severe risk factors, she strongly recommended that I start taking a statin drug.

Relevance for young adults. I started teaching my son Alex about healthful living when he was 2½ years old. Fortunately, he now, at 39, has an excellent healthful lifestyle and great health. So, it is nearly never too young to start learning about healthful living.

There are major problems regarding the health-related practices and outcomes of young adults in the U.S. Far too many young adults are sedentary and are developing significant cardiovascular health problems (Lee, 2008). Like other age groups, they are experiencing the epidemic of opioid addiction and overdoses.

Proposal of an undergraduate course on healthful living. A two- or three-hour course about healthful living should include much of the most important information about what a person should and shouldn't do in order to achieve and retain excellent health. This would involve coverage of selected important content of some existing three-hour courses and some content from the 17 chapters of this book that concern health. **It would be possible for students to be exposed to wonderful and, I think, "dynamite" information during nearly every class.** Unfortunately, I doubt that many health-area professors would be willing to teach much of the wonderful information in the first 17 chapters of this book, such as a safe, healthful alternative to taking a statin drug.

Decisions about content of this chapter. Sixteen of the other chapters of this book concern health and emphasize prevention and even reversal of health problems. It wouldn't make sense for that information to be repeated in this chapter. I have decided, instead, to focus on ways to reduce cancer risk. Fortunately, anti-cancer approaches turn out to be very similar to those to reduce risk of cardiovascular disease and brain disease. I'll provide also very current information about prevention of Parkinson's disease.

Ways to lower your cancer risk. You can find on the WebMD website an article with the title "8 ways to lower your cancer risk." Very similar information is on the Mdanderson.org website with the title "8 ways to reduce your cancer risk," and another similar article is on the prevention website. I will paraphrase that information.

Ways to Reduce Your Cancer Risk

1. **Don't smoke. Each year in the U.S., nearly 500,000 people die as a result of smoking.**

2. **Control your weight. Excess body fat is linked to the risk of developing nine types of cancer.**

3. **Exercise regularly.**

4. **Drink little or no alcoholic beverages.**

5. **Eat vegetables, especially broccoli.**

6. **Use sun screen.**

7. **Avoid getting over-stressed. Try to really relax regularly.**

8. **Have cancer-detection screenings done regularly.**

Prevention of Parkinson's disease. On the Institute of Natural Healing website, there is a short article, "5 simple ways to prevent Parkinson's." Here they are.

Eat peppers.

Drink white tea. Other teas help.

Take vitamin B6. They quote research confirming this benefit.

Consume healthy fats.

Take vitamin D3. I'll mention now, as discussed in other chapters, that the old RDA is far too low. I take 10,000 i.u. per day without ill effects. African Americans should get a physician's guidance about supplementation with D3, which, for them, can be dangerous.

Other important aspects of healthful living.

Have a primary physician. Though I believe in and have benefitted from several "alternative" health approaches, I believe it is very important for everyone to have a primary physician. Regular health checkups are important. Your physician can do blood tests to determine whether you have deficiencies, such as vitamin and mineral deficiencies.

Protect your dental health. Bad dental health can take ten years off of your life (McGuire, Thomas; BBC News). For many decades, I have used a tooth pick to entirely "pick" my teeth several times a day. Apparently this "does the job" as well as flossing. I brush after every meal and at bedtime. In my recent twice-yearly tooth cleaning, the hygienist was very impressed with my excellent dental health.

Several years ago, after I was diagnosed with prostate cancer, I learned that there are credible health experts who argue against having root canals. So, I had my three root canals removed. My overall health has been significantly better since having them removed.

Get enough high quality sleep. This supports good health in several important ways.

Identify a reliable source (probably on the Internet) of alternative, holistic approaches for dealing with health problems. Being able to find reliable information about alternative, holistic approaches for dealing with my health problems has helped me significantly numerous times, as discussed in chapter 5. Of course, I think a person should be very hesitant to ignore medical advice from a physician.

Protect home interior air quality. (Qinghua et al, 2010) During 2005, while living in a recently purchased house, I developed a cough that lasted for 11 weeks. Shortly after I installed an air-purification device, the cough ended.

Develop a written health-promotion plan for yourself. I have revised my heart- and brain-health routine many dozens of times over the years. This can include selecting recreational activities that will help you to be a happy and healthy person. I'll elaborate on this suggestion. You could get the list of suggested supplements near the end of chapter 4 and use information in this chapter to develop a VCR against heart and brain disease (including diabetes), cancer, and Parkinson's disease. (I suspect that this is the best suggestion I provide in this long book.)

Teach your children about the wonderful payoffs of healthful living. It's important to learn the payoffs of good health practices. Knowing the payoffs will help you to have enough health motivation.

Learn from the good and bad health examples and experiences of others. If several people related to you have had heart disease, Alzheimer's or dementia, or a type of cancer, you need to tell your doctor and try to prevent or at least detect that type of health problem early.

Regularly do some resistance training, such as weight lifting. Since the middle 1970s, I have done weekly limited resistance training, including some weight lifting, specifically to be strong enough to play golf reasonably well. I think this exercise has contributed significantly to my overall health and wellbeing.

Increase your sun exposure.

Flush toilets only after putting down the seat. Since I started doing this, my health has been better.

REFERENCES

BBC News: News, Health. "Key reason 'found' for gum and heart disease link." Available on Internet

Lee, Joyce (2008). Why young adults hold the key to assessing the obesity epidemic of children. *Archives of Pediatric and Adolescent Medicine*, Vol. 162, No. 7, pp. 682–7.

McGuire, Thomas. The relationship of oral to overall health and longevity: what every health professional needs to know. *BBC*. Available on Internet

Qinghua, Sun et al (2010). Contemporary reviews in cardiovascular medicine: cardiovascular effects of ambient particulate air pollution exposure. *Circulation*, Vol. 121, pp. 2755–2765.

Warren, Rick (2013). *The Daniel plan: 40 days to a healthier life.* Grand Rapids, MI: Zondervan.

—— CHAPTER 3 ——
Using Diet to Protect and Improve Your Heart and Brain Health

Elaboration. This chapter is primarily about foods we eat and beverages we drink. I hope it will provide helpful information for several categories of people: (1) people who want to achieve protection and improvement of heart and brain health without taking any (OK, maybe a few) supplements; (2) those who buy wonderful, expensive ingredients, cook and prepare them well, consume a great diet, and achieve excellent health benefits; (I suspect that even they can benefit from some high quality information about nutrition and supplements.) (3) people who have limited time and money but still want to cook and prepare meals that will meet their nutrition needs; and (4) people who acknowledge that they don't eat as good a diet as they would like, while hoping to improve the healthfulness of the foods and beverages they consume.

Those categories are distinguished because, for example, people in category 2 would want to buy wonderful ingredients and prepare Mediterranean diet meals, while people in category 4 might want to regularly eat reasonably healthful TV dinners.

Importance of information in this chapter for everyone. Please forgive this obvious point: To achieve good or excellent heart and brain health, everyone (even takers of many supplements, like me) need to implement suggestions of this chapter or some other credible source of information about good diet.

Discovering and dealing with nutritional deficiencies. "Macronutrients" in which a high percentage of Americans are deficient include vitamin D3, coenzyme Q10 (or ubiquinol, if you are over 45), magnesium, vitamin B12, vitamin K/K2, selenium, vitamin E, calcium, potassium, and iodine. My impression is that even a "fairly good" diet does not provide enough vitamin D3, coenzyme Q10 (or ubiquinol, if you are over 45), vitamin B12, or iodine. So, I think that all four of the groups listed above need to be careful to identify, with blood tests ordered by a doctor, and overcome nutritional deficiencies, even if this requires taking a supplement.

Though I have always taken a vitamin D3 supplement and have gotten a lot of sun exposure, I discovered several years ago that I was seriously deficient in vitamin D. My health and wellbeing have clearly been better since I started taking at least 10,000 iu of vitamin D3 per day. Some readers will be surprised to learn that I would take that much D3. You need to know that many highly qualified experts believe that the long-time RDA (recommended daily allowance) of D3 has been far too low.

The importance of regular moderate exercise for people who emphasize good diet. In several other chapters about health, I have given readers a recommended supplements-and-exercise routine (vascular cleansing routine, VCR). Though this chapter does not address supplements except in the two previous paragraphs above, readers who decide to emphasize good diet and minimize supplements clearly need to get regular moderate exercise. As discussed in chapter 6, there are advantages of getting the benefits of supplements and exercise at the same time. Though our society strongly discourages exercising shortly after eating, I recommend that you experiment concerning exercising not long after eating.

Money and time required to prepare excellent meals from raw ingredients. My assumption is that a substantial amount of money and time is required to prepare excellent meals from raw ingredients. I think there is need for information on how to prepare those types of meals without expending a lot of time and/or money.

Importance of this subject. As we all know, there are many ways that diet can impact a person's heart and brain health. Though much of the "expert" information about diet has been flawed in recent decades, I think we currently have reasonably good information available. This chapter tells about several physicians who emphasize good diet for health, whose patients very often achieve extremely positive results overcoming serious disease.

Some of the benefits of consuming a healthful diet, as suggested in this chapter. Not only will this be healthful from a heart health and brain health point of view: It will, to a very significant degree, be healthful from the cancer-prevention, anti-aging, and Parkinson's-prevention points of view.

An excellent article by an experienced heart surgeon that covers many of the points in this chapter. Dr. Dwight Lundell is the author of a 2012 article ("The great cholesterol lie exposed by Dr. Dwight Lundell") that is the most important and helpful statement by a cardiologist I have ever read or heard of. Much of it concerns heart-healthy diet.

Heart healthy fats. Recommendations of experts about fats have changed so much over recent decades that I want to address that very early in this chapter.

Dr. Josh Axe, who holds a doctoral degree in nutrition, recommends consumption of avocados, butter, coconut oil, extra virgin olive oil, and omega-3's (fish oil, DHA, flaxseed oil) in an article on the Internet: "The 5 best healthy fats for your body." On his website, he lists several other types of oils that can be healthfully consumed.

Dr. Walter Willett, Harvard School of Public Health, recommends getting about 40% of your calories from healthy fats. Dr. Mercola, who I believe is as credible as Dr. Willett, recommends getting between 50% and 70% of your calories from healthy fats ("To achieve optimal health, eat 50–70% of this frequently demonized food."). A person would have to work very hard to get 70% of calories from healthy fats. I buy a lot of very delicious SmartBalance with olive oil spread and put it on nearly everything I eat and have found that coconut oil tastes great with oatmeal, especially raisin/date/walnut oatmeal. I learned at the end of August 2018 that coconut oil has great benefits against low thyroid function, with is one of health problems.

A warning about trying to consume enough healthy fats. If a person simply adds more "healthy fats" to a diet that was not producing weight gain, it's obvious that weight gain will occur. I am trying to keep that from happening to me now.

Relevance for young adults. My impression is that the diet of young adults has gradually declined in quality during recent decades. Dr. Richard Isaacson and Christopher Ochner, PhD, have recently had an important book (2016) published on the prevention of Alzheimer's. They recommend that people undertake various types of Alzheimer's prevention, especially consumption of healthful foods and beverages, as early in life as possible.

Author's relevant experience. For years after graduating from law school in 1968, I would order at McDonald's a Big Mac, fries, Coke, and chocolate shake—a recipe for obesity. Since the early 1980s, I have very often ordered only a chicken sandwich at a fast food restaurant.

I buy a $2 package of mixed nuts at a convenience store about four or five times per week. My guess is that I buy about half of the $2 mixed nuts sold at three convenience stores in northeast Columbia, SC. Over the last 15 years, I have noticed substantial deterioration of the quality of foods and snacks sold in convenience stores.

Though I know about and take many nutritional supplements, I am very aware of many of the health benefits of excellent diet and have watched dozens of public television programs featuring outstanding physicians who emphasize excellent diet.

I know many people who "eat a better diet" than I do. I have, however, tried especially hard (and successfully) to avoid consuming foods and beverages that can have adverse health effects. For example, I have since 1982 nearly never eaten beef or processed meat, doughnuts, and other sugary "treats" and soft drinks. Fortunately, my less-than-perfect diet has not kept me from achieving excellent heart and brain health, in spite of extremely bad risk factors.

During 2016, I eliminated grains from my diet because of Dr. David Perlmutter's argument that consumption of grain foods is adverse for brain health and function. I have also moved far in the direction of eating low glycemic-index foods, because of concerns regarding type 2 diabetes risk. I am very happy with both of these major diet changes.

I like cheese-and-tuna omelets and, several years ago, often cooked and ate one. At some point, I sensed that eating them was adversely affecting my thinking and memory. So, I stopped eating them. Based on my recent reading about diet, I think the omelets were having bad health effects for me.

Integrative MDs and DOs who have diet as an important part of their practice. I recommend that young adults and others identify an excellent integrative MD or DO who emphasizes diet in his or her practice. Integrative MDs who have excellent dietary regimens include Dr. Mark Hyman, Dr. Russell Blaylock, Dr. David Perlmutter, Dr. Donald Levy, and Dr. Neal Barnard. I have been favorably impressed by Dr. Joel Fuhrman, who emphasizes consuming food that is sufficiently dense nutritionally, and have been favorably impressed with the work of an osteopathic physician (DO), Dr. Mercola, who has an excellent website. All of these physicians have had patients with one or more serious medical problems who, after complying with the physician's dietary regimen for some period of time, have entirely overcome one or more serious medical conditions.

During 2017 I bought off of the Internet Ultra Primal Lean weight-loss product developed and promoted by a physician. I took the product as indicated for about five days. Though I did not eat more than usual, **I actually gained about three pounds in five days**.

Good meals that don't take much money or time. Spending a lot of time and money cooking good food has not ranked high among my life priorities. For many years, I have eaten lots of Marie Callender's frozen dinners. During that period, my health has been steadily improving. When I am getting ready to eat a Marie Callender meal, I usually put SmartBalance spread made mainly with olive oil on the vegetables. That spread actually tastes better than butter.

Need for caution in eating "soy nuts." Eating soybeans, which are marketed as "soy nuts," is chemically similar to getting a shot of estrogen. I doubt that many men want to experience that regularly, if ever.

Weight loss and weight control. A good diet shouldn't produce weight gain. If a person becomes significantly overweight, the likelihood of developing high blood pressure, the metabolic syndrome, and even type 2 diabetes increases substantially.

Adverse health consequences of excess belly fat. There is no doubt that having excess belly fat has adverse health consequences, which can include higher blood pressure, development of metabolic syndrome, and increased risk of type 2 diabetes. Of course, risks of heart attack and Alzheimer's increase. Losing belly fat is very difficult. Here is an Internet article which claims to provide good information about that: "Synergistic diet and exercise for ridiculously fast fat loss," on the joshsgarage website.

Low risk of being slightly overweight for senior citizens. Christopher Wanjek is the author of an article, October 2, 2013, on the LiveScience website with the title "Weighty issue: Is it healthy for seniors to be a little overweight?" Based on two recent research studies, Wanjek answers that being slightly overweight is not dangerous for senior citizens.

An approach for losing and controlling weight. Dr. Oz is a very capable and accomplished integrative physician. To find a weight loss and control approach that may work for you, search for "Dr. Oz and student researcher discover $5 weight loss miracle." Apparently, the student lost 27 lbs. in three weeks. The method involves early on every day drinking tea with apple cider vinegar, followed by taking Slim Tech Cambogia.

The importance of emphasizing weight control. Because losing a lot of weight can result each time in loss of muscle tissue, it is extremely desirable to set a realistic weight limit for yourself and then work consistently to avoid gaining above that level. While some "experts" recommend against checking your weight every morning, I have found over many years that I need to check my weight every morning. If undesirable weight gain occurs, it's important to learn about it, stop it, and reverse it as soon as possible.

Apparent danger of the Atkins diet. Early in 2001, I acknowledged that I had gained far too much weight, reaching 212 pounds. Before going on the Atkins diet I could hit my golf 8 iron 150 yds. and my 5 iron 180 yds. After losing 40 lbs. on the Atkins diet, I had lost 30 yds. of distance on all of my irons. (In 2018 I met a strong golfer in his 60s who had exactly the same experience.) Obviously, that high-protein diet caused me to experience very undesirable loss of muscle tissue. Dr. Mercola mentions that emphasizing protein in your diet may have adverse consequences concerning hormones. It was during that weight loss that my troublesome increase in PSA started, resulting in my having prostate surgery.

Ideas about causes of major increase in obesity in the U.S. Several charts indicate that the major increase in obesity started occurring in the U.S. about in 1978. During and before the 1950s, many American teenagers attended a fairly small high school, and many of them played a varsity sport. In my very small-town high school, there was one substantially overweight person, who was a star basketball player. My guess is that, as American teenagers in the 1960s and 1970s attended progressively larger high schools and were progressively less likely to play a varsity sport, progressively more of them became overweight or obese. White males in high school had a better chance of playing varsity basketball or football before integration. The same applied to the likelihood that white females would be able to play varsity basketball.

The first statin drug was approved in 1987. Research has indicated that taking a statin results in the person being less likely to exercise. I believe that the fact that many millions of Americans take a statin drug has contributed substantially to the epidemic of obesity in the U.S.

Sufficiencies and deficiencies of nutrients. Every person who wants to eat responsibly should go to the Dr. Joel Fuhrman website and read an article with the title "nutrient density," which is only about 1½ pages long. Dr. Fuhrman focuses on the need for "micronutrients" or "phytonutrients." While an extremely high percentage of Americans are woefully deficient in these micronutrients, persons who eat according to Dr. Fuhrman's plan (information provided in the "nutrient density" article) should not be deficient in micronutrients.

Recent research about fats to minimize and fats to select. Research findings released in 2012 indicate that, among 6,183 women over 65 tracked for four years, consumption of saturated fat (animal fat) was associated with decline in "memory and abstract thinking," while consumption of monounsaturated fat (major source, olive oil) was associated with significantly less cognitive decline (Okereke, 2012). So, **there has been research indicating that consumption of a lot of saturated fat by older people, especially women, can result in cognitive decline.**

Whole grain eating. Several years ago, I became convinced that eliminating refined grain foods (and other refined carbohydrates and "white foods") and **shifting to whole grain eating helps with protecting and improving cardiovascular health.** (Of course, if you have celiac disease or other significant adverse reaction to gluten in your diet, you can't healthfully eat even whole grain foods.) Many heart- and brain-healthy nutrients are found in whole grain foods. It is a mistake, however, to eat a very great amount of whole grain foods. That will result in a high-carbohydrate diet, which is not healthful.

Dr. David Perlmutter ("Grain brain by David Perlmutter, MD (2013): brain health food list," on chewfo.com website) has an entirely different opinion regarding eating grains, even whole grains. He argues that eating a lot of whole grain foods can result in what he calls a "grain brain," which performs less well cognitively. Because I have very severe heart and brain disease risk factors, I accepted Dr. Perlmutter's advice to stop eating grains in about 2015 and am very happy with the results. Dr. Perlmutter argues also that going on a "low glycemic-index food" diet has great benefits regarding brain health and function and prevention of type 2 diabetes. As mentioned above, I accepted that recommendation also and am happy with the results.

Walnuts. One of the underlying causes of atherosclerosis is progressive endothelial dysfunction (blood vessels gradually functioning worse). Walnuts contain a variety of nutrients, including arginine, polyphenols, and omega-3 oils, that support the inner arterial lining and guard against abnormal platelet aggregation. These favorable biological effects explain why walnut consumption tends to protect against coronary-artery disease (Feldman, 2002).

The U.S. National Library of Medicine database contains 35 peer-reviewed published papers supporting a claim that ingesting walnuts improves vascular health and may reduce heart attack risk.

Alcoholic beverages. Very recent research has indicated that drinking of alcoholic beverages results in many deaths every year. Regular drinking of surprisingly few alcoholic beverages also results in many deaths. Of course, binge drinking causes deaths.

Fortunately, research (German & Walzem, 2000) has shown that drinking **red wine (men, no more than two glasses; women, no more than one**

glass) daily can help with heart health in at least two ways: provision of flavonoids and reduction of the tendency of blood to coagulate (clot).

Sugary soft drinks. The lead author of a research study (2007) by Boston University School of Medicine researchers has stated, "Even one soda per day increases your risk of developing metabolic syndrome by 50 percent." This is reported on the WebMD website.

Green tea and other tea. There is evidence that drinking green tea has heart health benefits ("Health benefits of green tea" at WebMD website). Drinking black, green, and white teas (all from the same plant) can be healthful.

A scientific study indicating that a "low carbs" diet can be effective and safe. Recently, there was an article on the Lifetime weight loss website with the title, "Low-carb vs low-fat—What does research show?", by Tom Nikkola, director of Nutrition and Weight Management. The author reviewed 14 random-dom controlled-diet trials. He found that low-carbohydrate (higher fat and protein) diets do a better job in weight loss and keeping the weight off than low-fat, high-carbohydrate diets. He found no evidence that a low-carbs diet increases CVD (cardiovascular disease) risk.

I include this article because of my clear impression that "nutrition experts" have misled the general public several times over the last 50 years. There has been recommendation of a "high-carbs" diet, which apparently has contributed significantly to the increases in obesity and type 2 diabetes. Nearly everything "experts" have said about oils/fats has been at least partly wrong. Responsible experts tell us now, among other things, that we need a small intake of animal saturated fat, such as real butter. Because of the findings of Okereke study mentioned above, I do not intentionally introduce saturated fat into my diet.

Heart disease risk of consuming canned and frozen foods. An author, Tamara Galloway, PhD, of a study (Melzer et al, 2012) in the journal *Circulation*, reports that consumption of BPA, which is found in many containers of canned foods and frozen foods, appears to be associated with an increase in occurrence of cardiovascular disease.

Achieving regression of atherosclerosis with diet. There is no doubt that reversal of atherosclerosis (hardening of the arteries) can be achieved with a program that mainly involves careful adherence to a rigorous diet. This has been accomplished by Dr. Ornish, Dr. Pritikin, and others. President Clinton, who has had serious cardiovascular health problems, including having a heart attack, has adopted a plant-based diet that is extremely restrictive, excluding meats and even fish. There is strong scholarly support for that approach (Esselstyn, 2001). If one of these approaches is appealing to you, you can easily find information on the Internet about those diets and about books describing the diet you are interested in. Chapter 9 of this book provides information about reversal of atherosclerosis through diet, supplements, and exercise.

Two recommended diet approaches. After reading about many dietary approaches for healthful eating, weight loss, and weight control, I have decided to provide some information about two approaches. Regardless of the particular diet approach you adopt, you should remember that **it is important to eat fresh vegetables and fruits to prevent heart disease**.

The Fuhrman healthful eating program. Dr. Joel Fuhrman, who was mentioned earlier, has developed excellent approaches to achieve disease reversal and **weight loss** which rely heavily on consuming enough of the right micronutrients. Dr. Oz is a true believer in Dr. Fuhrman and his ideas. (Of course, it's easy to find Fuhrman approaches on the Internet. To read an article that provides information about Dr. Fuhrman's methods, search for "Dr. Oz: I believed I was on a track for early death. Dr. Fuhrman saved my life" on the anewdayanewme.com website.) Adhering to the Fuhrman diet should eventually result in normal BP (blood pressure) without medication.

Dr. Fuhrman suggests eating lots of the foods listed below in order to get enough micronutrients, which are insufficient in nearly everyone's diet. He argues persuasively that, if you consume enough of crucial micronutrients, **you will be much less likely to have appetite-control problems**.

G greens and garlic
O onions
M mushrooms

B beans and berries
S seeds and nuts

When I eat at a restaurant with a salad bar, I eat only the salad bar items and work on making it a GOMBS meal. If you eat subs, you can ask for all of the available GOMBS vegetables on your sub. Based on newly acquired information about "healthy fats" that is near the start of this chapter, I am going to supplement any GOMBS meals with healthy fats.

In chapter 7, you will find a recipe I developed for a low blood pressure soup (**LBP** soup). If you decide to make the **LBP** soup, you can experiment with adding to the recipe some of the GOMBS ingredients, which will make your soup a genuine "super food" by improving nutrition and flavor. The recipe in chapter 7 includes simple suggestions for converting the recipe to turkey chili, which should also have bp-control benefit.

The Mediterranean diet. Very large-scale research has consistently shown that persons consuming a Mediterranean diet tend to have vastly better health and weight control outcomes than Americans in general. An Internet article, "Mediterranean Diet Guidelines," states that a Mediterranean diet emphasizes consumption of plant foods, is low in saturated fat and rich in monounsaturated fat (usually olive oil), low-to-moderate in consumption of dairy products, limited in consumption of fish, poultry, and red meat, and moderate in consumption of wine with meals. The article's author recommends also regular exposure to sunshine (for vitamin D), regular physical exercise, and reduction of stress.

Very important research, the Lyon Diet Heart Study, set out to mimic the Cretan diet, which is a version of the Mediterranean diet. The dietary change included 20% increases in fruit and bread and decreases in processed and red meat. **On this diet, deaths from all causes were reduced by 70%** (Kris-Etherton et al, 2001)**.**

<u>A variety of dietary approaches you can consider.</u>

Emphasizing consumption of "superfoods". Another good way to improve your diet is to increase your consumption of "superfoods". I obtained on the Internet 21 credible lists of superfoods, which contain lots of important nutrients, and counted times particular foods appeared on a list. While many foods were listed three or fewer times, the following foods were listed more, as indicated by the numbers in parentheses: avocado (7), beans/lentils (14), blueberries (11), broccoli (7), dark chocolate (7), salmon and other fish (17), garlic (7), spinach and other green leafy vegetables (12), milk (usually fat-free or 1%) (7), nuts, especially almonds and walnuts (16), oats and oatmeal (7), onions (4), sweet potatoes (5), tomatoes (7), and yogurt, especially low-fat (9). This list is very similar to a list on the WebMD website with the title "25 top heart-healthy foods."

Lists of foods to avoid and select.

Some suggestions about foods to avoid
Trans fats; partially hydrogenated oil
Fried foods
Hot dogs, processed meats
Pizza
Sausage
Processed cheese (the worst)
Doughnuts, hamburgers, cheeseburgers, chips & fries, ice cream
Croissants
Food containing MSG
Omega-6 oils—soybean, corn, peanut (Avoid heavy consumption.)
White foods (Limit white bread and pasta, potatoes, white rice, etc.)
High-sugar desserts (Avoid regular consumption.)
Saturated fat (e.g., fat in cheese and milk. Avoid heavy consumption.)
    (Though coconut oil is saturated, consuming it is healthful in many
    ways.)
Aluminum or copper in drinking water
Gluten in grains is very bad for people with Celiac disease and others
    with significant gluten sensitivity, which may be as high as 30% of
    people.
Sugary drinks
Avoid iron and copper in a multivitamin.
Soy nuts.

Some suggestions about foods you should eat

Fresh fruits and vegetables

Grape juice (two cups per day for anthocyanins) (Fruit juice can cause weight gain.)

Fish, especially wild salmon and sardines (Avoid fried fish.)

Dark chocolate

Avocado

Tomato

Chicken breast

Blueberries and other berries

Foods that are high in fiber, such as fresh fruits and vegetables and whole-grain foods

Fruits

Spinach

Soy sauce

Nuts, especially walnuts (which help with reversal of atherosclerosis), almonds, and seeds

Egg yolk

Apple juice

Coconut oil (as cooking oil or supplement); olive oil; palm oil (Olive and palm oils contain a lot of alpha-linolenic acid, a desirable omega-3 oil. These oils are much better to consume than peanut, soybean, sunflower, and safflower oils.)

Extremely high-quality cold-processed whey protein from health-food store (With exercise, it causes your body to produce glutathione, a very powerful antioxidant.)

Almond milk

Broccoli

Foods rich in antioxidants (e.g., vegetables)

Sweet potatoes

Garlic

Beets

Coffee (Drinking three cups of caffeinated coffee daily may help in prevention of Alzheimer's.)

Water (Sufficient hydration is crucial for brain health and function. Persistent dehydration can lead to brain shrinkage.)

Substituting healthful foods for unhealthful foods. You can move toward having a heart-healthy diet by substituting heart-healthy foods for ones that are not. Here are some suggestions:

Foods and beverages to avoid	Tasty, healthful substitute
Hamburgers	Turkey burger
Beef steak, unless grass-fed	Salmon, other fish
Beef chili	Turkey chili
Cow's milk and milk products	Goat milk and goat milk products
Cheese, especially processed cheese	Almond cheese
Candy, sugary desserts	Grapes, ripe fruit, watermelon, dark chocolate
Ordinary pasta (such as spaghetti)	Healthful pasta (whole wheat and others)
Macaroni and cheese	Really tasty vegetable casseroles
French fries	Slice potatoes, dip them in egg whites, then bake.
White potatoes	Sweet potatoes
White bread	Whole wheat or other whole-grain bread
Doughnuts, Danish, muffins	Whole-grain toast with preserves
White rice	Brown rice, wild rice
Whole milk	Skim milk, almond milk, almond/coconut milk
Fried foods	Foods that are fried in the most healthful ways possible, grilled foods
Soft drinks, like cola	Fruit juice, green tea with stevia sweetener and lemon
Butter (not bad in moderation)	SmartBalance spread or other healthful butter substitute; olive oil, coconut butter, coconut oil
Omega-6 oils (corn, soybean, sunflower, safflower oil); avoid cooking with canola oil	Omega-3 oil (flaxseed or algal oil); only coconut oil for high-heat cooking; olive oil OK for moderate-heat cooking

REFERENCES

Esselstyn, Caldwell et al (2001). Resolving the coronary artery disease epidemic through plant-based nutrition. *Preventive Cardiology*, Vol. 4, No. 4, pp. 171–77.

Feldman, Elaine (2002). The scientific evidence for a beneficial health relationship between walnuts and coronary heart disease. *Journal of Nutrition*, Vol. 132, No. 5, pp. 10625–11015.

German, J.B. & Walzem, R.L. (2000). The health benefits of wine. *Annual Review of Nutrition*, Vol. 20, pp. 561–93.

Isaacson, Richard S. & Ochner, Christopher (2016). *The Alzheimer's prevention & treatment diet.* Garden City Park, NY: Square One Publishers.

Kris-Etherton, Penny et al (2001). Lyon diet heart study. *Circulation*, Vol. 103, pp. 823–25.

Lundell, Dwight (2012). Heart surgeon speaks out on what really causes heart disease. On the Sott.net website.

Melzer, D. et al. (2012). Urinary bisphenol: a concentration and risk of future coronary artery disease in apparently healthy men and men. *Circulation*, Vol. 125, pp. 1482–90.

Okereke, Olivia et al (2012). Dietary fat types and 4-year cognitive change in community-dwelling older women. *Annals of Neurology*, Vol. 72, No. 1, pp. 124–34.

— SECTION 2 —
Alternative, Homeopathic, Holistic Medical Methods

CHAPTER 4
Health Benefits of Nutritional Supplements

<u>Elaboration</u>. Fully developed information about the efficacy of supplements in protection and improvement of human health can be covered in a three-hour undergraduate course but not in one chapter of this book. Therefore, I decided to provide in this chapter especially important information concerning the efficacy of supplements relating to heart and brain health.

Calculated cost per day of 15 carefully selected supplements. A little before the references at the end of this chapter, I report my careful calculation that those 15 supplements would have an average daily cost of less than $1. Taking many of those supplements, followed by exercise, since 1982 has given me astonishingly great health outcomes. Remember that you don't need to receive a substantial benefit from any of those supplements. If each provides a modest benefit, your total benefits can be substantial.

<u>Important research finding relating to supplementation with calcium</u>. On the Science Daily website, there is an article about research (Parag et al, 2017) concerning heart attack risk of amounts of calcium in artery plaque. A quote from the Science Daily article follows:

"Patients without calcium buildup in their coronary arteries had significantly lower risk of future heart attack or stroke despite other high risk factors such as diabetes, high blood pressure, or bad cholesterol levels, new research shows."

This study strongly suggests several things. (1) To learn a great deal about your heart-attack risk, you can get a calcium scan of your arteries. (2) A person should be very cautious about supplementation with calcium. (3) Traditionally considered heart-disease risk factors appear to be less predictive than once thought. (4) Specifically, elevated LDL is apparently not as serious of a risk factor as generally believed. (5) There is, therefore, even less justification for taking a statin drug.

Author's relevant experience. I have been taking nutritional supplements regularly since attending law school (1965–68). I recently counted that I take about 38 supplements either regularly or occasionally. Fortunately, I am aware of only one adverse consequence for me, which I will tell you about. In about 2013, I stopped taking vitamin E, an anti-coagulant, started taking vitamin K2, a coagulant, and developed a dangerous deep vein thrombosis (DVT) (blood clot) near the knee of my left leg. Taking Xarelto eliminated the DVT. Later, I shifted to Eliquis and plan to take that drug every morning for the rest of my life. The point is that a person needs to be cautious about using nutritional supplements, especially coagulants and anti-coagulants. Later in this chapter there is a section about suggested caution relating to many supplements.

The fact that I take many supplements either regularly or occasionally suggests that I may need nutritional assistance regarding a fairly large number of health vulnerabilities. Maybe it suggests that I don't do a good job of obtaining important nutrition in my diet. The truth is probably somewhere in between.

Some people may experience problems taking as many supplements as frequently as I do. I believe that it would be prudent for a person to gradually add to the number of supplements she or he takes daily.

How much prudence is needed in taking supplements? Late in October 2017, I was talking to a physician friend about nutritional supplements. Though he is an excellent physician and person, he, like an appallingly high percentage of physicians, knows very little about nutrition. He emphasized that people need to be careful about taking supplements. Having studied supplements since the early 1980s, I believe that the benefits from excellent supplements are so numerous and great that better advice from a physician would be, "Get information about supplements that you have good reason to believe was written carefully and honestly by a capable, honest, and responsible person using available scientific information. Then, don't hesitate to use that information in selecting supplements to take." I frankly believe that, for nearly everyone, it would be very **imprudent** to fail to take carefully selected nutritional supplements.

There can be tradeoffs concerning taking a particular supplement. For example, one of my favorite supplements, lecithin, has significant cognitive functioning benefits and benefits in fighting hardening of the arteries. Unfortunately, taking lecithin can increase prostate cancer risk among men. You may assume that, since I have had prostate cancer probably since the early 2000's, I must regret having taken lecithin twice a day since 1982. Wrong! I think lecithin was crucial in my victory over heart disease. Also, I expect to eventually defeat prostate cancer.

Quality of nutritional supplements. Occasionally, a significant problem regarding supplement quality emerges somewhere in the U.S. Therefore, it is prudent to be careful about quality of supplements you take. There is an informative document about this: "Natural v. synthetic: the shocking truth about vitamins," published in 2011 by Easy Health Options—Nature and Wellness Made Simple. On the nutritionaltree.com website, you can find "Nutritional supplement buying guide," which may be helpful.

A precaution about taking several types of pills. Fortunately, I'm not aware of having had any problems regarding interaction of supplements and prescribed drugs. Still, I try to take vitamin and mineral supplements together, herbs together, and prescribed drugs together. I wait at least 30 minutes after taking one type of pills before taking another type of pills. It's important to be careful to drink enough water when taking pills. When I take a lot of supplements at one time (about once a day), I drink more than a large glass of water.

<u>Importance of this subject</u>. For many years, the Alzheimer's Foundation has announced that Alzheimer's cannot be prevented or reversed. The fact that Dr. Dale Bredesen utilized 31 supplements in successful Alzheimer's-reversal research (2014) indicates the importance of supplements in the protection and improvement of health. The supplements included in the Bredesen patient programs are listed below. I take many of them.

Nutritional supplements included in Dr. Bredesen's Alzheimer's-reversal customized programs. Vitamin B12, MTHF, P5P (active form of B6), l-tryptophan, melatonin, TMG, methylcobalamin, curcumin, vitamin D3, DHA, EPA, ashwagandha (herbal supplement), bacopa monneira (herbal supplement), magnesium-threconate, vitamin K2, acetyl-l-carnitine, citico-line, vitamin E (tocopherols and tocotrienols), selenium, n-acetyl cysteine, ascorbate, alpha-lipoid acid, CoQ10 (presumably ubiquinol for persons over 45), zinc, resveratrol, thiamine, PQQ (pyrroloquinoline quinone, an enzyme taken as a supplement), pantothenic acid, coconut oil, Axona

In his excellent recent book, *Memory Rescue* (2017), Dr. Daniel Amen mentions 53 nutritional supplements.

Widespread ignorance of U.S. physicians regarding nutrition and nutritional supplements. Unfortunately, a high percentage of physicians have grossly inadequate knowledge about nutrition and nutritional supplements. I believe that this should be viewed as scandalous by Americans. Most individuals need to acquire information about nutritional supplements on their own. Of course, I hope this chapter and book will help readers in meeting this need.

Resistance of drug companies and, I regrettably think, many physicians to individuals contributing to solution or reduction of their medical problems by taking nutritional supplements. I believe that this gives us clues concerning the widespread fear of professors regarding express-ing criticism of statins or support for adoption of a supplement-and-exercise routine as an alternative to taking a statin.

Misleading articles about nutritional supplements. Occasionally I encounter an article (often in *Reader's Digest*) by or quoting a health professional to the effect that money spent on nutritional supplements is nearly entirely wasted. I very strongly believe that the people who provide those opinions either are not competent or are speaking dishonestly. During November of 2017, the widely distributed AARP monthly publication included a statement to the effect that there is no evidence that nutritional supplements help with prevention of Alzheimer's or other dementia. I suspect that AARP receives important monetary support from drug companies.

Need for good diet of persons who "take a lot of supplements." While I certainly "take a lot of supplements," I strongly believe that there is important information for us "big-time supplement takers" in chapter 3. For example, everyone needs to consume a lot of high quality fats.

Relevance for young adults. Many young adults do not have a nearly balanced and healthful diet. Because of this, it is very important for young adults to develop strong information about nutritional supplements.

Nutrients that are often deficient in individuals. Vitamin D3, coenzyme Q10 (or ubiquinol, if you are over 45), magnesium, vitamin B12, vitamin K/K2, selenium, vitamin E, calcium, potassium, and iodine are "macronutrients" in which a high percentage of Americans are deficient. My impression is that even a "fairly good" diet does not provide enough vitamin D3, coenzyme Q10 (or ubiquinol, if you are over 45), vitamin B12, and iodine. It is very important to know that taking a statin drug tends to very dangerously reduce a person's level of coenzyme Q10. Though African Americans tend to be deficient in vitamin D3, supplementation with D3 can be dangerous. The common deficiency in vitamin B12 can result in a shrunken brain.

If you want to make better decisions about supplements, it makes sense to request your doctor to conduct tests to detect nutritional deficiencies.

Sources of high quality information about the benefits and side effects of nutritional supplements. I have researched, mainly on the Internet, concerning the benefits and dangers of all of the nutritional supplements I mention in this book. If you do a search for "benefits and side effects of _____," my experience is that you will find information that will answer your questions.

I list below some of the sources on the Internet with credible information about nutritional supplements. If you want more information about a particular supplement, you can go to the first website listed (U. of MD) and find an article with references to relevant scientific research.

University of Maryland Medical Center Complementary and Alternative Medicine Guide

Office of Dietary Supplements in the NIH National Center for Complementary and Integrative Health

"The nutrition source." On the website of the Harvard T. H. Chan School of Public Health website

"Nutrition 101: finding good help and information." On the "thedoctorwillseeyounow" website.

American Society for Nutritional Sciences at www.nutrition.org/nutinfo

National Center for Biotechnology Information

Balch, Phyllis (2^(nd), ed., 2010). *Prescription for nutritional healing: A to Z guide to supplements.* NY, NY: Avery.

Discussion of particular supplements, including citations to supporting scientific research. The information below is primarily limited to supplements that apparently tend to help regarding heart and brain health. Of course, it is not necessary to take all of these supplements to achieve and maintain excellent heart and brain health and function. I think, however, that it will help a person with high heart disease risk factors to learn much of this information. It's important to know that, if you have high heart disease risk factors, you also have high brain disease risk factors.

Alpha-linolenic acid. This is an omega-3 polyunsaturated fatty acid found in some plants and fish. Research (Albert et al, 2005) has indicated that consumption of alpha-linolenic acid (ALA) tends to reduce the incidence of sudden cardiac death (SCD) in women. This may result from some anti-arrhythmic properties of ALA.

Alpha-lipoic acid (600 mg). Research has shown that mice receiving supplementation with alpha-lipoic acid developed fewer atherosclerotic lesions and gained less weight than control groups which did not receive that supplementation (Zhang et al, 2008). Alpha-lipoic acid is included in some commercially marketed weight loss products. After consuming alpha-lipoic acid or a special form of whey protein, the body produces glutathione, which Dr. Oz rates as the "Superhero of Antioxidants."

Chondroitin. Decades ago, scientific research about the heart health benefits of supplementation with chondroitin produced very promising findings (Izaku et al, 1968; Morrison et al, 1972). Chondroitin helps with production in the body of collagen, which is important for blood vessel health. My impression is that taking a chondroitin supplement tends to help with joint problems. This supplement is sometimes available as chondroitin-sulfate A.

Cinnamon. An excellent source on heart health and other health benefits of cinnamon is an Internet article (including numerous cites to scientific studies) on the World's Healthiest Foods website, which is sponsored by the George Mateljan Foundation. The article is titled "Cinnamon, Ground." Research cited in the article indicates that cinnamon reduces blood clotting. Apparently, consuming cinnamon can help with control of blood sugar. Cinnamon has anti-inflammatory effects also. With all of these benefits, cinnamon certainly should be consumed by a person who elects not to take a statin drug.

Coconut oil (1000 mg. More is OK.). Coconut oil, an important "healthy fat," is excellent for cooking with tomatoes because this increases the bioavailability of the lycopene in the tomatoes. Lycopene has benefits regarding endothelial (blood vessel) function. There is an excellent article on the Dr. Mercola website with the title "Which oil will help you to absorb nutrients better?" Dr. Mercola gives the answer to this question—coconut oil—and discusses several health benefits of coconut oil. There are five cites to scientific research articles.

Co-enzyme Q10 and ubiquinol (Coenzyme Q10 100 to 300 mg; ubiquinol 100 mg). There is extensive scientific literature documenting the benefits of supplementation with co-enzyme Q10 regarding cardiovascular health (Langsjoen & Langsjoen, 1999). Co-enzyme Q10 is converted in the bodies of younger persons into another form of co-enzyme Q10, ubiquinol. Unfortunately, the bodies of older persons (possibly persons as young as in their early 40s) lack this function, so we are likely to fail to receive the benefits of ordinary co-enzyme Q10 supplements. Since ubiquinol became available as a supplement only recently, it appears that there is little published literature available through Google Scholar concerning the effectiveness of ubiquinol regarding cardiovascular health.

Fortunately, an Internet article in *Life Extension Magazine* entitled "Pfizer abandons heart drug development" addresses the benefits of supplementation with ubiquinol. Research discussed in that article has clearly shown that ubiquinol can have very great benefits for persons with **serious heart disease**. Therefore, it should follow that ubiquinol supplementation can be beneficial for older persons wanting to prevent atherosclerosis.

DHA (300 mg). DHA is an omega-3 oil found in fish oil. Research shows that taking DHA prompts growth of new brain cells in the hippocampus, which is referred to as the memory center of the brain. The following is a quote from a review of scientific research articles:

> "DHA has a positive effect on diseases such as hypertension, arthritis, atherosclerosis, depression, adult-onset diabetes mellitus, myocardial infarction, thrombosis, and some cancers (Horrocks et al, 1999)."

This is the most impressive sentence about benefits of nutrition I have found in any scientific article. Fish oil contains EPA and DHA. I believe that, regarding heart and brain health, DHA is much more important than EPA.

DHEA (50 mg for men; 25 mg or as suggested by a physician for women). A study showed that men with high levels of DHEA tended to have greater protection against aortic atherosclerosis progression (Hak et al, 2002). Similarly, a study of Japanese men with type 2 diabetes found that those with the highest circulating levels of DHEA-sulfate (the form of DHEA commonly measured in blood tests) were much less likely to have carotid atherosclerosis (Fukui et al, 2005).

DMG. DMG is close in composition to the B vitamins. I have only recently learned that Balch & Balch, the authors of the most influential book about supplements, recommend DMG for 48 different health conditions.

As a person ages, her or his body gradually loses the ability to produce DMG. I have not yet found convincing evidence of these benefits.

Fiber supplement. To have a healthy brain, it helps to consume a lot of fiber. Obviously, you can eat a lot of fresh fruits and vegetables and whole grain foods. Of course, it won't hurt to regularly take a fiber supplement. I have read reports that eating apples or pears regularly can have great heart health benefits.

Fish oil (1000 mg. Some benefit from more.). Perciavalle Health News has a comprehensive article on the Internet about the use of fish oil with the title "Fish oil/omega-3 supplements: Benefits, side effects, and dosage." There are 165 citations to scholarly articles. (See also Herold & Kinsella, 1986; Gebauer et al, 2006) An important study on the effects of fish oil supplementation includes the following language:

> "In our study, patients with coronary artery disease who ingested approximately 1.5 g of omega-3 fatty acids per day for 2 years had less progression and more regression of coronary artery disease on coronary angiography than did comparable patients who ingested a placebo." (von Schacky et al, 1999)

A scholarly Internet article by Dr. Jay S. Cohen has the title "A preventative for Alzheimer's disease: another powerful study shows a markedly reduced risk of Alzheimer's with fish oils (Omega-3 oils)." This adds another benefit of supplementing with fish oil. I believe that the weight of the evidence indicates that supplementation with **fish oil** reduces heart attack risk (Leon et al, 2008).

There are problems regarding the quality of fish oil supplements. The NatureMade fish oil supplement, which contains a substantial amount of DHA, is highly recommended. I may decide to buy OmegaKrill 5X produced by BioTrust Nutrition. They claim to be using several expensive technologies which result in the best possible fish oil/krill/DHA product. The cost is slightly less than $1 per day.

A study published in 2012 (Rizos et al) found no association of omega-3 supplementation with heart attacks and other major adverse cardiovascular events. My guess is that there are methodology problems with that study. Still, because DHA is apparently substantially more important to human health than EPA (both being found in fish oil), I think it makes sense to focus on taking a DHA supplement, rather than a fish oil supplement.

Flavonoids. Three Italian scientists have reported research findings concerning benefits of ingesting flavonoids in an article entitled "Flavonoids: antioxidants against atherosclerosis." (Grassis et al, 2010) Dietary sources of flavonoids include citrus fruit, tea, wine (especially red wine), dark chocolate, and grapes, especially muscadine grapes. Flavonoids are found in resveratrol and grape-seed extract.

Folic acid (400mcg). In the past, researchers have recommended supplementation with folic acid (folate) to reduce homocysteine levels because elevated homocysteine is associated with occurrence of cardiovascular disease. Recent research, however, has indicated that, at least for men, **supplementation with folic acid can be associated with adverse heart-health consequences**. Also, research shows that the reduction of homocysteine level with supplements does not protect or improve cardiovascular health (Lonn, 2008). Therefore, supplementation with folic acid by men is not recommended in this book, except for men having cognitive decline problems. It is surprising, therefore, that a 14-year study of 80,082 female nurses suggested that **higher-than-usual supplementation with folic acid, alone or in combination with vitamin B6, is associated with substantially lower risk of coronary-heart disease in women** (Rimm, 1998). If I were a woman, I would take supplementary folate or folic acid beyond the amount in a multivitamin.

Garlic. The dosage will depend on the form of garlic supplement you take. My impression is that, to obtain the optimum benefits from garlic supplement, one should take aged garlic extract, which is expensive. This is a quote from a scholarly article about health benefits of aged garlic extract:

> "Oxidative modification of DNA, proteins and lipids by reactive oxygen species (ROS) plays a role in aging and disease, including cardiovascular, neurodegenerative and inflammatory diseases and cancer. Extracts of fresh garlic that are aged over a prolonged period to produce aged garlic extract (AGE) contain antioxidant phytochemicals that prevent oxidant damage." (Borek, 2001)

The website of the University of Maryland Medical Center has an article entitled "Garlic" that does an excellent job of reviewing the scientific studies concerning effects of garlic supplements. The following is a quote from that article:

> "Garlic can prevent and treat plaque buildup in the arteries. It is typically taken in capsules, but fresh garlic is also effective. Clinical trials have found that consuming fresh garlic or garlic supplements can lower cholesterol levels, prevent blood clots and destroy plaque.
>
> "Both the main active component of garlic, called allicin, and the constituent ajoene are responsible for preventing blood clots by reducing the 'stickiness' of blood platelets (University of Michigan Health System)."

Taking a garlic supplement might be more beneficial to women than to men in preventing and treating atherosclerosis (University of Michigan Health System).

Ginkgo biloba (60 mg). Ginkgo biloba is included in some high-priced cognitive functioning supplement formulas. Egyptians considered it to be an aphrodisiac.

GliSODin. GliSODin is an ingeniously designed, patented antioxidant with important anti-inflammatory effects. The cost is about $.55 per day. It is a supplement formula derived partly from cantaloupes. A substantial amount of scientific research has been done regarding health effects and benefits of GliSODin. If I wanted to achieve some regression of atherosclerosis (I don't need to, having done so decades ago.), I would very seriously consider taking GliSODin. Below is a quote from the evercare BrilliantBrightBrain website:

> "Oxidative stress is known to significantly contribute to the process of inflammation, which underpins conditions like rheumatoid arthritis, metabolic syndrome, and diabetes, as well as to neurodegenerative diseases like Alzheimer's."

Green tea extract, green tea. Even though I am not aware of conclusive research proof, there is a strong suggestion that green tea extract and green tea have a wide variety of cardiovascular health benefits. Given that it is established that tea—black, white, and green—is beneficial to your health and wellbeing, I sometimes take a green tea supplement, which helps with weight control.

If a man concludes that he is at risk of developing prostate cancer and atherosclerosis (hardening of the arteries), he could regularly take a four-ingredient formula, POMI-T, which includes pomegranate, green tea, tumeric, and broccoli, which should help with preventing each disease.

Hawthorn. Hawthorn is an herb with a variety of heart health benefits ("Three great heart-boosting herbs," by Victor Marchione, MD on the Doctorshealthpress.com website).

Iodine. Dr. David Brownstein reports that a high percentage of persons are deficient in iodine and that this deficiency contributes to the development of atherosclerosis.

L-arginine (500 mg). L-arginine causes the production of nitric oxide in the body. Nitric oxide is extremely important for human health.

There has been research suggesting that, for people over 40, l-arginine is not effective in causing production of nitric oxide. There is an expensive lozenge, CircO2, which is reported to efficiently cause production of nitric oxide.

I recently bought an l-arginine/citrulline complex supplement and immediately received much better benefit in preventing an elevated pulse. Because of this, I now recommend that persons over 45 take l-arginine/citrulline complex or CircO2 instead of l-arginine. **For men over 45 and women past menopause, I think that shifting to l-arginine/citrulline complex or CircO2 instead of l-arginine may be important regarding the prevention of heart attacks**.

L-carnitine. L-carnitine has very positive effects regarding **cardiovascular health, cognitive function, and even athletic performance** (Sinatra & Sinatra, 1999). Persons experiencing heart failure often are l-carnitine-deficient (Sole & Jeejeebhoy, 2002). Unfortunately, l-carnitine may contribute to buildup of plaque in blood vessels. I think more work needs to be done on the benefits and drawbacks of l-carnitine. Fortunately, I have won the heart disease prevention fight. Therefore, I regularly take alpha-lipoic acid/l-carnitine before exercise for benefits concerning brain health and function and athletic performance.

L-carnosine (500 mg). L-carnosine is a dipeptide that is ordinarily produced in sufficient amounts in the bodies of young people. As with ubiquinol, not enough is produced in the bodies of elderly people. Various types of research have suggested that l-carnosine tends to prevent aspects of aging. Some researchers believe that it prevents the major aging phenomenon, glycation.

L-tyrosine (500 mg). This is an amino acid that apparently helps with problems relating to stress. Many discussions of effects of l-tyrosine are available on the Internet.

Lecithin (1200 mg. More is OK.). Though there are problems with the consumption of soybean products, I believe that the consumption of lecithin is safe. Lecithin works to move fat and LDL ("bad cholesterol") through the blood stream, which prevents LDL adherence to artery walls.

Because of this, lecithin helps to keep arteries from clogging up, promoting improved cardiovascular health (Wilson et al, 1998). A quote from a 2009 article on the ScienceDaily website, "Food additive may one day help control blood lipids and reduce disease risk," describes promising research about the heart health benefits of lecithin. Lecithin contains phosphatidylcholine, from which the body makes acetylcholine, an important substance for brain health and function. Phosphatidylserine, which is extremely important regarding brain health and function, is also derived from lecithin.

Researchers at the Washington University School of Medicine (2009) found that lecithin may help to keep the liver functioning properly, which in turn lowers the risk of developing heart disease and diabetes (August issue of *Cell*).

Lycopene. A team of Korean scientists have recently published findings of important research concerning the positive effects of lycopene supplementation regarding blood vessel health and function (Kim et al, 2010). Two Canadian scientists have authored a review of research showing, among other things, that lycopene in tomatoes tends to have positive effects regarding cardiovascular health (Agarwal & Rao, 2000).

Magnesium (200 to 400 mg). Avoid magnesium-oxide. Magnesium-citrate is fine. Magnesium's usefulness in lowering atherosclerosis risk has been discussed for many years. Some evidence of this potential benefit surfaced in a long-term study called the "Atherosclerosis Risk in Communities Study" (ARIC). In it, nearly 14,000 men and women were examined regularly for seven years. One study found an association of lower magnesium with high blood pressure (Peacock et al, 1999). In the ARIC study, those who routinely had lower magnesium levels in their blood had higher rates of developing coronary heart disease, which develops from atherosclerosis (Liao et al, 1998). The fact that the ARIC study has been the basis for the publication of more than 800 scholarly articles indicates the study's importance.

Very significantly, two highly qualified scholars (Rosanoff & Seelig, 2004) have in recent years **recommended that supplementation with magnesium be used as an alternative to statin drugs for cholesterol control**. One reason this suggestion is that statin cholesterol-control and BP medications **eliminate important co-enzyme Q10 and ubiquinol in the human body**.

There is some controversy regarding whether the current magnesium RDA (400 mg) is sufficient. There is concern regarding the particularly high incidence of magnesium deficiency among the elderly (Durlach, 1993).

Researchers publishing in 2011 found that, for women, higher dietary and body content of magnesium were associated with **lower** occurrence of SCD (sudden cardiac death) (Chiuve et al, 2011).

Melatonin. Research has indicated that melatonin has benefits against Alzheimer's (Pappolla et al, 2003; Srinivasan et al, 2006), stroke (Reiter et al, 2005), and hypertension of men (Scheer et al, 2004).

Nattokinase (100 mg). Nattokinase is obtained from a type of soy cheese. It has been shown to be effective in dissolving blood clots. It may contribute to the reversal of atherosclerosis.

Niacin. Dr. William B. Parsons, Jr., is the author of a book (2000), *Cholesterol control without diet!: the niacin solution*. While I take 1000 mg of niacin per day, I continue to have elevated LDL and low HDL. Still, I believe that taking niacin twice a day for 35 years has provided me with some type of health benefit. I suspect that it involves the artery dilation that niacin causes.

The recommended dosage depends on your lipids profile. The worse the lipids profile, the higher the dosage of niacin supplementation. A top Duke lipidologist, Dr. John R. Guyton, recommended that I take 1500 mg of niacin per day as an alternative to taking a statin. People without a lipids problem might take 200 mg daily.

A major review of research regarding the effects of niacin on athero-sclerosis and vascular function (Ruparelia et al, 2011) indicates that niacin should be of great positive interest to persons with CVD problems, physicians, and scientists. So, that review confirms the wisdom of the advice I received from Dr. Guyton.

The type of niacin for non-diabetics to take for circulatory problems is niacin (nicotinic acid), **not niacinamide**. Diabetics should take niacinamide. An Internet article by William Davis, MD, in *Life Extension Magazine* (2007) entitled "Using niacin to improve cardiovascular health" provides extremely helpful information about the uses and benefits of niacin. There are citations to four scholarly articles. "The benefits of niacin in atherosclerosis" is an article in *Current Atherosclerosis Reports* (Tavantharan & Kasyap, 2001) which describes effects of niacin against atherosclerosis. (See also Knopp, 2000).

Phosphatidylcholine. Lecithin contains phosphatidylcholine. There is evidence that phosphatidylcholine stimulates growth of new brain cells. The body converts phosphatidylcholine to acetylcholine, which has brain health benefits.

Phosphatidylserine. This is a very important supplement in dealing with problems regarding brain health and function. It is the most important ingredient in many cognitive function formulas.

Pomegranate. "Pomegranate: reverses atherosclerosis and slows the progression of prostate cancer" is the title of a 2007 *Life Extension Magazine* Internet article with extensive scholarly discussion and citations. A three-year study involving drinking pomegranate juice showed that this consumption had several significant heart health benefits (Aviram, 2004).

Potassium. The article that convinced me that potassium is an important nutrient regarding cardiovascular health is titled "Potassium and your heart." Robert J. Byrg, MD, reviewed the article in 2010, and it includes a list of credible references. It is found on the WebMD web site.

Potassium may be involved in slowing the process of atherosclerosis and preventing the thickening of the walls of arteries, which can lead to cardiovascular disease. Recently, a high-potassium diet was shown to exert a protective effect against the development of vascular damage induced by excess salt intake, thus counteracting, to some extent, the dangerous effects of eating too much salt. This body of evidence from experimental studies provides biological plausibility to the protective effect of dietary potassium against cardiovascular events (D'Elia et al, 2011).

Quercetin (100 to 250 mg. Don't exceed 1000 mg). Quercetin, an important nutrient in muscadine grapes, is an important bioflavonoid (Lee, 2005). Quercetin can reduce blood clots and scavenge harmful free radicals and phenolic acids, which may help prevent heart disease (Hayek et al, 1997).

Resveratrol (250 mg). This is a flavonoid antioxidant. Though recent research questions whether taking resveratrol has health benefits, I do not believe that there is sufficient evidence to "abandon" resveratrol.

Silica. Research has shown that **silica**, which is available in many vegetables and grains and as a supplement tablet, is important for blood vessel health (Seaborn et al, 1993).

Taurine. Research has shown that persons who have a heart attack, in addition to tending to be **deficient in magnesium** (Baker, 1991–1992), tend to be deficient in the amino acid **taurine**. Supplementation with taurine helps with recovery of heart health after a heart attack (Sole & Jeejeebhoy, 2002) and in recovery from congestive heart failure (Azuma, 1983).

Tocotrienols. Tocotrienols are one of the two types of vitamin E. (The more common type is tocopherols.) A recent scholarly research review describes many benefits of tocotrienols regarding cardiovascular health (Prasad, 2011). Unfortunately, they have not been found to be helpful regarding established ischemic heart disease. "Cardiovascular benefits of tocotrienols" is the title of an article at the A.C. Grace Company website which discusses and cites **many scientific research studies** that have demonstrated the amazing benefits of desmethyl tocotrienols against atherosclerosis. A similar article, which is on the Wellness Resources website, is "Tocotrienols: twenty years of dazzling cardiovascular and cancer research" (2000). Apparently, it is good for the tocotrienols to be "palm-derived."

Turmeric/curcumin (500 mg). Research is suggesting that taking curcumin and vitamin D3 at bedtime can cause some reduction of beta-amyloid plaques in the brain. Those plaques are an important aspect of the development of some dementias.

Vitamin B6 (1.3 to 1.7 mg). Vitamin B6 has significant heart- and brain-health benefits. Supplementation of more than 2000 mg per day may cause neurological damage.

Vitamin B12 (1000 mcg). A high B12 status helps you to maintain a healthy brain. In very important University of Oxford research, **older people with lower-than-average B12 levels were found to be six times more likely to show signs of brain shrinkage**, as a possible forerunner to impaired cognitive function and Alzheimer's disease (Vogatzoglou et al, 2008). Vitamin B12 is important regarding the formation and health of blood cells (NIH, 2011c).

Vitamin C (1000 mg). Along with lowering your BP, vitamin C ensures proper dilation of blood vessels, which can prevent such diseases as atherosclerosis, congestive heart failure, and angina pectoris (severe chest pains that are caused by inadequate supply of blood to the heart). An Internet article in *Life Extension Magazine* entitled "Newly discovered health benefits of vitamin C" discusses these and other benefits. There are 58 citations to scholarly journal articles. If you would like to see one of the most powerful websites against statins, check out "Statin drug alert" on the Vitamin C Foundation website. Of course, they promote the benefits of vitamin C against CVD.

Vitamin D3 (2000 to 5000 iu, or as recommended by a physician). Recent research done by Ibhar Al Mheid, MD, and colleagues revealed that there is a protective effect of vitamin D against arterial stiffness and impaired blood vessel relaxation (Al Mheid, 2011). Vitamin D is protective against elevation of BP (Vimaleswaran et al, 2014).

Recent research is indicating that a high percentage of persons in the U.S. are vitamin D-deficient (Holick, 2007). For several reasons, older persons are especially likely to be vitamin D-deficient (NIH, 2011a). Reinhold Vieth, PhD, at the University of Toronto, says the toxicity of vitamin D doesn't begin until 40,000 units are consumed (*American Journal of Clinical Nutrition*, Vol. 69, pp. 842–56, 1999). Of course, not nearly that level is suggested in this book. I take 10,000 i.u. of vitamin D per day and don't have adverse effects. There is disagreement among experts regarding safe daily intake of vitamin D. The present recommended daily allowance is 400 iu. Scientists reporting in the *American Journal of Clinical Nutrition* (Vieth et al, 2001) conclude that a daily intake of 4000 iu is sufficiently safe.

Unfortunately, vitamin D from a supplement is not as effective in carrying out important functions in the body as vitamin D resulting from sun exposure.

While supplementation with vitamin D3 for persons not of African descent who are deficient can provide cardiovascular health benefits, recent research indicates that supplementation for Black persons who appear to be "deficient" in D3 can have adverse health consequences.

Avoid synthetic vitamin D2.

Vitamin E (tocopherols). Important recent research has shown that 2000 mg daily of vitamin E significantly helps persons with early Alzheimer's to retain important functioning.

Vitamin K2 (180 to 200 mcg). Recent research indicates vitamin K2 helps dramatically in prevention of calcification in blood vessel plaque. (There is more calcium than LDL in this plaque.) Any person who supplements beyond a multivitamin with calcium should seriously consider taking vitamin K2. Vitamin K2 increases the tendency of blood to clot.

Walnuts. (Though walnuts are not a supplement, consuming them is so beneficial that I will cheat and include them here.) One of the underlying causes of atherosclerosis can be progressive endothelial dysfunction (blood vessels gradually functioning worse). Walnuts contain a variety of nutrients, including arginine, polyphenols, and omega-3 oils, that support the inner arterial lining and guard against abnormal platelet aggregation. These favorable biological effects explain why walnut consumption tends to protect against coronary-artery disease (Feldman, 2002).

The U.S. National Library of Medicine database contains 35 peer-reviewed published papers supporting a claim that ingesting walnuts improves vascular health and may reduce heart- attack risk.

Zinc. Dr. David Brownstein reports that zinc supplementation helps in prevention of atherosclerosis.

Patented heart-health formula. I have found only one such product which I think I should make readers aware of.

OmegaQ Plus with resveratrol and turmeric. Dr. Stephen Sinatra, a prominent cardiologist, developed and markets this formula. It includes B6, folate, B12, squid oil, DHA, EPA, turmeric, l-carnitine, coenzyme Q10, and resveratrol. Taking one capsule before your VCR and another at bedtime will cost $50 per month. If I were to decide to take it, I would also take D3, DHEA, l-arginine, garlic, lecithin, niacin, magnesium-citrate, and potassium.

Patented cognitive functioning supplement formulas. I believe that any person who has significant concerns about cognitive decline should very seriously consider taking one of these formulas.

Brain Ammo. Sold by Life Essentials. While Procera AVH and Cognizin have been shown in research to have cognitive functioning benefits, I believe that Brain Ammo has the best selection of ingredients, based on recent research. Those ingredients are phosphatidylserine (most important), gingko biloba, acetyl-carnitine, St. John's wort, l-glutamine, DMAE, bacopin, and vinpocetin. The cost per day is slightly less than $2.

Procera AVH

Cognizin IQ 150

Cresceo

Advanced Memory Formula. There are excellent ingredients, and the cost is only $1 per day. I have been taking this for several years and believe the benefits for me have been substantial.

Prevagen. I take this and believe there are significant benefits.

Several of the following supplements are in one or more of the patented formulas above: caprylic acid, huperzine A, tramiprosate, bacopa monieri, vinpocetine, acetyl-ocysteine, DHEA, fish oil, gingko, ginseng, panax, iron, pycnogenol, vitamin B6, vitamin B12

Supplements for eye health. Two companies that sell supplements to help with eye health and good vision are Ocuvite and PreserVision.

Precautionary information about taking supplements for heart- and brain-health benefits. It is important to be cautious regarding taking nutritional supplements. Vitamin and mineral supplements ordinarily contain nutrients that have for eons been found in foods regularly eaten—without ill effects—by humans. It is not surprising that these vitamins and minerals are not very likely to have adverse side effects. Still, we should exercise caution concerning anything we ingest into our bodies. That applies to nutritional supplements.

You need to know that increasing anti-coagulant supplements (fish oil, vitamin E, nattokinase) can result in a tendency to bleed. Reducing anti-coagulant supplements and starting to take vitamin K2, which is a co-agulant (increases blood clotting) can lead to dangerous blood clotting.

Before taking a DHEA supplement, it would make sense for a woman to have a sex- hormone test. Obviously, if she presently has more testosterone than desired in her blood, she should not take DHEA.

You should ensure that niacin can be safely taken along with medications you take. There is support for the idea that **diabetics should take niacinamide instead of niacin (nicotinic acid)**.

Though supplementation with vitamin D3 can be extremely beneficial for persons not of African descent, supplementation with vitamin D3 of apparently vitamin D-deficient persons of African descent can be very dangerous. Everyone should avoid taking synthetic vitamin D2.

There is a possibility that excessive supplementation with ordinary vitamin E (tocopherols) can adversely affect health (NIH, 2011b).

I think there are good reasons to be cautious about consuming soy foods and supplements. (I continue to think that lecithin from soy is safe to consume. You can, however, buy non-soy lecithin.) Information on this is available in a book by Kaayla T. Daniel, PhD: *The Whole Soy Story*. There is a convincing review of this book on the credible Mercola.com website: "Soy myth exposed: soy is not a health food."

Men need to know that eating soybeans may adversely affect male hormones. If I were a woman, I would occasionally eat roasted soybeans.

Recent analyses of more than ten clinical trials involving about 12,000 patients found **calcium supplementation to be associated with a 20% to 30% increase in heart-attack risk**. The lead researcher argues that it is time to reassess the role of calcium supplementation for the treatment and prevention of osteoporosis (Reid et al, 2010).

Dr. Stephen Seely of the University of Manchester contends that, contrary to recommendations of nutritional authorities in the U.S. and other countries, young adults need only 300–400 mg of calcium daily and that older adults need even less. He writes,

> "First, the general observation can be made that, in countries where the daily calcium intake is 200–400 mg, arterial diseases are non-existent. Blood pressure does not increase with age. In countries where the daily intake is 800 mg, arterial disease is the leading cause of mortality" (Seely, 1991).

Some excellent multivitamins include 300mg of vitamin C, which is 500% of the recommended daily allowance. Though some physicians have recommended mega-doses of vitamin C, I do not in this book recommend daily supplementation with vitamin C beyond a multivitamin. (When I want to stop a cough or cold from developing, I take a vitamin C (500 mg) and a zinc (50 mg) supplement, both of which have heart health benefits.)

In the past, researchers have recommended supplementation with folic acid (folate) to reduce homocysteine levels because elevated homocysteine is associated with the occurrence of cardiovascular disease. Recent research, however, has indicated that, at least for men, **supplementation with folic acid can be associated with adverse heart health consequences**. Also, research shows that the reduction of homocysteine level with supplements does not protect or improve cardiovascular health (Lonn, 2008). Therefore, supplementation with folic acid by men is not recommended in this book, unless the man is having brain function problems. As discussed earlier, one study suggested that supplementation with folic acid can have **substantial heart-health benefits for women** (Rimm, 1998).

While vitamin B6 has some heart health benefits, supplementation with more than 2000 mg per day can cause neurological damage.

Selenium clearly has some heart health and general health benefits. I am convinced, however, that supplementation beyond what is ordinarily found in a multivitamin is not warranted.

Consuming a melatonin supplement and drinking an alcoholic beverage together definitely has adverse consequences, including a "hangover" type of headache. Melatonin should be consumed shortly before going to bed.

Several supplements discussed above, including fish oil, can thin human blood. Therefore, there can be health risks of taking high doses of fish oil. You should ensure with your physician that taking this dose would be safe and healthful for you. Since several blood thinning supplements are taken together in most routines in this book, persons with problems concerning inadequate blood clotting should consult with their physician to ensure that performing a supplement-and-exercise program is sufficiently safe.

Promotion of healing. During my adult years, I have had a giant amount of physical activity, including walking more than 22,000 miles while playing golf. Many dozens of times, I have developed pain of a joint, including nearly all of my major joints. I have noticed that, when I have joint discomfort, if I take MSM and a supplement containing chondroitin, it is very likely that the discomfort will be gone the next day or very soon thereafter.

A poster listing likely or possible health benefits of particular nutritional supplements. I will again state that I am not a health expert. Therefore, I cannot prescribe any of these supplements to prevent or cure a disease or other health problem. Also, the supplements listed below have not been evaluated by the Food and Drug Administration regarding provision of health benefits.

I have reviewed research concerning effects of these supplements and believe that it is likely or possible that particular supplements will provide indicated benefits.

OVERVIEW OF BENEFITS OF NUTRITIONAL SUPPLEMENTS

The letters to the right of the supplements listed below indicate the conditions the supplement does or probably will help with. Here is the letter code: **AC**=anti-coagulant; **AI**=anti-inflammatory; **AO**=antioxidant; **AP**=athletic performance; **B**=brain and thinking; **BP**=blood pressure control; **BS**=help with blood sugar control; **C**=cancer; **CoAg**=coagulant; **EF**=promotes good endothelial (blood vessel) function and health; **H**=heart health; **I**=immune system; **J**=joint health; **MH**=mental health; **NO**=nitric-oxide production; **PA**=prevention of atherosclerosis; **Sl**=sleep; **Sx**=sexual enjoyment; **WC**=weight control; Percentages in parentheses are the percentage of "daily value" in the Equate Complete Multivitamin Men's 50+.

Alpha-lipoic acid **B, C, MH, BP** (Take before exercise to produce glutathione (**AO**).)

Arginine (l-arginine) **C, H, Sx, WC, EF, NO, PA, BP**

Chromium piccolinate **WC, H, BS** (50% of chromium)

Chondroitin **J, H, EF**

Cinnamon **H, AC, AI, BS**

Co-enzyme Q10 **B, C, H, PA**

(Ubiquinol is the better form of co-enzyme Q10 for persons over 45.)

Curcumin (turmeric) **B, C, J, AI, PA**

DHA **B, H, AC, C, MH, PA**

DHEA **B, Sx, H** (Take with melatonin for sex/testosterone benefit.) Fish oil **AI, B, C, H, AC, J, MH, PA, BP** (Flaxseed oil has some of these same benefits.) (Fish oil may increase prostate cancer risk.)

Folate, folic acid (for women only) **H, EF, B** (75%) (Some experts recommend none for men.)

Garlic **C, H, I, AC, PA, BP**

Gingko biloba **AC**

Green tea extract **B, C, WC, PA**

Iodine **C, WC, H** (100%)

L-carnitine **B, AP**

L-taurine **H, EF, PA**

L-theanine **MH,** normal pulse

L-tyrosine **B, MH, Sx, WC, H**

Lecithin **B, H, MH, Sx, PA**

Lycopene **H, EF, AO**

Magnesium **H, B, MH, BS, PA, BP** (**not** magnesium-oxide; magnesium-citrate is OK) (13% Deficiency is common, harmful.)

Melatonin **B, C, MH, Sl, H**

Nattokinase **H, AC**

Niacin **C, H, EF, J, MH, Sx, PA** (niacinamide for diabetics; nicotinic acid for non-diabetics) (100% Especially for heart-health benefit, much more can be taken safely.)

Pomegranate extract **H, PA**

Probiotic **C, I**

Quercetin **C, H, PA** (stroke prevention)

Resveratrol, Grapeseed Extract **AI, C, H, AO, PA** contain flavonoids

Selenium **C, MH, Sx, H, AO** (143%. Additional supplementation probably not needed.)

Taurine **H, PA**

Vitamin B6 **B, C, BS, EF** (300%. For brain health benefit, much more is sometimes recommended.)

Vitamin B12 **B, EF** (prevents shrunken brain)**, H, BS** (1667%. Deficiency is common and very harmful.)

Vitamin C **B, C, H, J, Sx, AO, PA, BP** (200%. There is controversy concerning optimum supplementation.)

Vitamin D3 **C, H, D, BS, PA** (150%. Deficiency is very common and harmful. Some physicians recommend very much more than "daily value.")

Vitamin E (tocopherol) **B, C, J, Sx, AC, AO** (Ordinary vitamin E. 200%)

Vitamin E (tocotrienols) **H, C, PA**

Vitamin K2 **CoAg**

This poster is primarily intended to make people aware of possibilities, not to provide the best possible, most complete information about how to deal with health problems.

<u>Calculated minimum cost of 15 supplements for a basic heart-health routine</u>. If I were starting supplement use at age 25 to 45, had my "bad lipids profile," and knew what I now know, I would buy and take daily (a few twice daily) the following nutritional supplements. Supplements I would take twice daily would be curcumin, fish oil, lecithin, magnesium-citrate, niacin, vitamin B6, and vitamin D3. That would increase cost by $.30 per day.

I carefully searched for the best price on the Internet and ended up with Puritan's Pride and Swanson's supplements. Remember: I looked carefully for the best buy on the desired dosage. Obviously, your cost for "premium quality" supplements from other companies will be higher. I have mainly

bought supplements from Puritan's Pride for about 20 years, which has not
kept me from having excellent results.

Alpha-lipoic acid, 600 mg, Swanson	$.17
Coenzyme Q10, 200 mg, Puritan's Pride	.09
Curcumin/turmeric, 800 mg, Puritan's Pride	.035
DHA, 300 mg, Puritan's Pride	.092
DHEA, 50 mg, Puritan's Pride	.064. Women should take less, maybe 25 mg, as recommended by doctor.
Fish oil, 1000 mg, Puritan's Pride	.04
Folic acid, 400 mcg, Puritan's Pride	.014. Men should not take unless they are having "senior moments."
L-arginine, 500 mg, Puritan's Pride	.104
Lecithin, 1200 mg, Swanson	.064
Magnesium-citrate, 200 mg, Puritan's Pride	.062
Niacin (nicotinic acid), 500 mg, Swanson	.042
Potassium-gluconate, 99 mg, Swanson	.029
Vitamin B6, 50 mg, Puritan's Pride	.03
Vitamin B12, 1000 mcg, Puritan's Pride	.02
Vitamin D3, 5000 iu, Puritan's Pride	.03 Taking much more than the long-time recommended daily allowance is safe.

Daily cost	$.886
Monthly cost	$26.58
Yearly cost	$323.39

For a person, like me, who would take several supplements twice daily,
the cost per day would be about $1.20. For less than the cost of a sugary

soft drink or sugary treat, a person can take these very carefully selected supplements.

It saves money, time, and bother to buy about a year's supply of supplements from one of the companies mentioned above.

As I mention far too many times in this book, for me, the results of taking these supplements, followed by exercise 4 or 5 days per week over 36 years have provided, in spite of extremely bad heart and brain disease risk factors, unbelievably excellent heart and brain health.

High-cost, special-function supplement formulas. Supplement manufacturers market a wide variety of multi-ingredient supplement formulas. If you think of a significant health problem that many people would like to get rid of, you can probably find a supplement formula that is marketed to deal with that problem.

Fortunately, I can afford to buy a good number of these products, and I do take Advanced Memory Formula (cognitive function), LunaFlex-PM (sleep and joint comfort), Elysium (anti-aging), and Prevagen (memory), with a combined cost of $7 per day. I take several additional supplements that cost about $1 per day. Given the excellent health outcomes I'm experiencing, I do not regret incurring this expense in the slightest.

REFERENCES

Agarwal, Sanjiv & Rao, Akkinappally Venketeshwer (2000). Tomato lycopene and its role in human health and chronic diseases. *Canadian Medical Association Journal*, Vol. 163, No. 6., pp. 739–744.

Al Mheid, I. et al (2011). Vitamin D status is associated with arterial stiffness and vascular dysfunction in healthy humans. *Journal of the American College of Cardiology*, Vol. 58, No. 2, pp. 186–192.

Albert, C.M. et al (2005). Dietary alpha-linolenic acid intake and risk of sudden cardiac death and coronary disease. *Circulation*, Vol. 112, pp. 3232–3238.

Ames, Bruce (2006). Low micronutrient intake may accelerate the degenerative diseases of aging through allocation of scarce micronutrients by triage. *Proceedings of the National Academy of Sciences*, Vol. 103, No. 47, 17589–17594.

Anthony, M.S. et al (1998). Effects of soy isoflavones on atherosclerosis: potential mechanisms. *American Journal of Clinical Nutrition*, Vol. 68, No. 6, 1390S–1393S.

Aviram, M. et al (2004). Pomegranate juice consumption for 3 years by patients with carotid artery stenosis reduces common carotid intima-media thickness, blood pressure and LDL oxidation. *Clinical Nutrition*, Vol 23, No. 3, p. 423.

Azuma, J. et al (1983). Therapy of congestive heart failure with orally administered taurine. *Clinical Thereutics*, Vol. 5, No. 4, pp. 398–408.

Baker, S.M. (1991–1992). Magnesium deficiency in primary care and preventive medicine. *Magnesium and Trace Elements*, Vol. 10, pp. 251–262.

Borek, Carmia (2001). Antioxidant health effects of aged garlic extract. *Journal of Nutrition*, Vol. 131, pp. 1010S–1015S.

Chiuve, Stephanie E. et al (2011). Plasma and dietary magnesium and risk of sudden cardiac death in women. *American Journal of Clinical Nutrition*, Vol. 93, pp. 253–260.

Chobanian, Aram V. (2001). Control of hypertension—an important national priority. *New England Journal of Medicine*, Vol. 345, pp. 534–535.

Daniel, Kaayka T. (2005). *The whole soy story: the dark side of America's favorite health food*. Warsaw, IN: New Trends Publishing.

D'Elia, Lanfranco et al (2011). Potassium intake, stroke, and cardiovascular disease: a meta-analysis of prospective studies. *Journal of American College of Cardiology*, Vol. 57, No. 10, pp. 1210–1219.

Durlach, J. et al (1993). Magnesium and ageing. II. Clinical data: aetological mechanisms and pathophysiological consequences of magnesium deficit in the elderly. *Magnesium Research*, Vol. 6, No. 4, pp. 379–394.

Edwards, R.L. et al (2003). Quercetin reduces blood pressure in hypertensive subjects. *Journal of Nutrition*, Vol. 137, pp. 2405–2411.

Enstrom, E.E. et al (1992). Vitamin C intake and mortality among a sample of the United States population. *Epidemiology*, Vol. 3, No. 3, pp. 194–202.

Feldman, Elaine B. (2002). The scientific evidence for a beneficial health relationship between walnuts and coronary heart disease. *Nutrition*, Vol. 132, No. 5, pp. 1062S–1101S.

Fuhrman, J. (2011). *Super immunity: the essential nutrition guide for boosting your body's defenses to live longer, stronger, and disease free.* NY, NY: HarperCollins.

Fukui, Michiaki et al (2005). Serum dehydroepiandrosterone sulfate (DHEA) concentration and carotid atherosclerosis in men with type 2 diabetes. *Atherosclerosis*, Vol. 181, No. 2, pp. 339–344.

Gebauer, Sarah K. (2006). N–3 fatty acid dietary recommendations and food sources to achieve essentiality and cardiovascular benefits. *American Journal of Clinical Nutrition*, Vol 83, No. 6, pp. S1526–1535S.

Gey, K.F. (1995). Cardiovascular disease and vitamins. Concurrent correction of 'suboptimal' plasma antioxidant levels may, as important part of 'optimal' nutrition, help to prevent early stages of cardiovascular disease and cancer, respectively. *Bibl Nutr Dieta*, Vol. 52, pp. 75–91.

Grassis, David et al (2010). Flavonoids: antioxidants against atherosclerosis. *Nutrients*, Vol. 2, pp. 889–902.

Haffey, Thomas A. (2009). How to avoid a heart attack: putting it all together. *Journal of the American Osteopathic Association*, Vol. 109, No. 5, supp. 1, pp. 14–20.

Hak, A.E. et al (2002). Low levels of endogenous androgens increase the risk of atherosclerosis in elderly men: the Rotterdam study. *Journal of Clinical Endocrinology and Metabolism*, Vol. 87, No. 8, pp. 3632–3639.

Hayek, T. et al (1997). Reduced progression of atherosclerosis in apolipoprotein E-deficient mice following consumption of red wine, or its polyphenols quercetin or catechin, is associated with reduced susceptibility of LDL to oxidation and aggregation. *Arteriosclerosis, Thrombiotic, and Vascular Biology*, Vol. 17, pp. 2744A–2752.

Herold, P.M. & Kinsella, J.E. (1986). Fish oil consumption and decreased risk of cardiovascular disease: a comparison of findings from animal and human feeding trials. *American Journal of Clinical Nutrition*, Vol. 43, pp. 566–598.

Holick, Michael F. (2007). Vitamin D deficiency. *New England Journal of Medicine*, Vol. 357, pp. 266–281.

Holmquist, Christina et al (2003). Multivitamin supplements are inversely associated with risk of myocardial infarction in men and women—Stockholm Heart Epidemiology Program (SHEEP). *The American Society for Nutritional Sciences Journal*, Vol. 133, No. 8, pp. 2650–2654.

Horrocks, L.A. et al (1999). Health benefits of docosahexaenoic acid (DHA). *Pharmacological Research*, Vol. 40, No. 3, pp. 211–225.

Husain, S.et al (1998). Aspirin improves endothelial dysfunction in atherosclerosis. *Circulation*, Vol. 97, No. 8, pp. 716–720.

Isaacsohn, J.L et al (1998). Garlic powder and plasma lipids and lipoproteins. *Archives of Internal Medicine*, Vol. 158, pp. 1189–1194.

Izuka, K. et al (1968). Effects of chondroitin sulfates on serum lipids and hexosamines in atherosclerotic patients: with special reference to thrombus formation time. *Japanese Heart Journal*, Vol. 9, pp. 453–460.

Jimenez, Guallar E. et al (2001). The association of chromium with the risk of a first myocardial infarction in men. The EURAMIC Study (abstract). *Circulation*, Vol. 103, p. 1366.

Kendrick, Malcolm (2007). *The cholesterol con: the truth about what really causes heart disease and how to avoid it.* London: John Blake Publishing.

Kim, J.Y et al (2010). Effects of lycopene supplementation on oxidative stress and markers of endothelial function in healthy men. *Journal of Atherosclerosis*, Vol. 11, p. 36.

Knopp, Robert H., 2000. Evaluating niacin in its various forms. *American Journal of Cardiology*, Vol. 86, Issue 12, Supp. 1, pp. 51–56.

Koscielny, J. et al. Latza (1999). The antiatherosclerotic effect of allium sativum. *Atherosclerosis*, Vol. 144, pp. 237–249.

Langsjoen, Peter H. & Langsjoen, Alena M. (1999). Overview of the use of CoQ10 in cardiovascular disease. *Biofactors*, Vol. 9, Issue 2–4, pp. 273–284.

Lee, Joon-Hee et al (2005). Identification of ellagic acid conjugates and other polyphenolics in muscadine grapes by HPLC-ESI-MS. *Journal of Agricultural and Food Chemistry*, Vol. 53, No. 15, pp. 6003–6010.

Leon, Hernando et al (2008). Effect of fish oil on arrhythmias and mortality: systematic review. *British Medical Journal*, Vol. 337, p. 2931.

Liao, F. et al (1998). Is low magnesium concentration a risk factor for coronary heart disease? The Atherosclerosis Risk in Communities (ARIC) Study. *American Heart Journal*, Vol. 136, pp. 480–490.

Lonn, E. (2008). Homocysteine-lowering B vitamin therapy in cardiovascular prevention—Wrong again? *Journal of the American Medical Association,* Vol 299, pp. 2086–2087.

Luo, G. et al (1997). Spontaneous calcification of arteries and cartilage in mice lacking matrix GLA protein. *Nature,* Vol. 386, pp. 78–81.

Meilahn, Elaine N. (1995). Low serum cholesterol: hazardous to health? *Circulation,* Vol. 92, pp. 2365–2366.

Memory, John & Evatt, Lynn (2012). *Vascular cleansing routines: safe and effective heart health programs for women (and men).* Winston-Salem, NC: Wakexpress (digital publishing at Wake Forest University).

Mertz, W. (1993). Chromium in human nutrition: a review. *Journal of Nutrition,* Vol. 123, No. 4, pp. 626–633.

Morrison, L.M. et al (1972). Prevention of vascular lesions by chondroitin sulfate A in the coronary artery and aorta of rats induced by a hypervitaminosis D, cholesterol-containing diet. *Atherosclerosis,* Vol. 16, pp. 105–118.

Morrison, L.M. & Enrick, N.L. (1973). Coronary heart disease: reduction of death rate by chondroitin sulfate A. *Angiology,* Vol. 24, pp. 269–287.

Napoli, C. et al (2004). Long-term combined beneficial effects of physical training and metabolic treatment on atherosclerosis in hypercholesterolemic mice. Proceedings of the National Academy of Sciences, online early edition, May 24, 2004.

National Institutes of Health, Office of Dietary Supplements (2011a). Dietary supplement fact sheet: vitamin D.

National Institutes of Health, Office of Dietary Supplements (2011b). Dietary supplement fact sheet: vitamin E.

National Institutes of Health, Office of Dietary Supplements (2011c). Dietary supplement fact sheet: vitamin B12.

Pappolla, Miguel A. et al (2002). The neuroprotective activities of melatonin against the Alzheimer B-protein are not mediated by melatonin membrane receptors. *Journal of Pineal Research*, Vol. 32, No. 3, pp. 135–142.

Parag, H.J. et al (2017). The 10-year prognostic value of zero and minimal CAC. *JACC: Cardiovascular Imaging*, Vol. 10 (No. 8), p. 957.

Parsons, W.B. (2000). *Cholesterol control without diet!: the niacin solution.* Chicago, IL: Lilac Press.

Peacock, J.M. et al (1999). Relationship of serum and dietary magnesium to incident hypertension: the Atherosclerosis Risk in Communities (ARIC) Study. *Annals of Epidemiology*, Vol. 9, pp. 159–165.

Prasad, K (2011). Tocotrienols and cardiovascular health. *Curr Pharm Des*, Vol. 17 (21), pp. 2147–54.

Rautiainen, Suzanne et al (2010). Multivitamin use and the risk of myo-cardial infarction: a population-based cohort of Swedish women. *American Journal of Clinical Nutrition*, Vol. 92, No. 5, pp. 1251–1256.

Reiter, R.J. (2005). When melatonin gets on your nerves: its beneficial actions in experimental models of stroke. *Experimental Biology and Medicine* (Maywood), Vol. 230, No. 2, pp. 104–107.

Rimm, E.B. et al (1998). Folate and vitamin B6 from diet and supplements in relation to risk of coronary heart disease among women. *Journal of the American Medical Association*, Vol. 279, No. 5, pp. 359–364.

Rizos, E.C. et al (2012). Association between omega-3 fatty acid supplementation and risk of major cardiovascular disease events: a systematic review and meta-analysis. *Journal of the American Medical Association*, Vol. 308 (No. 10), pp. 1024–33.

Rosanoff, A. & Seelig, M.S. (2004). Comparison of mechanism and functional effects of magnesium and statin pharmaceuticals. *Journal of the American College of Nutrition*, Vol. 23, No. 5, pp. 5015–5055.

Rudman, D. et al (1990). Effects of HGH in men over 60 years old. *New England Journal of Medicine*, Vol. 323 (No. 1).

Ruparelia, N. et al (2011). Effects of niacin on atherosclerosis and vascular function. Curr Opin Cardiol, Vol. 26 (1), pp. 66–70.

Scheer, F.A. et al (2004). Daily nighttime melatonin reduces blood pressure in male patients with essential hypertension. *Hypertension*, Vol. 43, No. 2, pp. 192–197.

Schroeder, H.A. et al (1970). Chromium deficiency as a factor in atherosclerosis. *Journal of Chronic Diseases*, Vol. 23, No. 2, pp. 123–142.

Schurgers, L. J. et al (2001). Role of vitamin K and vitamin K-dependent proteins in vascular calcification. *Journal of Cardiology*, Vol. 90, No. 15.

Seaborn, C.D. et al (1993). Silicon: a nutritional beneficence for bones, brains and blood vessels? *Nutrition Today*, Vol. 28, No. 4, pp. 13–18.

Seely, Stephen (1991). Is calcium excess in western diet cause of arterial disease? (Editorial). *International Journal of Cardiology*, Vol. 33, No. 2, pp. 191–198.

Sesso, Howard D. et al (2008). Vitamins E and C in prevention of cardiovascular disease in men: the Physicians' Health Study II randomized controlled trial. *Journal of the American Medical Association*, Vol. 300 (18), pp. 2123–2133.

Shea, M.K. et al (2009). Vitamin K supplementation and progression of coronary artery calcium in older men and women. *American Journal of Clinical Nutrition*, Vol. 89, No. 6, pp. 1799–1807.

Sinatra, Stephen T. (2008). *The Sinatra Solution: metabolic cardiology*. Laguna Beach, CA: Basic Health Publications, Inc.

Sinatra, Stephen T. & Sinatra, Jan (1999). *L-carnitine and the heart: how the powerful combination of l-carnitine and coQ10 can have a positive impact on one's health and well being*. NY, NY: Keats Publishing (McGraw-Hill)

Sole, M.J. & Jeejeebhoy, K.N. (2002). Conditioned nutritional requirements: therapeutic relevance to heart failure. *Herz.*, Vol. 27, No. 2, pp. 174–178.

Srinivasan, V. et al (2006). Melatonin in Alzheimer's disease and other neurodegenerative disorders. *Behavioral and Brain Functions*, Vol. 2, No. 1, p. 15.

Tavintharan, A. & Kasyap, Moti, L. (2001). The benefits of niacin in atherosclerosis. *Current Atherosclerosis Reports*, Vol. 3, No. 1, pp. 74–82.

Vieth, Reinhold et al (2001). Efficacy and safety of vitamin D3 intake exceeding the lowest observed adverse effect. *American Journal of Clinical Nutrition*, Vol. 73, No. 2, pp. 288–294.

Vimaleswaran, K.S. et al, 2014. Association of vitamin D status with arterial blood pressure and hypertension risk: a mendelian randomisation study. *The Lancet Diabetes & Endocrinology*, early online publication 26 June 2014.

Vogiatzoglou, Anna et al (2008). Vitamin B12 status and rate of brain volume loss in community-dwelling elderly. *Neurology*, Vol. 71, No. 11, pp. 826–832.

Von Schacky, Clemens et al (1999). The effect of dietary omega-3 fatty acids on coronary atherosclerosis: a randomized, double-blind, placebo-controlled trial. *Annals of Internal Medicine*, Vol. 130, pp. 554–562.

Walsh, Judith M. E. & Pignone, Michael (2004). Drug treatment of hyperlipidemia in women. *Journal of the American Medical Association*, Vol. 291, pp. 2243–2252.

White, Lon R. et al (2000). Brain aging and midlife tofu consumption. *Journal of the American College of Nutrition*, Vol. 19, No. 2, pp. 242–255.

Wilson, T.A. et al (1998). Soy lecithin reduces plasma lipoprotein cholesterol and early atherogenesis in hypercholesterolemic monkeys and hamsters: beyond linoleate. *Atherosclerosis*, Vol. 140, pp. 147–153.

Wu, A. et al (2008). Docosahezaenoic acid dietary supplementation enhances the effects of exercise on synaptic plasticity and cognition. *Neuroscience*, Vol. 155, pp. 751–759.

Young, Robert O. & Young, Shelly Redford (2002). *The pH miracle: balance your diet, reclaim your health*. NY, NY: Warner Books, Inc.

Zhang, W. J. et al (2008). Dietary alpha-lipoic acid supplementation inhibits atherosclerotic lesion development in apolipoprotein E-deficient and apo-lipoprotein E/low-density lipoprotein receptor-deficient mice. *Circulation*, Vol. 117, No. 3, pp. 421–428.

—— CHAPTER 5 ——
Solution of Health Problems with Alternative and Holistic Medical Methods

<u>A cautionary statement for persons with health problems</u>. **I am not a physician or other type of health expert and am not discouraging people from taking advantage of the availability of conventional medical practitioners**. A person should decide not to follow a doctor's advice only when she or he has strong scientific and/or research information or assistance of an integrative or holistic physician or a naturopathic doctor (ND).

<u>Elaboration</u>. "Alternative" medical treatment does not involve use of conventional medical methods and FDA-approved drugs. "Complementary" medical treatment involves the same methods as alternative medical treatment but is offered together with ordinary medical treatment by MDs and DOs. "Holistic" medical treatment involves emphasis on the whole person. An MD can take that approach and be referred to as a holistic physician. Holistic treatment can involve many of the methods of alternative medical treatment.

There are many competent holistic, integrative MDs, DOs, and NDs (naturopathic doctors) in the U.S. Unfortunately, if their treatments are not conventional medical treatment, their services probably will not be covered by health insurance. There are several excellent books about alternative and holistic medical methods. Below, I tell you about five of these books. Information about a list of outstanding practitioners is also given below.

Dangers resulting from the deification of doctors. About 2.5 years ago, I developed a very painful kidney stone. I searched on the Internet for a product that would solve the problem. I discovered Cleanse Drops, bought them, got pain relief 15 minutes after drinking drops in water, and passed the stone without pain two hours later. Six months later, I offered to give an unopened bottle of Cleanse drops to a man with an extremely painful kidney stone. Though mine had been very painful, I'm confident his was much more painful. He refused my offer because the drops had not been approved by his urologist. That astonished me.

I had several fraternity brothers who were, as far as I could tell, not much smarter than me, who attended and completed medical school and have practiced medicine for many years. Although many tens of thousands of U.S. physicians are significantly smarter than me, I don't view a doctor as any type of god, which has helped me very greatly regarding health.

Importance of this subject. Many people have the impression that, if you believe you have a health problem, the only rational thing to do is to go to an MD practicing conventional medicine. That is not correct. I think that many of the "cures" described in the books listed below can be successful. While I believe that some alternative-health practitioners exaggerate the potential benefits of some remedies he or she is promoting, I know from research reports and my own experience that many of these cures do work.

Deficiencies concerning conventional medical methods. Gary Null, PhD and a team of mainly MDs have a book (Null et al, 2011) in which they report that annually about one million Americans die as a result of some type of medical mistake or treatment. The point is that there are giant adverse human consequences of failures of traditional medicine in the U.S. Terry A. Rondberg reports in a book (1998) that 60% of surgeries in the U.S. are unnecessary. My experiences have been consistent with that statistic.

Relevance for young adults. Young adults need to acquire information about the availability of effective approaches for dealing with health problems. As discussed above, there are several types of fully licensed medical specialties which utilize alternative, holistic medical methods. For example, many nurse practitioners use integrative, holistic medical approaches.

Books on the subject of this chapter which I believe were competently developed and written. Instead of listing them in the reference section, I will provide full information here. All of the authors, except for Jenny Thompson, hold an MD, PhD, or ND. I have not confirmed what Jenny Thompson's educational qualifications are, but she has done much impressive work on this subject. Dr. Julian Whitaker practices alternative medicine and has a major presence on the Internet.

Health Sciences Institute (2011). *Today's greatest alternative medicines*. Baltimore, MD.

Hoffman, Ronald & Barry Fox (2007). *Alternative cures that really work*. NY, NY: Rodale, Inc.

Stengler, Mark, & James F. Balch, Robin Young Balch (2016). *Prescription for natural cures*. NY, NY: Turner Publishing Co.

Thompson, Jenny (2013). *Miracles from the vault: anthology of underground cures*. Baltimore, MD: Institute of Health Sciences.

Wright, Jonathan V. (2013). *Treasury of natural cures*. Baltimore, MD: NewMarket Health Publishing, LLC.

A list of prominent physicians who use integrative medicine approaches. To obtain a list of these physicians, you can search for "Newsmax health's top 100 physicians who embrace integrative medicine." Many of these physicians provide regular updates on developments in their medical areas, often for $35 to $50 per year. You can buy books on health/medical subjects from some of these physicians.

There is an excellent integrative MD, Dr. Connie Casebolt in Greenville, SC. Several years ago, she and I co-facilitated a discussion about statin drugs. Near the end, she said that she had agreed with everything I had said. Of course, I was very glad to hear that comment from an excellent MD.

Author's relevant experience. I do not have qualifications or expertise needed to provide full information about this subject while teaching a college course.

Fortunately, I have several times, utilizing available scientific information, "figured out" how to solve a health problem that a conventional physician had been unable to solve. Also, I have several times declined to follow medical advice from an MD. I always had scientific information or another sound reason for these refusals and am not aware that any of my refusals have resulted in an adverse health outcome for me. In several cases, I got "pointed in the right direction" by doing an Internet search. Below is a list of health problems I have dealt with successfully by non-medical means.

Examples of my utilization of non-medical approaches to solve a health problem. I did not obtain treatment by a non-physician health practitioner in any of these situations.

Problem	Non-medical remedy	Outcome
Middle 1970s. Diagnosis of hand arthritis	Hand exercise at home	Symptoms overcome in one year. Have lived since about 1978 with very strong, pain-free hands.
Early 1980s. MD recommended taking a statin.	I developed my own routine for heart-disease prevention.	My program has been remarkably successful.
1980s. Told I would soon need left-hip replacement	Stretching (First doctor's diagnosis was wrong.)	Complete recovery

About 2008. Developed hip discomfort. Learned from a friend what exercises strengthen muscles supporting a hip joint.	I did those exercises for about two days.	This eliminated the hip discomfort and made the hip feel stronger.
2008. Told by MD rotator cuff tear required surgery. Friend convinced me not to have surgery.	Gradual strengthening of muscles around rotator cuff at home.	Complete, pain-free recovery
2013. Very painful tennis elbow. Physical therapists wouldn't teach me "eccentric" exercises.	Found "eccentric" exercises on the Internet. Did those exercises at home.	Once I started the exercises, problem ended in 10 days.
2015. Kidney stone with severe pain	Cleanse Drops (available on Internet)	Stopped pain in 15 minutes. Stone passed later that day.
2018. Severe lower leg pain	Since I knew pain could result from a vein blood clot, I took a nattokinase supplement, which is an excellent anti-coagulant.	Pain ended within 30 min.

If one person can achieve this many excellent outcomes using non-medical approaches, without consulting with an alternative medicine practitioner, how great is the overall potential for alternative, holistic health approaches in the U.S.?

My receipt of alternative medical treatments for aggressive recurrent prostate cancer. Though my recent PSA results have not been as high as 1, my PSA increased by 825% during 2017, which I believe indicates that my cancer is very aggressive. As I report in the essay that follows this chapter, I during 2018 received simultaneously the following alternative anti-cancer treatments: Salicinium, EWOT, and PEMF. A PSA test result I obtained in August, 2018 suggested that those treatments had stopped the advance of my cancer. I am hoping that those treatments together will eliminate my cancer. Of course, you can find information on those treatments on the Internet.

<u>My impressions concerning protection and improvement of joint health</u>. My impression is that fairly often a person with joint pain caused by physical activity will start taking an NSAID (non-steroidal anti-inflammatory drug), such as aspirin, ibuprofin (Advil and Motrin), or Naproxen, and then resume physical activity. While I am not a physician or health expert, I strongly disagree with this practice, because there is a danger that significant damage to the joint will occur.

My practice when I have joint pain is to stop the aggravating physical activity, rest the joint, strengthen the muscles supporting the joint, and, in some cases, do stretching to extend the range of motion. If you plan to use weight(s) in an effort to strengthen muscles around a joint, you should start with low weight and then add weight very carefully. Now 74, I have had a giant amount of physical activity and exercise and have had significant pain in my hands, hips, shoulders, wrists, knees, elbows, neck, and back. My routine has worked on everything until the summer of 2017. On July I developed fairly sharp right hip pain. I used too much weight in my strengthening routine, and the pain got worse. I was afraid I was headed for hip surgery. I bought a supplement formula, Lunaflex PM, which is claimed to help you sleep better, which is said in turn to allow the cartilage in the formula to achieve joint repair. Fortunately, both of those things have occurred for me so far. I expect to protect my right hip from excessive exertion for the rest of my life.

If you have arthritic joint pain, I suggest that you read an article on the WebMD website, "Alternatives and supplements for arthritis joint pain." I have taken chondroitin-sulfate for many years and believe it has helped me greatly. Recently, I started taking MSM, which is specifically for joint pain.

It definitely helps me. Though I am nearly 75, I can walk 18 holes of golf and play reasonably well.

To find exercises that easily ended my serious tennis elbow, search on the Internet for "eccentric exercise for tennis elbow."

Overview of my experiences with physicians and with non-medical measures. I have respect for the medical profession and for many MDs. However, the many MDs who have insisted that I take a statin were wrong in suggesting that such a decision was my only safe and responsible option. (I strongly believe that would not have been a responsible option for me.) The heart- and brain-health program I developed has been extremely safe and effective. The one time I went along with a physician regarding major surgery (prostate surgery), the side effects were extremely bad. (Experiencing general anesthesia can cause serious brain function problems for the patient.) Having read extensively about prostate surgery recently, I believe that there are expensive (no insurance coverage) integrative physicians who could have provided fully satisfactory treatment for my prostate cancer without surgery.

I will note that, over the years, a good number of physicians have provided to me very helpful treatment for a variety of other problems, such as dangerous blood clotting.

Can this chapter lead to a career for you? I believe that alternative, holistic, and complementary medical approaches are the "wave of the future" relating to health in the U.S. They often are the best ways to attempt to prevent disease and illness, which is something nearly every person needs.

REFERENCES

Null, Gary et al (2011). *Death by medicine*. Mt. Jackson, VA: Praktikos Books.

Rondberg, Terry A. (1998). *Under the influence of modern medicine*. Chiropractic Journal.

AN ESSAY ABOUT MY EXPERIENCES FIGHTING PROSTATE CANCER

In 2001, I weighed too much (212 lbs.) and took the advice of Dr. Robert Atkins and followed the Atkins (very high protein, extremely low carbohydrate) diet for several months. I lost 40 pounds. Because I lost 30 yards on my "full" golf shots, I think I lost a significant amount of muscle tissue. About that time, my PSA (prostate specific antigen) began to rise. I have read that the Atkins diet can increase your risk of developing cancer. So, I extremely strongly advise against the Atkins diet.

From 2001 to 2007, I used non-medical approaches to slow increase of PSA. In 2007, I was diagnosed with prostate cancer. I worked extremely hard trying to beat it by non-medical means. (My bet is that, if a family has a **lot of money**, a man can beat prostate cancer by non-medical means.) In 2007, I started taking supplements, including l-lysine, which are said to prevent metastasis of prostate cancer. It is possible that this has kept me alive so far. Below, I list these supplements.

Because of sharp increase of PSA late in 2008, I gave up on beating the cancer by non-medical means and arranged to have prostate surgery conducted by an internationally prominent robotic-surgery physician at Johns Hopkins. His robotic surgery was touted as nearly certain to protect nerves important for male sexual response. My nerves were not protected. He did not advise me (which I should have discovered on my own) that research does not show that people who have prostate surgery live longer than people who don't have surgery and don't have other major treatment. He did not advise me that there would be a major risk of cancer recurrence after surgery, which did occur. So, I strongly advise against prostate surgery.

Three years after my prostate surgery, a prostate cancer recurrence occurred. I had 49 radiation treatments in 2014 ordered by an Asheville, NC, oncologist, who did not warn me about the risk of recurrence of prostate cancer after radiation treatments.

In 2015, a second recurrence started. Since learning this, I have been taking a supplement formula, Pomi-T, which is supposed to either kill or slow the growth of prostate cancer. My PSA was 0.04 late in 2016 and 0.37 late in 2017. Pomi-T apparently can't affect cancer as aggressive as mine.

In about 2013, I co-facilitated a discussion about statin drugs with Greenville, SC, integrative physician Dr. Connie Casebolt. Because I was very impressed with her knowledge concerning alternative approaches against heart disease, I have obtained her medical treatment services against my second recurrence of prostate cancer. A test in February of 2018 showed that I did have active cancer. She recommended that I implement and follow the Salicinium protocol for totally eliminating cancer. It is credibly reported on the Internet that Salicinium is extremely successful against stage-four metastatic prostate cancer. I started following the protocol in March of 2018. It involves taking four pills three times a day, drinking alkaline water all day, and drinking milk with a Salicinium liquid in the morning and evening. Though Dr. Casebolt recommended that I follow the routine for two months, I followed it for six weeks, which is recommended in an article on the Internet. Unfortunately, my cancer-indicator test after six weeks indicated that my cancer had not been reduced. Here is information about my PSA.

My PSA was .04 on January 4, 2017.

My PSA was .37 on January 9, 2018.

So, during 2017 my PSA (and prostate cancer) increased by 825%.

At that rate of increase, it would be predicted that my PSA in early May 2018 would be about 1.56.

In fact, my PSA on May 2, 2018 (end of Salicinium) was .4.

This suggests that Salicinium was to some extent effective against growth of my prostate cancer.

Because Salicinium did not eliminate my cancer, I arranged to start PEMF treatments by a chiropractor in Charlotte, NC. I also started doing EWOT (exercise with oxygen training/therapy/treatment) at home every day. It involves setting an oxygen concentrator between 5 and 10 on the gauge and getting 15 minutes of nearly strenuous exercise. Because I very strongly believe that EWOT has major benefits, I plan to do it on every day I don't play golf for the rest of my life. During August of 2018, I had a PSA result that strongly suggested that Salicinium, EWOT, and PEMF have stopped the advance of my cancer. I am optimistic that I will be able to obtain treatments that will keep prostate cancer from killing me.

Here is a list of mainly supplements that are said to help with prevention of cancer metastasis: DMG, folic acid, B6, B12, vitamin C, lysine, proline, DHA, quercetin, ellagic acid, turmeric, resveratrol, green tea extract, digestive enzymes. If cancer never metastasizes, it may not succeed in killing its host.

— SECTION 3 —
Cardiovascular Health

An Essay about the Complexity of Causation

In my graduate studies in criminology and in my doctoral dissertation on work-related stress (1981), thinking about causation tended to be very complex. As a Criminal Justice professor, I sometimes gave students a hypothetical situation involving a 15-year-old girl living in South Carolina who runs away from home and becomes a street prostitute in Atlanta. Dozens of circumstances and factors could contribute to causation of those behaviors. There are many factors that can wholly or partially cause the physiological stress reaction (fight-or-flight reaction). I believe that a chapter 27 addendum shows that the causes of a crime can be extremely complex.

When I learned in 1982, as described in chapter 6, that I have very severe heart- and brain-disease risk factors, I assumed that there were many possible contributing causes of those diseases. So, I used available scientific information and developed my own supplement-and-exercise routine, which I have improved many times and have followed since then. I had the impression that each of the about eight supplements and the exercise could help with at least one possible cause of heart and brain disease. That was before statin drugs came on the scene in the U.S.

In 1987 the first statin drug, Mevacor, was approved by the FDA for sale to reduce a patient's LDL cholesterol. Drug companies wanted to convince Americans that the following simple story is true: "'Bad cholesterol' (LDL) is the cause of heart disease. If you take Mevacor, it will reduce your LDL, which will prevent your development of heart disease." Also, they wanted to persuade Americans that the supporting research was done with the rigorous research methods of the "hard sciences." It is interesting that models of causation in the "hard sciences" relating to efficacy of drugs are much less complex than causation models tend to be in the social and behavioral sciences.

Americans believed the drug companies' story, and those companies made and are still making billions.

There are, however, several problems with their story. To be healthy, a person needs to have enough LDL. Also, it is likely that any heart disease prevention benefits of a statin drug result from the anti-coagulant, anti-inflammatory, anti-oxidant, and pro-endothelial (blood vessel) function effects of the statin drug, not from the reduction of LDL. The drug companies' "simple-causation model" research did not look at those possibilities.

So, was the drug companies' simple model of causation or my very complex model of causation correct? (It's important to know here that nearly all of the things that cause brain disease also cause heart disease.) Research by UCLA professor Dr. Dale Bredesen (2014) definitively answered that question.

The Alzheimer's Association has always said that Alzheimer's cannot be prevented or reversed. In recent years, Dr. Bredesen did Alzheimer's/dementia-reversal research (2014) with ten subjects, each of whom had either Alzheimer's or severe dementia. Nine of the ten patients improved significantly, and two were able to return to work.

Dr. Bredesen utilized a very complex model of causation. He identified 25 aspects of metabolism and body function that can be involved in development of Alzheimer's or dementia and developed a custom treatment program for each patient. Dr. Bredesen lists thirty-one supplements as available treatments. If, for example, a patient took 10 supplements and exercised, it was not necessary for any one supplement to have a major benefit. Instead, 10 modest positive effects could together "get the job done." Also, a synergism of effects probably occurred, making the effects of the supplements and exercise together greater than the sum of their effects occurring separately.

I think it should be medical malpractice for physicians to convince patients that all they need to do to prevent cardiovascular disease is take a statin drug to reduce LDL. Obviously, the Bredesen type of complex-causation model corresponds very much more closely to the realities of human body metabolism and function than the drug companies' story. As detailed in chapter 6, my quite complex approach against cardiovascular and brain disease has never included taking a statin or reducing LDL by other means. I now take about 38 supplements regularly or occasionally. Screenings done in 2017 showed that I have excellent cardiovascular health.

REFERENCES

Bredesen, D. (2014). Reversal of cognitive decline: a novel therapeutic program. *Aging*, Vol. 6, pp.707–717.

Memory, J.M. (1981). *Work-related stress of state criminal trial court judges.* Unpublished doctoral dissertation, Florida State University, Tallahassee, FL.

—— CHAPTER 6 ——
Non-Drug Prevention of Atherosclerosis (hardening of the arteries)

Cautionary statement regarding adopting a non-statin heart health approach. **The author is not a physician and is not a health expert. Therefore, he cannot diagnose or treat illness or disease or prescribe medication to cure disease.** Especially if you have advanced cardiovascular disease (high heart attack, stroke, SCD risk, very high blood pressure, congestive heart failure, or other serious heart disease), you should not do anything discussed in this book relating to heart and brain health. A person with minor heart disease should consult with a physician before doing one of the supplement-and-exercise routines described in this book. The routine in this chapter is absolutely not for persons with serious heart disease problems, unless they have medical supervision while implementing the routine. The VCRs (routines) in this book are absolutely not intended for anyone who is taking a statin drug for control of cholesterol or BP.

Clarification. This chapter describes a basic supplement-and-exercise routine for heart and brain health which is mainly intended for people, like me (the author), who have a "bad lipids profile," but not more than minor cardiovascular disease.

Among other things, this chapter tells about **an extremely successful heart and brain health routine I developed in 1982 to deal with my very severe heart and brain disease risk factors.** As I report too often, now at 74 years old, I have **excellent cardiovascular health and excellent brain**

function. To accomplish this, I have had to be very well informed about health (especially heart and brain health), motivated, determined, and consistent in performing my routine. I have also been prudent about diet.

Here's a question I often hear: "Why are you so glad that you have regularly done your own supplement-and-exercise routine since 1982, instead of taking a statin drug?"

Of course, the main reasons are the excellent heart health and brain health and function I am able to enjoy at 74 years of age, in spite of very severe heart and brain disease risk factors.

While a statin drug at best slows the development of atherosclerosis (hardening of the arteries), I am confident that, especially in the 1980s, my routine actually reversed atherosclerosis I had previously developed. A CT scan in 2005 and Life Line screenings done in 2017 showed that my arteries are remarkably free from occlusion.

Taking a statin drug tends to reduce willingness to exercise (Thompson, 2012). Because I have done my routine more than 8000 times, I have received wonderful benefits from exercise, benefits from the gradually improving selection of supplements, and synergistic benefits of supplements and exercise together more than 8000 times. (I want to clarify that, if a person wants fairly quick help against atherosclerosis, the person can, with medical supervision, carry out the atherosclerosis-reversal approach described in chapter 9 of this book.)

Adverse side effects of a statin drug (Roberts, 2012) I might have experienced include the following: type 2 diabetes, which risk has been shown to be increased by 46% by taking a statin drug (Cederberg et al, 2015); muscle damage, kidney damage, heart failure, immune suppression, decreased mental function, increased cancer risk (Blaylock, 2012); major reduction of enjoyment of sex (Gorman, 2012); possible failure to be able to do strong scholarly work during my career since 1982. Research (Meilahn, 1995) has shown that low LDL level can be associated with bad health consequences. If I had taken a statin drug since 1987, the resulting low level of LDL and probable reduction of quality of my cognitive functioning during my 60s and 70s would have kept me from writing this book and doing other challenging and rewarding writing and musical creativity in recent years. Taking a statin drug nearly certainly would have greatly reduced my enjoyment of golf, bridge, and dancing. I probably would have developed Alzheimer's disease long before my current age of 74.

Increase in urgency of ads concerning danger of a "bad lipids profile." If you are concerned about your elevated LDL, you may know that, during April of 2018, Amgen, which makes and markets Repatha, a non-statin cholesterol-control drug, has introduced two TV ads which increase the urgency of the message that failure to sufficiently control your LDL greatly increases danger of having a heart attack or stroke. As I communicate in this chapter, the supplement, exercise, and diet approaches I adopted in 1982 and have improved many times since then have apparently dealt with any possible problems regarding elevation of LDL and have freed me entirely from anxiety about my "bad lipids profile." Instead, I have worked very hard on other heart and brain health matters.

How you can skip to the recommended supplement-and-exercise routine (VCR)? It is very important for me to provide in this chapter many types of research, scientific, and medical information prior to recommending a routine you can follow. If you would like to go on and get to the recommended routine, you can skip to "a suggested supplement-and-exercise routine (VCR)" that includes recommended supplements. I must warn you that, if you do that, you will not obtain important information.

Another cautionary statement. If you don't have the motivation to eat a reasonably heart-healthy diet, buy and take supplements, and then get meaningful exercise very often and consistently for years, it might be better for you to take the route recommended by your doctor, which probably involves taking a statin drug and expecting it to do the work for you.

Good news for discouraged persons with minor atherosclerosis. You may feel discouraged to learn that I have done my routine (VCR) about 8000 times since 1982. Within one or two years of starting my VCR, my blood pressure decreased so much that it seemed obvious that the VCR had achieved some reversal of my minor atherosclerosis. So, you can do the VCR in this chapter and monitor results. If you want to make quicker progress than that, you can read chapter 9 and consider using more advanced supplements recommended in that chapter.

The reason a statin drug is so often suggested or prescribed. Stated as simply as I can, if a physician's patient is shown to have a "bad lipids profile" and the doctor suggests and/or prescribes a cholesterol-control drug and if the patient later suffers a very adverse consequence of a heart attack, the doctor will be able to successfully defend a law suit brought by the patient. If the doctor doesn't suggest and/or prescribe a cholesterol-control drug and if the patient suffers a very adverse consequence of a heart attack, the doctor will probably lose when sued by the patient.

Very important research findings concerning one of the risks of taking a statin drug. In deciding whether you will take a statin drug, I suggest that you strongly consider recent excellent research which showed that taking a statin drug was associated with a 46% increase in risk of developing type 2 diabetes (Cederberg et al, 2015).

In a major research study (Culver et al, 2012), long-term use of statins by women was shown to produce a 50% increase in risk of developing diabetes The Culver study was, at that time, at least the fourth major study to find a link between statin use and increased incidence of diabetes.

Results of a major study of patterns of prescription of cholesterol-lowering drugs. A major study (Savole & Kazanjian, 2001) of patterns of prescription of cholesterol-lowering drugs in Canada produced this conclusion:

> "This study concludes that statins prescribing practices need to be realigned with research evidence. This implies refocusing utilization away from women and the elderly, toward men with CHD."

> This medical language discourages use of a statin by women or the elderly.

FDA warnings about statin drugs. **To learn about FDA warnings about risks of taking a statin drug, you can read an article, "Statin risks: what you need to know after new FDA warnings," March 1, 2012, Newsmaxhealth.com website.**

Negative effect of taking a statin drug on willingness to exercise. Dr. Paul D. Thompson reports in an article (2012) on the Newsmaxhealth.com website, "Statin side effects can stop you from exercising," that several types of research have shown that taking a statin drug can cause muscle damage that can make exercising painful.

Taking a statin drug can induce complacency about health and life style.

Possible effects of taking a statin drug for Donald Trump. When inaugurated, Donald Trump regularly took a statin drug. My impression is that competent physicians believe that taking a statin helps nearly no person over 65. Research has shown that taking a statin drug can have an adverse effect on cognitive functioning, which seems to be occurring for Trump. (Dr. Duane Graveline has several books about these adverse side effects.) I believe, also, that Donald Trump satisfies many of the criteria for the metabolic syndrome, which is the subject of chapter 7.

Several of many books that are critical of statin drugs.

Bowden, Jonny & Sinatra, Stephen (2012). *The great cholesterol myth: why lowering your cholesterol won't prevent heart attacks—and the statin-free plan that will.* Lions Bay, BC, Canada: Fair Winds Press.

Kendrick, Malcolm, MD (2007). *The cholesterol con: the truth about what really causes heart disease and how to avoid it.* London: John Blake Publishing, Ltd.

Roberts, B. (2012). *The truth about statins: risks and alternatives to cholesterol-lowering drugs.* NY, NY: Pocket Books.

Rosch, Paul J. (2016). *Fat and cholesterol don't cause heart attacks and statins are not the solution.* Yakima, WA: Columbia Publishing.

Deceptive use of statistics in research concerning statin drugs. In an article cited above, Dr. Blaylock says:

"[O]ne commonly sees ads saying that Lipitor, for instance, lowers the incidence of heart attack death by 30 percent. In actual numbers, it is lowering the risk from 6 percent to 4 percent in an individual—that is, an actual 2 percent reduction. But mathematically, 4 percent is about 30 percent lower than 6 percent."

A dangerous extension of guidelines concerning taking a statin drug. A 2014 article on the CBSNews website, "13 million more Americans would take statins if new guidelines followed: study," reports that "[a]lmost half of Americans ages 40 to 75 and nearly all men over 60 qualify to consider cholesterol-lowering statin drugs." It was reported in a 2015 article on the website of the American Council on Science and Health that 33.3 million Americans were at that time taking a statin. This book and especially this chapter are intended to provide a safe and effective alternative to taking a statin drug.

Availability of credible information about non-conventional approaches concerning heart disease. To let you know that the information in this chapter and other chapters of this book relating to cardiovascular health is consistent with important information in the health field, I'll give you information about a short book and four websites:

> *Hushed up natural heart cures and deadly deceptions of popular heart treatments* by Michael Cutler, MD (2013). If cardiovascular health is a major concern for you, this would be a good short book to buy and read.

> Website and publications of Dr. David Brownstein

> **jonbarron.org** "Heart health program: learn how to reverse heart disease and problems naturally." Though Barron is not a physician, he is extremely successful in providing non-conventional health information.

> **holisticonline.com** "Commonsense care for cardiovascular health and heart disease." Dr. George Jacobs

Lifeextension.com. There are articles on many subjects relating to heart and brain health.

Difference of the routines (VCR's) in this book and non-statin approaches of many physicians who practice alternative, complementary, integrative, and/or holistic medicine. In this chapter I provide information about many physicians who successfully use non-drug approaches against heart disease. Unlike most of their heart health routines, the routines in this book involve taking carefully selected supplements, waiting 30 minutes, and then getting 20 to 40 minutes of moderate exercise. This allows synergy of the supplements with each other and with the exercise. If you decide to use a non-drug heart health routine obtained from a physician, which I do not discourage, I encourage you to implement it with that sequence: take supplements, wait 30 minutes, exercise. As discussed later in this chapter, there is research support for that sequence.

Detailed information concerning heart- and brain-health benefits of particular supplements. For detailed information about heart- and brain-health benefits of particular nutritional supplements, refer to chapter 4.

Apparent ineffectiveness of l-arginine. For humans up to some age, l-arginine promotes the production of nitric-oxide in blood vessels, which has cardiovascular health benefits. On the Internet, there are statements to the effect that l-arginine does not provide this benefit after some age. I recently bought l-arginine/citrulline complex supplement and immediately received much better benefit concerning preventing an elevated heartbeat. Because of this improvement, I am now recommending that persons over 45 take l-arginine/citrulline complex instead of l-arginine. For men over 45 and women past menopause, I think that taking l-arginine/citrulline complex instead of l-arginine may be important regarding prevention of heart attack.

Author's relevant professional activities and experience. During 2012, Wake Forest University's digital publisher released a book by me and a co-author (Memory & Evatt, 2012) that is primarily about prevention of heart disease by women. The title of the book is *Vascular cleansing routines: safe and effective heart health programs for women (and men)*.

As mentioned earlier, in 1982 I learned for the first time that I have several severe cardiovascular disease risk factors. In later years, I have learned about many additional heart- and brain-disease risk factors I am subject to. Because readers can reasonably want to have detailed information about this, I have placed that information here.

Heart (and Brain) Disease Risk Factors of John Memory

Substance measured	Number of tests since 1983	Average	Heart disease risk
LDL ("bad" cholesterol)	21 (2018, 182, high risk)	149.4	High in borderline range
Total cholesterol	27 (2018, 317, high risk)	234	6 from "high risk" level
Triglycerides	27 (2018, 696, high risk)	292	High risk
HDL ("good" lipid)	22	38.9	High risk
C-reactive protein (inflammation indicator)	small number	4.34	High risk
Homocysteine	small number	14	Top of intermediate risk level
Blood sugar	small number	96	Nearly elevated
Ratio of total chol. and HDL	(Total cholesterol divided by HDL)	6.1	High risk

My LDL particles are pattern B (small), which significantly increases heart-disease risk. I have extremely small HDL particles, which significantly increases heart-disease risk.

An older brother had a heart attack in his 50s. In her 70s, my mother had hypertension. She died at 81 from a burst aortal aneurysm. A pathologist told me she had a genetically transmitted blood vessel disease.

My waist circumference has for several years been more than 40", which is high enough to satisfy a criterion for the metabolic syndrome. The metabolic syndrome is a serious risk factor for heart disease, type 2 diabetes, and Alzheimer's.

In my only such test, I was indicated to be highly insulin resistant, which is associated with high heart disease and type 2 diabetes risk. A physician found in 2018 that I am "pre-diabetic."

I have low thyroid functioning, which has adverse health effects. (I have been taking remedial medication since about 2009.)

All of my life, I have awakened often (usually between 6 and 8 times) during sleep to urinate. Failure to get long periods of high quality sleep tends to have adverse consequences concerning heart and brain health.

My dissolved oxygen is low enough that I use an insurance-paid oxygen machine at night. Low dissolved oxygen can have adverse health consequences. My brain function is compromised when I do not have a machine that works well.

Information about my current health status. The results of the five standard Life Line Screening tests I mentioned earlier were as follows:

Carotid artery disease: left, mild; right, normal
Arterial fibrillation: normal
Abdominal aortic aneurysm: normal
Peripheral arterial disease: left, normal; right, normal
Osteoporosis: low risk

Since the numerical results regarding carotid artery disease of my right and left sides were the same, I don't understand why the left carotid artery risk was "mild".

Late in October 2017 I had a two-hour brain function evaluation by a

PhD neurologist at the Medical University of South Carolina (MUSC) in Charleston. He concluded that there was no evidence of problems regarding my brain health and function. (I believe that my determined efforts concerning brain health and function have made this result possible.) In 2005, a Columbia, SC, cardiologist performed a CT scan on me. He was astonished by how free my arteries were from occlusion.

My development of my own non-statin heart and brain health routine. In 1982, having recently written a doctoral dissertation (Memory, 1981) on a health subject (work-related stress), I was able to find credible scientific information and use it in developing my own supplement- and-exercise routine to prevent heart and brain disease. I've performed some version of the routine more than 8000 times. The results above buttress my opinion that a non-statin heart health routine utilizing supplements and exercise can produce startlingly positive results. Later in this chapter I describe in detail my supplement-and-exercise routine, which I call a "vascular cleansing routine" (VCR), because it has done that extremely well for me.

I have rejected the recommendations of many physicians that I take a statin drug and, of course, hope that reading related chapters of this book will help people to make well informed decisions about taking a statin drug.

I am confident that, if I had gone the route of taking a statin drug, I would not have heart and brain health that would be nearly as good as I have now. Instead, I would have suffered many of the adverse side effects of taking a statin drug that were listed earlier in this chapter. A highly qualified and experienced cardiologist, Dr. Peter H. Langsjoen, argues that statins are causing an epidemic of heart failure in the U.S. (Newsmaxhealth.com website, "Is your statin drug killing you?", March 29, 2012). This epidemic stems from the statin drug's depletion of coenzyme Q10 in the body, an enzyme which is crucial for heart health.

Importance of this subject. An epidemic of cardiovascular disease is currently occurring in the developing world (Gersh, 2010) and among young adults in the U.S. (Lee, 2008).

Americans know that conventional physicians nearly always suggest taking a statin drug to patients who have "a bad lipids profile," which can include elevated LDL ("bad cholesterol"), elevated triglycerides, and low

HDL ("good cholesterol"). I assume, also, that many people do not realize that there is excellent research support for a non-statin heart health routine by persons with a "bad lipids profile." The fully licensed health practitioners who recommend these non-statin programs include holistic and integrative medical doctors (MDs) and osteopathic physicians (DOs) and naturopathic doctors (NDs). Unfortunately, though a patient can have insurance pay for a doctor's visit and for a statin drug, insurance nearly never pays for an office visit with one of these other practitioners, who might recommend a non-statin heart health program.

Actual benefits of taking a statin drug. It is likely that any benefit from a statin drug, instead of resulting from reduction of LDL (bad cholesterol), results from anti-coagulant effect, anti-inflammatory effect, and anti-oxidant effect, and support of blood vessel health and function of the statin drug (Roberts, 2012). Those four benefits can be obtained fully and adequately in a supplement-and-exercise heart and brain health routine, such as mine.

Most importantly, using diet, supplements, and exercise to promote heart and brain health, especially if you start fairly early, will probably also prevent hypertension, prevent metabolic syndrome, prevent type 2 diabetes, prevent heart attack, greatly reduce your Alzheimer's/dementia risk, and greatly improve many other aspects of your life and health. I will repeat: That is what has happened for me.

Importance for people who, for some reason, cannot take a statin drug or other cholesterol-control drug. Such a person's doctor probably will suggest that the person use supplements to overcome a "bad lipids profile." **Such an approach would fail to, as discussed two paragraphs above, achieve anti-coagulant, anti-inflammatory, anti-oxidant, and pro-endothelial function effects**. I recommend that persons in this situation implement the routine (VCR) given later, which will provide all of those benefits.

The danger of taking aspirin to prevent heart attacks. The Food and Drug Administration (2014) has released a statement warning about the tendency of aspirin to cause dangerous bleeding in the brain and in other parts of a human body. Because of this, I do not include aspirin in any supplement-and-exercise routine (VCR) recommended in this book. Fortunately, there are several supplements that can provide a safe level of anti-coagulant effect (blood thinning). It is important for persons who perform a VCR to achieve a safe balance of coagulant (causing a tendency of blood to clot, which is possible with vitamin K2) and anti-coagulant effects.

Relevance for young adults. This is important for university and college students because, even at that age, a medical examination can disclose a "bad lipids profile," including elevated LDL. In many situations, the attending doctor will recommend using diet and exercise to reduce LDL and triglycerides and increase HDL. If this does not solve the "bad lipids profile" problem, the doctor nearly always will recommend that the individual start taking a statin or other cholesterol-control drug.

Another reason why this is important for "college age persons" is that there is currently an epidemic of heart disease among young adults in the U.S. In the 1990s, a major increase in child obesity occurred, which has been associated with major increase in type 2 diabetes, hypertension, and cardiovascular disease among that group when they are young adults (Lee, 2008).

Health benefits of physical exercise. **I expect that this amazing information will help you to be motivated to exercise regularly performing a VCR to protect and improve your heart and brain health.** In some cases, I was able to provide reference to a research article. Based on extensive reading about this since 1982, I have a high degree of confidence concerning the accuracy of this information. I'll now list the astonishing benefits of physical exercise I have become aware of.

Deterrence of cardiovascular disease and related conditions hypertension, type 2 diabetes, obesity, and problems with endothelial function (function of blood vessels) (Okabe et al, 2006)
Strengthening of the heart
Improvement of blood circulation (Thompson et al, 2003)
Most effective way to build brain power (Ratey, 2008)
Combined with Mediterranean diet, reduction of Alzheimer's risk by 60% (Scarmeas et al, 2009)

For older persons with serious depression, as effective as taking an anti-depressant drug in depression control (Blumenthal et al, 1999)

Reverses detrimental effects of the physiological stress reaction (Salmon,2001).

Helps with troublesome anxiety

Moderate exercise produces growth of new brain cells in the hippocampus.

Improvement of brain function

Promotion of production of DHEA

Improvement of sex life

Helps with achieving healthful sleep

Promotion of production of human growth hormone (HGH)

Promotion, after taking alpha-lipoic acid, of production of glutathione

Helps with delivery of nutrients and oxygen to body tissues

Promotion of production of serotonin and dopamine

Promotion of release of endorphins

Reduction of risk of coronary artery disease, type 2 diabetes, osteoporosis, obesity, depression, and cancer of breast and colon (Thompson et al, 2003)

Some types of exercise that work well in a supplement-and-exercise routine (VCR). At nearly 74, I find that very brisk walking after taking just the right supplements allows me to feel great and think well. Swimming, jogging, bicycling, and riding a dual-action exercise bike can provide enough exercise. Of course, other types of exercise also will "get the job done." As mentioned earlier, during 2018 I decided to do exercise with oxygen therapy (EWOT) at home on every day I don't walk golf. This is the first exercise I have been willing to do strictly for health benefits.

Importance of doing moderate exercise. Many times in this book I mention that strenuous exercise makes blood platelets stickier, and moderate exercise makes them less sticky. During the 1980s and early 1990s, the exercise I did in my VCR often was strenuous, with my pulse rate getting to 175 bpm. I think it is important for me to inform readers that, starting in the middle 1980s to sometime in the early 1990s, I had several instances of very uncomfortable chest pain. Though I went to a cardiologist several times, none of the visits resulted in diagnosis of any type of heart health problem. Once I settled on doing only moderate exercise, I have had nearly no instances of chest pain.

CDC recommendation regarding exercise. The Centers for Disease Control and Prevention recommend that persons get at least 150 minutes of moderate intensity exercise per week. Each segment of exercise should be at least 10 minutes long. This tends to support my impression that I receive substantial benefits from walking very briskly for 17 minutes after taking numerous supplements.

Seeking synergy of effects of supplements and exercise. Synergy is achieved when doing two activities together provides greater benefits than the combination of the two activities done separately. I believe that health and exercise experts have failed to do sufficient research concerning whether there are synergistic effects of supplements and exercise operating simultaneously. Having done my VCR over 8000 times since 1982, I have shown that it can be very safe to take carefully selected supplements, wait 20 to 30 minutes, and then get at least 20 minutes of exercise that is at least as strenuous as brisk walking. I am aware of substantial benefits and no risks from utilizing this sequencing for persons with good cardiovascular health but a "bad lipids profile." Very importantly, doing this causes your body to convert alpha-lipoic acid into glutathione, which is a very important antioxidant.

Scientific support for supplement-and-exercise routines (VCR's). There is scientific support for the most unusual aspect of my routine—taking carefully selected supplements, waiting 30 minutes, and then getting about 30 minutes of moderate exercise. **Research has shown that taking nutritional supplements, followed by moderate exercise, can result in removal of small particles of blood vessel plaque (Napoli et al, 2004). The researchers used vitamin C, ordinary vitamin E, and arginine supplements.** They concluded that, to achieve beneficial effects, attention needs to be on the right degree of exercise (graduated and moderate) and the ideal mixture of supplements. In a recent review of brain research, Henriette van Praag (2009) reported that taking certain supplements or eating particular foods and then exercising has a variety of brain health benefits. She states unequivocally that doing this has substantial health potential. The following quote strongly supports the approach of combining taking supplements and exercising:

> "Concordance between the health benefits of exercise and nutrition and a compensatory role of antioxidant nutrients against the potentially harmful effects of exercise suggests that nutrition and exercise should form important components of any regimen for prevention of chronic diseases and/or promotion of optimal health." (Singh, 1992)

Medical approval of my supplement-and-exercise routine. In about 2000, I had a 45-minute medical appointment with Dr. John R. Guyton, a Duke medical professor who was later the president of the National Lipid Association. He concluded our appointment by approving my supplements (especially niacin) and exercise program for me as an alternative to taking a statin drug. Of course, Dr. Guyton must have known that research had shown that the things I settled on in 1982—niacin (nicotinic acid), fish oil, garlic, lecithin, potassium, magnesium-citrate—all in different ways tend to prevent and, in some cases, reverse cardiovascular disease and prevent heart attacks.

Even though Dr. Guyton approved for me the version of my VCR I was doing in about 2000, I don't think it would be responsible for me to represent that his recommendation and approval should extend to other people doing some version of my VCR. Readers might want to tell their physician about Dr. Guyton's approval of the routine for me.

Why hasn't research been done on the effectiveness of the author's approach? Clinical trials, which often cost hundreds of millions of dollars, determine whether a drug has measurable, statistically significant benefits. Since my routine utilizes nearly 20 different supplements, no supplement manufacturer would want to pay for research that would not show that their one supplement has benefits. This is complicated by the fact that a VCR involves supplements, followed by exercise. As previously discussed, there undoubtedly are synergistic effects of supplements and exercise.

Of course, I would be delighted if the publication of this book leads to research concerning the efficacy of one or more of the routines described in this book.

Again I will emphasize that it is very important for readers to understand that heart health approaches similar to mine are advocated for by many integrative and holistic medical doctors (MDs) and osteopathic doctors (DOs) and by virtually all naturopathic doctors (NDs). Integrative physicians often utilize non-traditional, non-drug approaches in dealing with health problems. Here are the names of several of the top integrative cardiologists in the U.S.: Dr. Mehmet Oz, Dr. Mimi Guarneri, Dr. Chauncey Crandall, Dr. Arthur Agatston, and Dr. Stephen Sinatra. Many of these physicians have websites where you can obtain further information.

I will briefly compare the experiences of one of these very prominent cardiologists, Dr. Chancey Crandall with my own. He finished medical school at Yale in the early 1980s. After decades of practice as a cardiologist, he had a "widow maker" heart attack and was fortunate to survive. In 1981, I earned my PhD in criminology; soon thereafter learned I had serious heart disease risk factors, developed my own non-statin program, and at 74 have excellent cardiovascular health. So, I ask you, "Why should cardiologist Dr. Crandall have vastly more credibility concerning the **prevention of cardiovascular disease** than non-physician John Memory?" My guess is that my heart disease risk factors have been much more severe than those of Dr. Crandall. I know of an 80-year-old cardiologist who, even without adverse heart disease risk factors, had to have a double bypass operation during his 70s.

A **program** is every part of a plan, including supplements, exercise, diet and stress coping, to protect and improve an aspect of health. A **routine**, which can be part of a program, refers in this book to taking carefully selected supplements, waiting 30 minutes, and then getting at least 20 minutes of moderate exercise. As mentioned earlier, because my routine has very effectively cleansed my blood vessels, I refer to my routine as a "vascular cleansing routine" or VCR. As you're walking out the door on Saturday morning, you can announce, "Honey, I'm doing my VCR. I'll be back in 30 minutes." Strangely enough, calling a routine a VCR would probably help it to work for you.

Persons for whom this information and the routine below are intended. It is primarily intended for people who have been told by a physician or other health profession that they have a "bad lipids profile" or that they "have an elevated risk of developing cardiovascular disease." Though I believe that implementation of the VCR below by a person with minor occurrence of atherosclerosis should be safe, I think that persons with more than minor cardiovascular disease or risks should get the assistance of a physician before implementing a supplement-and-exercise routine (VCR).

If your risks are even nearly as serious as mine, as given earlier in this chapter, I think you should consult with a physician before implementing the VCR below.

Important facts about blood pressure. Your BP is "normal" if it is less than 120/80 mmHG. A November 2017 change in hypertension guidelines has converted to hypertension what previously was previously classified as "**pre-hypertension**". **Now, y**ou have **high BP (hypertension)** if your top (systolic) BP number is usually 130 or higher, or your bottom (diastolic) number is usually 80 or higher.

If your blood pressure is often as high as 130–139/80–89, I think it would be prudent for you to consult with a physician before implementing the VCR below.

I believe that if your goals are achieving excellent cardiovascular health and retaining excellent cognitive functioning, it makes sense to have a goal of maintaining an average BP which is somewhat lower than 120/80. When I started my VCR in 1982, I often had blood pressure around 125/75. Probably within a year, I had reduced my blood pressure to around 90/60.

If your BP is usually above 120/80, I encourage you to go to the website of Optimal Naturals and select "blood pressure." You will find an excellent, professionally prepared article about high blood pressure, which provides information detail which is not included in this chapter.

Health risks of elevated blood pressure. Research has shown that having high blood pressure can have very adverse health consequences (Chobanian, 2001). This can include damage to the lining of blood vessels (the endothelium), which can lead to buildup of plaque in blood vessels. Of course, very high blood pressure (hypertension) can trigger rupture of plaque, which can lead to a heart attack. Even moderately high BP during middle age can have adverse effects on brain health and cognitive function (Reitz et al, 2007).

Because of these risks, it is very important to prevent even moderately elevated BP.

Years ago, I read a credible statement that controlling BP **does not** prevent the development of underlying cardiovascular disease. Because of this, I think it is a mistake for a person to have **just** controlling blood pressure as her or his heart-health goal. My guess is that people who continue to implement a VCR will achieve some regression of atherosclerosis and reduction of BP. As mentioned earlier, I am confident that occurred for me.

A "quick fix" to reduce inflammation. For some people, the following will be an easy fix regarding elevated BP. Some instances of BP elevation result from inflammation in the blood vessels. You may have had a blood test (C-reactive protein) to detect problematic inflammation. To reduce inflammation, you can take turmeric and a cinnamon supplement or put plenty of cinnamon on your cereal or oatmeal. (By the way, turmeric is so important regarding brain health that everyone with any concerns whatsoever in that area should take it.) It is possible that taking turmeric and cinnamon will reduce your inflammation and, consequently, overcome your hypertension.

Supplements which help with BP control. Very important recent research (Vimaleswaran et al, 2014) showed that the higher your Vitamin-D status, the lower your risk of hypertension. Many of the primary supplements in the routine below (e.g., magnesium-citrate, fish oil, taurine, arginine) help with BP control. Other supplements which, according to WebMD, may help with BP control are alpha-lipoic acid, coenzyme Q10/ubiquinol for people over 45, DHA, potassium, and vitamin C. Calcium and garlic also can help with BP control. (As discussed later, taking a calcium supplement can actually increase CVD risks.)

Stroke prevention, especially my approaches for preventing a stroke. As you know, having a stroke can result in death or severe disability. As previously mentioned, I am not a physician or other health expert and cannot diagnose or treat illness. If you have heart disease (atherosclerosis), elevated BP, or even a "bad lipids profile," I think you should talk to your physician about stroke prevention.

My situation regarding vulnerability to stroke is probably quite unusual for a 74-year-old man with a "bad lipids profile." Performance of my VCR routine frequently since 1982 has resulted in my arteries being nearly entirely free from occlusion (plaque buildup). So, even when my heart races in the 175-185 range during tachycardia, I apparently don't need to worry about arterial plaque breaking off, resulting in a stroke or heart attack. During a long tachycardia occurrence, I developed a dangerous deep vein thrombosis (DVT), possibly because fast pulse can increase risk of blood clotting. During another one, I developed a pulmonary embolism (blood clot in a lung). So, I try very hard to prevent tachycardia and to stop it, if it occurs. I intend to take Eliquis and several supplement blood thinners (anti-coagulants) for the rest of my life.

Why I am **not** recommending supplements to deal with a "bad lipids profile" by lowering LDL, lowering triglycerides, etc. Since 1982, my goal has been preventing atherosclerosis, providing anti-coagulant effect, preventing oxidation of LDL, preventing inflammation, and improving the health and function of my heart and blood vessels, not improving my lipids "numbers." **Since my cardiovascular health has been excellent, and my blood pressure has been fine, the fact that I have continued to have a very "bad lipids profile" since 1982 hasn't worried me at all.**

Information from several sources about supplements that help with prevention of atherosclerosis and heart disease. Dr. Russell Blaylock, a neurosurgeon and expert on health benefits of nutrients, has been quoted on the Internet as saying that "curcumin, quercetin, ellagic acid, mixed tocopherols, mixed tocotrienols, vitamin C, magnesium, and mixed carotenoids all safely reduce the risk of strokes and heart attacks and are far more effective than statins" ("Statins: big dangers, little benefit" on the Newsmax health web site.).

Cardiologist Dr. Ray Sahelian in an Internet article, "Atherosclerosis natural treatments with vitamins, herbs, and supplements," recommends flavonoids, fish oil, pomegranate, resveratrol, green tea extract, and grape seed extract. Dr. Sahelian, in a different article, "Heart disease treatment with foods, herbs, vitamins, supplements," lists fish oil, psyllium fiber, vitamin C, B complex vitamins, curcumin, garlic, and magnesium as helpful against heart disease. In the same article, he lists vitamin E and coenzyme Q10 as specifically useful to reduce inflammation in heart disease.

On the WebMD website, the following were reported to be "possibly effective" against atherosclerosis: alpha-linolenic acid, black tea, garlic, niacin, vitamin B6, vitamin C. In a different article on the WebMD website, "6 supplements for heart health," the following are recommended: fiber (sterols and stanols), coenzyme Q10, fish oil, garlic, and green tea.

On the naturallysavvy.com website, there is an article, "5 key nutrients for cardiovascular health," that lists vitamin C, B vitamins (B6 and B12), vitamin D, magnesium, and l-arginine, with extensive citations to scientific studies. It is noted that the benefits of vitamin D probably depend on supplementation much higher than the 200–600 i.u. dosage.

An article titled "Lecithin benefits" on the herbwisdom.com website says that "[l]ecithin provides lubrication that prevents large fatty deposits from adhering." Researchers at the Washington University School of Medicine (2009) found that lecithin may help to keep the liver functioning properly, which in turn lowers the risk of developing heart disease and diabetes (August issue of *Cell*). My "guess" is that conventional and non-conventional medical practitioners have generally failed to discover and disseminate information about the heart health benefits of lecithin. Because lecithin provides acetyl-choline, phosphatidylcholine, and phosphatidylserine, it is extremely helpful regarding brain health and function.

To improve my information about this subject, I reviewed brief descriptions of 200 recent research studies relating to cardiovascular disease late in 2017. None of them concerned prevention of atherosclerosis.

I regret that this information doesn't produce a generally accepted list of supplements to use in preventing atherosclerosis and achieving other heart health benefits.

An approach for making your own selections of supplements to include in your VCR. **Of course, you can do the VCR as described below.** You may, however, want to select supplements yourself to economize or to get particular benefits. Here are the main effects which you want to achieve relating to heart health. Immediately below this is a poster that is also in chapter 4 of this book. Using the codes on the poster, you can select supplements that provide the following benefits.

Prevention of atherosclerosis (PA)
Prevention of blood clotting in your blood vessels (AC)
Prevention/control of inflammation (AI)
Prevention of oxidation of LDL (AO)
Support of blood vessel health and function (EF)
Support of heart health and function (H)
Prevention/control of hypertension (BP)

OVERVIEW OF BENEFITS OF NUTRITIONAL SUPPLEMENTS

The letters to the right of the supplements listed below indicate the conditions the supplement does or probably will help with. Here is the letter code: **AC**=anti-coagulant; **AI**=anti-inflammatory; **AO**=antioxidant; **AP**=athletic performance; **B**=brain and thinking; **BP**=blood pressure control; **BS**=help with blood sugar control; **C**=cancer; **CoAg**=coagulant; **EF**=promotes good endothelial (blood vessel) function and health; **H**=heart health; **I**=immune system; **J**=joint health; **MH**=mental health; **NO**=nitric-oxide production; **PA**=prevention of atherosclerosis; **Sl**=sleep; **Sx**=sexual enjoyment; **WC**=weight control;

Percentages in parentheses are percentage of "daily value" in the Equate Complete Multivitamin Men's 50+.

Alpha-lipoic acid **B, C, MH, BP** (Take before exercise to produce glutathione (**AO**).)
Arginine (l-arginine) **C, H, Sx, WC, EF, NO, PA, BP**
Chromium piccolinate **WC, H, BS** (50% of chromium)
Chondroitin **J, H, EF**
Cinnamon **H, AC, AI, BS**
Co-enzyme Q10 **B, C, H, PA**
(Ubiquinol is the better form of co-enzyme Q10 for persons over 45.)
Curcumin (turmeric) **B, C, J, AI, PA**
DHA **B, H, AC, C, MH, PA**
DHEA **B, Sx, H** (Take with melatonin for sex/testosterone benefit.)
Fish oil **AI, B, C, H, AC, J, MH, PA, BP** (Flaxseed oil has some of these same benefits.) (Fish oil may increase prostate cancer risk.)

Folate, folic acid (for women only) **H, EF, B** (75%. Some experts recommend
  none for men.)

Garlic **C, H, I, AC, PA, BP**

Gingko biloba **AC**

Green tea extract **B, C, WC, PA**

Iodine **C, WC, H** (100%)

L-carnitine **B, AP**

L-taurine **H, EF, PA**

L-theanine **MH,** normal pulse

L-tyrosine **B, MH, Sx, WC, H**

Lecithin **B, H, MH, Sx, PA**

Lycopene **H, EF, AO**

Magnesium **H, B, MH, BS, PA, BP** (**not** magnesium-oxide; magnesium-citrate
  is OK) (13%. Deficiency is common, harmful.)

Melatonin **B, C, MH, Sl, H**

Nattokinase **H, AC**

Niacin **C, H, EF, J, MH, Sx, PA** (niacinamide for diabetics; nicotinic acid
  for non-diabetics) (Especially for heart-health benefit, much more
  can be taken safely.)

Pomegranate extract **H, PA**

Probiotic **C, I**

Quercetin **C, H, PA** (stroke prevention)

Resveratrol, Grapeseed Extract **AI, C, H, AO, PA** contain flavonoids

Selenium **C, MH, Sx, H, AO** (143%. Additional supplementation probably
  not needed.)

Taurine **H, PA**

Vitamin B6 **B, C, BS, EF** (300%. For brain health benefit, much more is
  sometimes recommended.)

Vitamin B12 **B, EF** (prevents shrunken brain), **H, BS** (1667%. Deficiency is
  common and very harmful.)

Vitamin C **B, C, H, J, Sx, AO, PA, BP** (200%. There is controversy concerning optimum supplementation.)

Vitamin D3 **C, H, D, BS, PA** (150%. Deficiency is very common and harmful.
  Some physicians recommend very much more than "daily value.")

Vitamin E (tocopherol) **B, C, J, Sx, AC, AO** (Ordinary vitamin E. 200%)

Vitamin E (tocotrienols) **H, C, PA**
Vitamin K2 **CoAg**
This poster is primarily intended to make people aware of possibilities, not to provide the best possible, most complete information about how to deal with health problems.

A suggested supplement-and-exercise routine (VCR). You should do this VCR at least four or five times per week. You may want to take additional supplements described above. I think it is good to take supplements also on non-exercise days.

Even though this VCR as given below is for women, there are very few changes needed for it to be appropriate for men. Instead of taking 25 mg of DHEA, men can take 50 mg. It is especially important for women to take folate instead of folic acid. Unless a man is experiencing troubling "senior moments," it would probably be better for him not to take folic acid.

As indicated above, this VCR is primarily for people who have been told that they have a "bad lipids profile." For them, taking the indicated levels of niacin and lecithin is appropriate. (I have taken niacin and lecithin twice a day for 36 years and strongly believe that I have received substantial benefits.) If a person does not have elevated cardiovascular-disease risk factors, it will be appropriate to take the lower dosages of niacin and lecithin.

BASIC HEART- AND BRAIN-HEALTH ROUTINE (VCR) FOR WOMEN
(I encourage you to select additional supplements discussed above to include.)

Supplements to take> > > > > Wait 30 minutes> > > > Get 20 to 40 min. of
with large gl. water   moderate exercise.
magnesium-citrate (200–400 mg)   Another time in the day,
fish oil (1000 mg)   take w/ lrg. glass of water
taurine (500 mg)   vitamin D3 (2000 to 5000 iu or
l- arginine (500 mg)   as directed by an MD)
alpha-lipoic acid (600 mg)   vitamin B12 (1000 mcg) & B6
coenzyme Q10 (200 mg) or, if   (100 mg)
over 45, ubiquinol (100 mg)   DHEA (25 mg or as directed by
DHA (300 mg)   MD) (50 mg for men)

potassium (100 mg)
vitamin C (200 mg)
lecithin (1300 mg)
garlic (Dose according to type.)
coconut oil (3 capsules)
If "bad lipids profile,"
niacin (500 mg)
If not "bad lipids profile,"
niacin (200 mg)

folate (not folic acid) (Men may
take folic acid.)
garlic (Dose according to type.)
If "bad lipids profile,
niacin (500 mg)
lecithin (1300 mg)
No exercise after this.

You should take alpha-lipoic acid (maybe also with l-carnitine) before exercising because this causes your body to produce glutathione, which is an antioxidant with excellent benefits.

Just as the body loses the ability to obtain benefit from ordinary coenzyme Q10, the body loses the ability to have l-arginine achieve production of nitric oxide. So, if you are as old as 45, instead of taking l-arginine, you should take an arginine/circulline supplement.

You should take vitamin D3 with turmeric/curcumin before bedtime. This assists your brain in removing beta-amyloid plaques, which are found in the brains of persons with Alzheimer's disease. If you take D3 before bedtime, you can forego taking it "at another time in the day," as indicated above.

Maybe an hour after the exercise, you can take your BP to see if there has been any effect.

As you know, the supplements in this routine have a wide variety of heart and brain health benefits.

Two alternative ways to implement a VCR.

Selection of supplements at the end of chapter 4. Very close to the end of chapter 4, there is a list of 15 supplements which would be sufficient for a person between 25 and 45 years old who has a "bad lipids profile." The cost per day, including taking several twice per day, would be about $1.20. That is a much better list that I used for several decades.

Another way to implement a VCR, involving use of a major formula and additional supplements. Instead of performing the routine given above, you can take **OmegaQ Plus with resveratrol and turmeric,** which is a formula developed and marketed by prominent cardiologist, Dr. Stephen Sinatra. It includes B6, folate, B12, squid oil, DHA, EPA, turmeric, l-carnitine, coenzyme Q10, and resveratrol. Taking one before your VCR and one at bedtime will cost $50 per month. If I were to decide to take it, which I may decide to do, I would also take DHEA, l-arginine, garlic, lecithin, niacin, magnesium-citrate, and potassium before my VCR. I would take D3 at bedtime with the other capsule.

Exercise as part of your program. It is recommended that you perform the VCR above at least four times, maybe more, per week.

As mentioned earlier, strenuous exercise actually makes your blood platelets stickier, and moderate exercise makes your blood platelets less sticky (Wang et al, 1994). Also, strenuous exercise causes creation of "free radicals." If you decide to do strenuous exercise, it will be especially important for you to take supplements that have enough anti-coagulant and antioxidant effects before that exercise.

Of course, you can do exercise in addition to your VCR exercise. Getting at least 30 minutes of moderate exercise every day is a good goal.

Increasing your stamina by gradually increasing the intensity of your exercise. One way to do this is to buy adjustable wrist and ankle weights (You can buy Gold's Gym adjustable weights at Walmart.) and gradually increase the amount of weight you use while walking or jogging. Now, instead of carrying weights, I walk as briskly as I can, while "pumping" my arms vigorously in coordination with my leg movements. I use all of my weights doing EWOT, as described earlier.

Some experimentation by you. Since people vary in many important ways, it may help you to experiment to see which supplements and how much of what types of exercise seem to work best for you.

A way to quickly get in shape and stay in shape. If you walk golf either pushing or pulling a small cart, you can try jogging between shots. Doing this for nine holes provided extremely good exercise for me. Because of the hazards of strenuous exercise, you can jog fast enough to nearly be exercising strenuously.

Diet to help with heart and brain health. Chapter 3 is about "using diet to protect and improve your heart and brain health." Of course, it would be a mistake for you to follow the VCR in this chapter and sabotage that work with bad eating.

REFERENCES

Blaylock, Russell (2012). Statins: big dangers, little benefit. Newsmaxhealth.com website. February 21, 2012.

Blumenthal, J. A. et al (1999). Effects of exercise training on older patients with major depression. *Archives of Internal Medicine*, Vol. 159, No. 19, pp. 2349–2356.

Cederberg, H. et al (2015). Increased risk of diabetes with statin treatment is associated with impaired insulin sensitivity and insulin secretion: a 6-year follow-up study of the METSIM cohort. *Diabetologia*, the journal of the European Association for Study of Diabetes.

Centers for Disease Control and Prevention (2007).

Chobanian, Aram V. (2001). Control of hypertension—an important national priority. *New England Journal of Medicine*, Vol. 345, pp. 534–535.

Culver, A. L. et al (2012). Statin use and risk of diabetes mellitus in post-menopausal women in the Women's Health Initiative. *Archives of Internal Medicine*, Vol. 172, No. 2, pp. 144–52.

Cutler, Michael (2013). *Hushed up natural heart cures and deadly deceptions of popular heart treatments*. Cullman, AL: Easy Health Options.

Food and Drug Administration (2014). FDA warns consumers of the dangers of aspirin therapy. NBC News.

Gersh, B.J. et al (2010). The epidemic of cardiovascular disease in the developing world: global implications. *European Heart Journal*, Vol. 31, pp. 642–648.

Gorman, M. (2009). Statin drugs may be dampening your sex life: new study: the greater the cholesterol drop from these drugs, the greater the drop in sexual pleasure. RodaleWell.com website. March 9, 2009.

Lee, Joyce (2008). Why young adults hold the key to assessing the obesity epidemic of children. *Archives of Pediatric and Adolescent Medicine*, Vol. 162, No. 7, pp. 682–7.

Meilahn, Elaine N. (1995). Low serum cholesterol: hazardous to health? *Circulation*, Vol. 92, pp. 2365–2366.

Memory, John M. (1981). *Work-related stress of state criminal trial court judges.* Unpublished doctoral dissertation, Florida State University, Tallahassee.

Memory, John & Evatt, Lynn (2012). *Vascular cleansing routines: safe and effective heart health programs for women (and men).* Winston-Salem, NC: Wakexpress (digital publishing at Wake Forest University).

Ratey, John J. with Hagerman, Eric (2008). *Spark: the revolutionary new science of exercise and the brain.* NY, NY: Little, Brown and Company.

Reitz, C. et al (2007). Hypertension and the risk of mild cognitive impairment. *Arch Neurol.,* Vol 64, No. 12, pp. 1734–40.

Roberts, Barbara (2012). *The truth about statins: risks and alternatives to cholesterol-lowering drugs.* NY, NY: Pocket Books.

Salmon, Peter (2001). Effects of physical exercise on anxiety, depression, and sensitivity to stress: a unifying theory. *Clinical Psychology Review*, Vol. 21, Issue 1, pp. 33–61.

Savole, I. & Kazanjian, A. (2002). Utilization of lipid-lowering drugs in men and women: a reflection of the research evidence. *Journal of Clinical Epidemiology*, Vol. 55, Issue 1, pp. 95–101.

Scarmeas, Nikolaos et al (2009). Physical activity, diet, and risk of Alzheimer's disease. *Journal of the American Medical Association*, Vol. 302, No. 6, pp. 627–637.

Taka-aki Okabe, B.M. et al (2006). Effects of exercise on the development of atherosclerosis in apolipoprotein E-deficient mice. *Experimental Clinical Cardiology*, Vol. 11, No. 4, pp. 276–279.

Thompson, Paul D. et al (2003). American Heart Association scientific statement: exercise and physical activity in the prevention and treatment of atherosclerotic cardiovascular disease. *Arteriosclerosis, Thrombosis, and Vascular Biology*, Vol. 23, pp. e42–49.

Walsh, J.M. & Pignone, M. (2004). Drug treatment of hyperlipidemia in women. *Journal of the American Medical Association*, Vol. 291, p. 2243.

Wang, J.S. et al (1994). Different effects of strenuous exercise and moderate exercise on platelet function in men. *Circulation*, Vol. 90, pp. 2877–2885.

— CHAPTER 7 —
Non-Drug Prevention and Control of Hypertension (elevated blood pressure)

A suggestion for people who are skeptical about this chapter. If you have low-level hypertension and are skeptical about the content of this chapter (and book), here's a suggestion: Go on and make some of the LBP (low blood pressure) soup according to the recipe at the end of this chapter. If, as I predict, you experience significant reduction of BP, I encourage you to read the rest of this chapter. Later, you can experiment with a supplement-and-exercise routine (VCR) to control and even reduce your underlying BP.

Cautionary statement. **The author is not a physician or health expert.** Very high blood pressure is extremely dangerous and can cause a heart attack or blood clotting that can result in a stroke, a deep-vein thrombosis (DVT), or a pulmonary embolism. As noted below, even moderately high BP during middle age can cause serious brain-health problems later in life. I believe persons with blood pressure higher than 120/80 should implement the routine in this chapter only with medical supervision. Persons with very high blood pressure should immediately consult with a physician.

A suggestion for people with problems and concerns relating to their blood pressure. Buy one or more wrist BP monitors. Mainly because of my need to monitor my pulse to prevent tachycardia, I keep one of them in my living room and one in my bedroom.

<u>Important recent changes of criteria for elevated blood pressure</u>. In November 2017 the American Heart Association and the American College of Cardiology converted the old **"pre-hypertension"** to constitute hypertension. Now, if your top (systolic) number is usually as high as 130 and/or your bottom (diastolic) number is usually as high as 80, you have hypertension according to the new guidelines. **Experts are emphasizing that people who are in the 139–140 and/or 80–90 range probably should not need to take blood pressure control medication. I believe this chapter can provide substantial help for many people in that situation.**

<u>Elaboration</u>. This chapter is not just about control of high blood pressure to a safe level: It is about reversal of the physiological conditions, including inflammation, weight gain, and atherosclerosis, that tend to cause hypertension.

<u>Importance of this subject</u>. Uncontrolled hypertension is likely to be associated with a variety of serious medical problems, including atherosclerosis, metabolic syndrome (syndrome X), type 2 diabetes, Alzheimer's or other dementia, heart attack, and heart failure. I strongly believe that it is a serious mistake for a person of any age to allow himself or herself to have hypertension for a significant period of time.

As discussed in several chapters, one of the worst and most preventable life sequences relating to health is, starting in your 20s or 30s and caused partly by bad diet and sedentary life style, gaining weight and an increase in blood pressure. This can produce the metabolic syndrome (syndrome X), which can involve insulin resistance. Unchecked, this can lead to development of type 2 diabetes. Unchecked, this can lead to Alzheimer's disease or other dementia. Though this sequence is easily prevented without medication, the result is horrific for the individual. For me, the activities needed to prevent that sequence have improved my health and life experiences astonishingly well.

There are a variety of non-medical, non-drug ways to control and possibly eliminate hypertension. These approaches include improvement of diet and, I believe, regular performance of a supplement-and-exercise routine (VCR) with moderate, not strenuous, exercise.

Author's relevant experience. I was very fortunate that my mother was an excellent "southern cook," who produced very healthful meals. During the summer, our lunches and dinners on the back porch often included three-to-five fresh vegetables. They were perfectly prepared and delicious. We never had a dessert. Maybe because of this excellent diet and my regular exercise as a teenager, my blood pressure during college tended to be low.

By the early 1980s, my blood pressure was significantly higher, often around 125/75. As you've read earlier, I discovered in 1982 that I have very serious heart disease risk factors. **I realized that, if I allowed my blood pressure to continue to rise, I would be in serious health trouble.** I hope you have read about the supplement-and-exercise routine (vascular cleansing routine) I developed in 1982. Within 1½ years after I started doing my routine regularly, my blood pressure had gone down, often to about 90/60.

Remarkable success in dealing with severe hypertension without medication. In chapter one you read about my friend Sarah. Years ago, she had type 2 diabetes and hypertension. She had a heart attack and was told that she died and had to be resuscitated. After the heart attack, she was on several drugs that were not controlling her hypertension. So, she obtained excellent science-based information about controlling her various medical problems. Gradually, she was able to stop taking all of the medications. She was able to control her blood pressure by non-medical, non-drug means and actually was told that she was no longer a type 2 diabetic. A person should try to do this only with medical supervision.

Undesirability of taking a statin BP medication. Many BP medications are statin drugs and tend to have many of the adverse side effects of a statin drug. This chapter contains extensive and detailed information about ways to control BP without medication. I strongly believe that, in 1982, I was definitely on a trajectory toward a lifetime of dangerously elevated BP. Just as I have had to be well informed, cautious, determined, and energetic for the last 36 years, persons who want to avoid taking a statin BP drug will need to be.

Important facts about blood pressure. High BP is called the "silent killer" because it usually has no signs or symptoms. Your BP is "normal" if it is less than 120/80 mmHG.

I believe that, if your goals are achieving excellent cardiovascular health and retaining excellent cognitive functioning as a "senior citizen," it makes sense to make average BP which is significantly lower than 120/80 a goal for yourself.

Even if your BP is as low as 120/80, I encourage you to go to the website of Optimal Naturals and select "blood pressure." You will find an excellent, professionally prepared article about high blood pressure, which provides information detail which is not included in this chapter. That company sells a BP-control product, Blood Pressure Essentials, which will cost something less than $.60 per day. Before buying that product, I encourage you to see if the supplements, exercise, and foods recommended in this chapter will do the job for you. An advantage of these supplements is that they should advance many aspects of your heart and brain health and function.

Health risks of elevated blood pressure. Research has shown that having high blood pressure (BP) can have very adverse health consequences (Chobanian, 2001). This can include damage to the lining of blood vessels (the endothelium), which can lead to a buildup of plaque in blood vessels. Of course, very high blood pressure can trigger plaque rupture, which can lead to a heart attack. Even moderately high BP during middle age can have adverse effects on brain health and cognitive function (Reitz et al, 2007). **Because of these risks, it is very important to prevent even moderately elevated BP.**

I have found no scientific evidence that controlling BP causes regression of underlying atherosclerosis. Because of this, I think it is a mistake for a person to have **just** controlling blood pressure as her or his heart health goal. My guess is that people who continue to implement the VCR provided below will achieve some regression/reversal of atherosclerosis (hardening of the arteries).

The connections of "stress" and blood pressure. The physiological stress reaction (fight or flight reaction) tends to cause a "spike" in blood pressure and elevation of BP while that reaction continues. Experts disagree on whether "stress" can contribute to causation of persistent hypertension. Fortunately, dealing with "stress" involves doing many of the same things you can do to deal with hypertension.

A "quick fix" to reduce inflammation. For some people, the following will be an easy fix for elevated BP. Some amount of BP elevation results from inflammation in the blood vessels. You may have had a blood test (C-reactive protein) to detect problematic inflammation. To reduce inflammation, you can take turmeric and a cinnamon supplement or put plenty of cinnamon on your cereal or oatmeal. (By the way, turmeric is so important regarding brain health that everyone with any concerns whatsoever in that area should take turmeric.)

Supplements which help with BP control. Very important recent research (Vimaleswaran et al, 2014) showed that the higher your Vitamin-D status, the lower your risk of hypertension. Several supplements, including, magnesium-citrate, fish oil, taurine, and arginine, help with BP control. Other supplements which, according to WebMD, may help with BP control are alpha-lipoic acid, coenzyme Q10/ubiquinol for people over 45, DHA, potassium, and vitamin C. Garlic can help with BP control.

Just as the body loses the ability to receive benefit from the consumption of ordinary coenzyme Q10, the body loses the ability to have l-arginine achieve production of nitric oxide in the blood vessels. So, if you are as old as 45, instead of taking l-arginine, you should take a combination of l-arginine and circulline.

Even though the routine as given below is for women, there are very few changes needed for it to be appropriate for men. Instead of taking 25 mg of DHEA, men can take 50 mg. It is especially important for women to take folate instead of folic acid. Unless a man is experiencing troubling "senior moments," it would be better for him not to take folic acid.

A suggested routine. Unless you have moderate-to-serious hypertension, implementing the VCR below and eating indicated foods should tend to achieve BP control without medication. You should do this VCR at least four or five times per week. I believe that it will be worthwhile for you to take the supplements also on no-exercise days.

BP-Control Routine (VCR) for Women

Supplements to take> > > > > Wait 30 minutes> > > > > Get 20 to 40 min. of
with large gl. water   moderate exercise.

magnesium-citrate (200–400 mg)	Another time in day,
fish oil (1000 mg)	take w/ lrg. glass of water
taurine (500 mg)	vitamin D3 (2000 to 5000 is or
arginine (500 mg)	as directed by MD)
alpha-lipoic acid (600 mg)	vitamin B12 (1000 mcg), B6 (100 mg)
coenzyme Q10 (200 mg) or, if	DHEA (25 mg or as
over 45, ubiquinol (100 mg)	directed by MD)
DHA (100 mg)	folate (not folic acid)
potassium (100 mg)	garlic (Dose according to type.)
vitamin C (500 mg)	If "bad lipids profile,
lecithin (1300 mg)	niacin (500 mg)
garlic (Dose according to type.)	lecithin (1300 mg)
coconut oil (3 capsules)	No exercise after this.
If "bad lipids profile,"	
niacin (500 mg)	
If not "bad lipids profile,"	
niacin (200 mg)	

It would be prudent to wear a wrist BP monitor during VCR exercise. You can check your BP during exercise to be able to stop exercise if troubling increase in BP occurs. Maybe an hour after the VCR exercise, you can take your BP to see if there has been any effect.

Happily, the supplements in this routine have a wide variety of heart and brain health benefits in addition to BP control.

Using a major formula and additional supplements. As an alternative to taking the supplements listed above, you can take **OmegaQ Plus with resveratrol and turmeric,** which is a formula developed and marketed by prominent cardiologist Dr. Stephen Sinatra. It includes B6, folate, B12, squid oil, DHA, EPA, turmeric, l-carnitine, coenzyme Q10, and resveratrol. Taking one as part of your VCR and one at bedtime will cost $50 per month. If I were to decide to take it, I would also take DHEA, l-arginine, garlic, lecithin, niacin, magnesium-citrate, taurine, and potassium before my exercise. At bedtime, I would take D3 with the other capsule.

Exercise as part of your program. As mentioned in the previous chapter, strenuous exercise actually makes your blood platelets stickier, and moderate exercise makes your blood platelets less sticky (Wang et al, 1994). While avoiding strenuous exercise, you can do exercise in addition to the VCR exercise. Getting at least 30 minutes of moderate exercise every day is a good goal. I have walked about 22,000 miles while playing golf and have no doubt that doing so has been very helpful regarding my heart and brain health.

Increasing your stamina by gradually increasing the intensity of your exercise. One way to do this is to buy adjustable wrist and ankle weights (You can buy Gold's Gym adjustable weights at Walmart.) and gradually increase the amount of weight you use while walking or jogging. Now, instead of carrying weights, I walk as briskly as I can while "pumping" my arms vigorously in coordination with my leg movements. I now use all of my weights while doing EWOT.

Some experimentation by you. Since people vary in many important ways, it may help you to experiment to see which supplements and how much of what types of exercise seem to work best for you. Since you can use a wrist BP monitor, you can easily check for results of your VCR even away from home.

Patented BP-control supplement formulas. There are many BP-control patented supplement formulas available for purchase on the Internet. Though I think the things included in this chapter will dramatically help most people with high BP, you may wish to buy one of those formulas. Earlier, I mentioned Blood Pressure Essentials from Optimal Naturals. There are, however, a good number of other products.

Foods and a beverage which help with BP control. Dr. Oz recommends regularly eating collard greens, consuming cocoa powder, consuming whey protein, and taking l-taurine for BP control. Research has suggested that purple potatoes, cooked and eaten plain (not fried), can lower BP. Dr. Julian Whitaker, a California cardiologist (with a website) who emphasizes non-medical approaches against CVD, recommends drinking V8 juice and taking potassium for BP control.

I have developed a low blood pressure soup (**LBP** soup) that has dramatically reduced my BP and the BP of several friends. The recipe is at the end of this chapter.

Everyone reading this knows it is important to limit salt intake. It is important, however, to get enough iodine when you consume very little iodized salt.

Can BP be too low? My blood pressure occasionally has been as low as 78/48, and my only negative symptom has been some dizziness when I stood up. Still, I think that, if a person is accustomed to having high BP, the person can have uncomfortable symptoms from suddenly having low BP. If you lower your BP significantly with these natural measures and really don't feel well, you should check with your physician. (I expect that most readers would love to have the problem of BP that is "too low.")

Blood pressure medication. MDs will prescribe one or more drugs to control hypertension. Dr. Chandra Gulhati states (Internet article, "Do anti-anxiety drugs help lower blood pressure?") that an anti-anxiety drug will help with BP control if the cause of the elevated BP is stress.

Many BP medications are statins. Therefore, a statin BP drug can have the wide variety of adverse side effects of a statin drug. One is serious depletion of coenzyme Q10 in the body. Many experts believe this is resulting in an epidemic of congestive heart failure deaths in the U.S. If you are currently taking a BP medication, you may decide, with approval of your physician, to go through several stages to see whether some combination of things mentioned in this chapter will achieve BP control for you without taking a BP medication. (Over the years I have many times refused—always with scientific basis—to do something directed by a physician and have never had an adverse outcome. My impression is that many physicians are reluctant to go along with a patient gradually going off of a statin BP med or some other BP med.)

<u>Ways to achieve BP reduction.</u>

Achieving some BP reduction through reduction of blood vessel occlusion (reversal of atherosclerosis). My experience was that, within one or two years of starting to do the earliest version of my heart and brain health routine (VCR) in 1982, my BP lowered from about 125/75 to usually being about 90/60. This suggests, I think, that some atherosclerosis regression had occurred. Remember: **I was not taking taurine, tocotrienols, pomegranate, arginine, or many of the other BP supplements and was not eating collard greens, purple potatoes, or the LBP soup or drinking V8 juice.** Here are some supplements and foods which have been shown to help with natural reversal of atherosclerosis (hardening of the arteries): tocotrienols (a form of vitamin E), pomegranate extract, nattokinase (derived from soy), and walnuts. Fish oil may help. A patented formula, GliSODin, may help. Chapter 9 is specifically about attempting to reverse atherosclerosis by alternative (non-drug) means.

Reducing BP through weight loss. Since there are so many well publicized weight-loss programs, I will not advocate an elaborate program here. I strongly discourage the Atkins diet, mainly because losing 40 pounds on that diet apparently caused me to suffer significant loss of muscle tissue, causing me to lose 30 yards on my golf iron and "wood" shots.

Unfortunately, nearly everyone who loses a lot of weight gains it back. I strongly believe that, realistically, succeeding in preventing undesirable weight gain is much more important than losing weight. My current weight "red line" is 205 pounds. If I reach that weight or higher, I then work on weight loss as long as necessary. It helps me to make just about my only food for the day a chocolate whey protein shake including two tablespoons of coconut oil and a teaspoon of green tea powder. I also find walking 9 holes of golf about every other day helpful for maintaining my weight.

<u>The danger of complacency.</u> I am **absolutely serious** in saying that it is possible that taking the VCR supplements, exercising, and eating collard greens, purple potatoes, and the **LBP soup** regularly will lower your BP enough for you to become **complacent** about protecting and building your heart and brain health and function. **I strongly believe that it is important to**

do as many sensible and healthful things as you can to protect and build your underlying cardiovascular health and brain health and function.

My low blood pressure (LBP) soup. In about 2007, I learned that lycopene (a carotinoid anti-oxidant) found abundantly in canned tomatoes can be made **much more** available for health purposes by cooking the tomatoes with oil. So, I developed a soup which includes broccoli and canned tomatoes pureed together and cooked with coconut oil. I soon noticed that eating that soup lowered my BP substantially.

Great results from eating LBP soup. I have already told about my friend Sarah's efforts to improve her cardiovascular health. During 2010, when she was not taking BP medication or a patented BP-control supplement, she took her BP. It was 169/97, which was dangerously high. I cooked a large pot of my soup and gave it to her. She ate two bowls of the soup per day for four days. She waited for two hours after eating a bowl of soup and then took her BP. She took her BP at least three times per day, including once each morning on the day after eating soup. For Saturday through the following Tuesday, her average BP reading was 117/70. After eating the soup regularly for several weeks, she often got even lower BP readings.

My guess is that the soup is remarkably healthful for blood vessels (endothelial health and function). Because lycopene, found abundantly in tomatoes, helps with the dilation and contraction functions (endothelial function) of blood vessels (Agarwal & Rao, 2000), it certainly can be included in a supplement-and-exercise routine. Chromium, which is also found abundantly in tomatoes, is also helpful regarding cardiovascular health (Jimenez et al, 2001).

Though readers are welcome to make the soup and send the recipe to friends and relatives, I hold a provisional patent (patent pending) on the recipe. Therefore, no one is welcome to attempt to obtain financial benefit from making or writing about the soup.

RECIPE OF LOW BLOOD PRESSURE SOUP (LBP Soup)

Blood pressure benefit. The impression of the inventor of this soup, John M. Memory, is that eating the soup has consistently lowered blood pressure for eaters. A person can experiment concerning how much soup to eat and when to eat it. If consistent BP control is needed, eating several small bowls during the day might be best.

Ingredients. The amount of each ingredient can be somewhat less or more than the amount indicated below. Coconut oil is added immediately before eating when the soup is very hot.

Two 30 oz. cans of cooked tomatoes; if not available, buy tomato pasta sauce, which is always available.

A can or jar of coconut oil. You may not know that coconut oil enhances the flavor of many foods. Eating this soup can help you to consume enough high-quality oil.

One 30-oz. can of cooked beans. Pork and beans enhance the flavor of this soup.

One large head of fresh broccoli

1 medium-size onion

1 green pepper

2 cloves of garlic

Preparation for cooking. Dice the onion. Remove hull from garlic. Cut the broccoli into at least four pieces. Cut the green pepper into several pieces.

Puree all vegetables into a can of tomatoes in a blender. Put this into a large cooking pot appropriate for cooking in a microwave. Puree the other can of tomatoes and add it to the pot.

Cooking. Cook on high for 10 minutes in a microwave oven. Remove pot and stir well. Cook on high for 10 more minutes.

When cooking is completed, remove pot and add beans. Add salt, garlic powder, and spices to taste. If needed, you can heat the soup including beans for two-to-five more minutes.

Adding coconut oil. If the entire pot has been heated to be served, add one tablespoon of coconut oil for every bowl of soup. If a bowl is heated separately, add an ample tablespoon of coconut oil after heating and stir until the coconut oil has melted.

Converting LBP soup recipe to turkey chili (with BP-control benefits). After pureeing ingredients and before cooking, add a large can of tomato paste and the desired quantity of ground turkey, ground without skin. Of course, you can add vegetables and spices to taste.

REFERENCES

Chobanian, Aram V. (2001). Control of hypertension–an important national priority. *New England Journal of Medicine*, Vol. 345, pp. 534-535.

Want, J.S. et al (1994). Different effects of strenuous exercise and moderate exercise on platelet function in men. *Circulation*, Vol. 90, pp. 2877-2885.

—— CHAPTER 8 ——
Non-Drug Prevention and Reversal
of Metabolic Syndrome

Precautionary statement. Persons with the metabolic syndrome can have dangerously elevated blood pressure or dangerous atherosclerosis. Such persons should consult with a qualified physician prior to taking action recommended in this chapter.

Elaboration. Many adults, including many young adults, have the metabolic syndrome (also known as syndrome X), which involves being overweight, having excess belly fat, high waist circumference, high blood pressure, high blood sugar, "unhealthy" cholesterol levels, and, often, insulin resistance. This is not a disease, but rather is a syndrome of several adverse health conditions. Unfortunately, many children are diagnosed as having the metabolic syndrome.

The metabolic syndrome concerns at least six different aspects of metabolism. Dr. Dale Bredesen distinguished 25 different aspects of metabolism and human body function in his successful Alzheimer's-reversal research, which is covered in chapter 12. The point is that human body functioning relating to heart and brain health is actually much more complex than suggested even by the metabolic syndrome.

Author's relevant experience. Since the late 1990s, I have satisfied several of the criteria for having the metabolic syndrome. Fortunately, I have not had elevated blood pressure or blood sugar. About two years ago, I had allowed my weight to get to 222 pounds, which was far too high. I started having what I thought were diabetic foot pains. To avoid full-blown type 2 diabetes, I lost 15–18 pounds, and the pains ended. That was an example of what a person may be able to do against metabolic syndrome and type 2 diabetes. Fortunately, I have kept that weight off by monitoring my weight very consistently.

Importance of this subject. If the metabolic syndrome is allowed to continue, it is likely that the person's health will deteriorate, with high risk of development of atherosclerosis, type 2 diabetes, and Alzheimer's or other dementia. It is likely that, eventually, premature death will occur. This sequence is the subject of the "heading to heart disease hell" motivation poster in chapter 1.

Percentage of African Americans who are obese. Elsewhere in this book, I provide information about research that indicated that about 48% of African Americans are obese. I suspect that virtually all of these people meet the criteria for the metabolic syndrome. Tragically, a high percentage of obese persons will move on to having type 2 diabetes and then to having Alzheimer's or other dementia.

Contribution of consumption of "soft drinks" to the risk of developing the metabolic syndrome. The lead author of a research study (2007) by Boston University School of Medicine researchers has stated, "Even one soda per day increases your risk of developing metabolic syndrome by 50 percent." This is reported on the WebMD website.

An all-too-common example of a person falling victim to this adverse health sequence. In other chapters, I have mentioned a young man I knew well during the 1960s. He was remarkably talented and enjoyed relationships with women. He took up golf during college. During his 30s, he won an amateur golf tournament, which was an astonishing athletic achievement. After college, he earned a doctorate and licensing in a health specialty. The "world was his oyster!" Unfortunately, he drank alcoholic beverages heavily, became an alcoholic, became severely overweight, possibly developed the metabolic syndrome, became a type 2 diabetic, lost the ability to practice in his specialty, and had his house foreclosed on. At the age of 70, he had a fall, which caused fatal injuries. I assume that it would have been possible for him to prevent all of these adverse health developments.

Relevance for young adults. Unfortunately, partly because of the catastrophic increase of childhood obesity, millions of children in the U.S. have the metabolic syndrome. So, there is no doubt whatsoever that this subject has great relevance for millions of young adults (Lee, 2008).

Information on the Internet about reversal of the metabolic syndrome. You can easily find information about "reversal of metabolic syndrome" on the Internet.

What should you do if you have or nearly have the metabolic syndrome? Here are several possibilities.

(1) Select and implement recommendations found on a credible website specifically about reversal of metabolic syndrome.

(2) Go to and read chapter 7 of this book about control of BP. Any actions by you should be consistent with the precautionary statement at the first of that chapter.

(a) Then, you can adapt the supplement-and-exercise routine (VCR) for hypertension prevention and control in that chapter. On the WebMD website, there is a list of nutritional supplements that may help with the reversal of the metabolic syndrome. They include several supplements with a variety of heart and brain health benefits. They are chromium (often taken as chromium-piccolinate), DHEA (more for men than for women), green tea, melatonin (taken at bedtime), pomegranate (apparently helps with the reversal of atherosclerosis), and vitamin D3 (which is crucial for heart and brain health). Implementing the VCR in chapter 6 would involve taking several supplements (including all or nearly all just listed), waiting 30 minutes, and then getting at least 20-to-30 minutes of at least moderately strenuous exercise. (Extra benefit: Doing this will probably improve your sex life.)

(b) Improve your diet to allow you to lose enough weight to reduce your waist measurement. It is especially important to lose belly fat. There is an Internet article that claims to help with this: "Synergistic diet and exercise for ridiculously fast fat loss," on the joshsgarage website.

(c) If you have or nearly have high blood sugar, it would be helpful to implement low glycemic-index eating. There are many excellent websites about this.

(d) A low glycemic-index diet should help in reduction of high triglycerides. It will also help in avoiding development of type 2 diabetes.

REFERENCES

Lee, Joyce (2008). Why young adults hold the key to assessing the obesity epidemic of children. *Archives of Pediatric and Adolescent Medicine*, Vol. 162, No. 7, pp. 682–7.

— CHAPTER 9 —
Reversal of Atherosclerosis by Non-Medical, Non-Drug Means

Cautionary statement for persons with serious cardiovascular health problems. I will repeat that I am not a physician nor an expert in any other health specialty. I am not qualified to diagnose or treat illness. **If you have had a heart attack, have been diagnosed with serious atherosclerosis (hardening of the arteries), or have major heart attack or sudden cardiac death (SCD) risk factors, you should consider the information in this chapter only with the assistance of a qualified MD, DO, or ND. You should implement the supplements-and- exercise routine (VCR) described in this chapter only under the supervision of a qualified physician.**

While I want to strongly discourage independent use of the information in this chapter by persons with the conditions listed above, I think it is important for people to know that atherosclerosis can be reversed. There have been many scientific studies which have shown that certain dietary and lifestyle approaches (e.g., those of Dr. Ornish, Dr. Pritikin, Dr. Esselstyn, and Dr. Fuhrman) can tend to reverse atherosclerosis.

Results of recent research about whether heart stents relieve chest pain. On the CBS Evening News on November 2, 2017, there was a segment that concerned recently released research results that indicate that there was no difference in the chest pains experienced by patients who have had a stent installed and control subjects who had not.

Author's relevant experience. Several times in recent years, I have felt what I thought were angina pains in the vicinity of my heart. Each time, I have taken several of the supplements listed below, waited 30 minutes, and then exercised. Each time, after doing this for several days, the pain has stopped. Of course, I do not know whether I was actually experiencing angina. I, obviously, am not suggesting that this would relieve the pain of patients who have had a stent installed. Also, I am not suggesting that anyone should do this without supervision of a physician.

Internet articles on the subject of this chapter.

Detailed heart disease reversal program by a physician. Dr. Jeffrey Dach, MD, has on his website an article, "Reversing heart disease without drugs."

Use of a cream to achieve chelation. You can find on the Internet information about Chelactiv, which is a cream that is claimed to cause chelation that will, among other things, remove arterial plaque, especially calcium plaque. Of course, a person should use that product only with medical supervision.

Information on a highly respected website. My impression is that Life Extension Magazine on the Internet provides excellent materials developed by competent and qualified professionals. On their website you can find an article on the subject of this chapter, "Natural methods for reversing atherosclerosis," published October 2008, by Joanne Nicholas. She provides extensive citations to scientific research. I believe my VCR is superior because it specifically involves taking nutritional supplements, waiting 30 minutes, and then getting 20 to 30 minutes or more of at least moderate exercise. I believe health experts of all sorts have failed to detect the important synergy achievable when supplements are taken not long before exercise.

Stay away from the Pauling Therapy Essentials Formula, which doesn't include any of the major atherosclerosis reversal supplements.

Importance of this subject. Several federal government reports estimate that about 25% of Americans have some type of cardiovascular disease.

Undoubtedly, a substantial percentage have atherosclerosis (hardening of the arteries), which involves occlusion of arteries with plaque.

Relevance for young adults. During the Korean War, autopsies of soldiers who died in combat indicated that many of them, in spite of being in their late teens or early 20s, had already started developing "hardening of the arteries." Unfortunately, the current bad diet and sedentary lifestyles of many young adults are leading to high frequency of high blood pressure and measurable atherosclerosis (Lee, 2008).

Cardiovascular disease risk factors. The conventional risk factors of cardiovascular disease include obesity, smoking, diabetes, elevated BP, and close relatives who have had a heart attack relatively early in life. Here is an extremely important risk factor to add. **If you have a coronary-artery calcium scan which shows you have a substantial amount of coronary-artery calcification, your heart attack risk is high** (Divakaran, 2015). Fortunately, if that scan indicates that you do not have coronary-artery calcification, the findings of the Silverman research indicate that your heart attack risk actually is low, even if you appear to be at high risk according to your conventional risk factor score.

Difference in time-of-life when men and women are most at risk regarding cardiovascular disease. Men are substantially more at risk regarding major CVD (cardiovascular disease) events, such as heart attacks, than women before the average age of female menopause. After that time, women are substantially more at risk regarding major CVD events than men.

This suggests that "crunch time" for improvement of cardiovascular health for men is substantially before the average age of female menopause. I started substantially improving my cardiovascular health when I was 38. It follows that the crunch time for women should be significantly before the age of menopause.

Consideration of the primary cause(s) of your atherosclerosis. Different people can have different combinations of causes of atherosclerosis. These causes can include stress (the physiological stress reaction resulting from stressors), calcification in arterial plaque, abnormally high

LDL, oxidation of LDL as a result of the operation of free radicals, smoking, physical inactivity, endothelial (blood vessel) dysfunction, inflammation, the metabolic syndrome (also known as syndrome X), exposure to toxins, diabetes or pre-diabetes, uncontrolled hypertension (high BP), and others.

Hopefully, your medical advisor will have excellent information and skill which will help her or him use the information in this chapter.

Why ordinary medical approaches won't achieve optimum results. My impression is that most MDs will use a statin drug and aspirin in secondary prevention, which is prevention with persons who have already had a heart attack or have severe diagnosed atherosclerosis. Research has shown that, in this type of situation, a statin drug can prevent some heart attacks. While aspirin therapy can help in the prevention of a second heart attack, taking aspirin can have substantial health risks (FDA, 2014). (As a result, aspirin is not included in the routines in this book.) My impression is that heart attack prevention by a physician does not have a goal of the reversal of the patient's atherosclerosis. For example, research has shown that Crestor, a statin drug, can at best slow the progress of development of atherosclerosis (Crouse et al, 2007).

Information about nutritional deficiencies of the heart. Scholarly articles and treatises emphasize that **the heart is extremely sensitive to nutritional deficiency**. So, it will be important to nourish your heart as part of an atherosclerosis-reversal program.

Researchers have found that chromium deficiency was associated with the occurrence of first heart attacks among male research subjects (Jimenez et al, 2001). There is research evidence that supplementation with chromium can increase HDL (Mertz, 1993), which is desirable. It is prudent to regularly consume a **whole food source of chromium, silica, magnesium, and selenium,** such as **whole grain foods.**

Research has shown that persons who have a heart attack, in addition to tending to be **deficient in magnesium** (Baker, 1991–1992), tend to be deficient in the amino acid **taurine**. Supplementation with taurine helps with recovery of heart health after a heart attack (Sole & Jeejeebhoy, 2002) and in recovery from congestive heart failure (Azuma, 1983). There is no doubt that supplementation with **fish oil** reduces heart attack risk (Leon et al, 2008). Persons under 45 should take **co-enzyme Q10**, and persons 45 and over should take **ubiquinol** (a more usable form of co-enzyme Q10 for older persons) (Langsjoen & Jangsjoen, 1999). Research has shown that **silica**, which is available in many vegetables and grains, is important for blood vessel health (Seaborn et al, 1993).

Ideas from Dr. Russell Blaylock about the prevention of heart attack and stroke. Dr. Russell Blaylock, a neurosurgeon and expert on health benefits of nutrients, has been quoted on the Internet as saying that "curcumin, quercetin, ellagic acid, mixed tocopherols, mixed tocotrienols, vitamin C, magnesium, and mixed carotenoids all safely reduce the risk of strokes and heart attacks and are far more effective than statins" ("Statins: big dangers, little benefit" on Newsmax health web site.)

A precaution before exercise. Though I am not worried about having a heart attack, I take an l-arginine/citrulline supplement (1.25 g) before exercise and at bedtime. It produces nitric oxide, which helps to prevent blood clotting in blood vessels.

Reversal of atherosclerosis with diet and lifestyle approaches. There have been many scientific studies which have shown that certain dietary and lifestyle approaches (e.g., those of Dr. Ornish, Dr. Pritikin, Dr. Esselstyn, Dr. Fuhrman) can tend to reverse atherosclerosis. If this interests you, you can do searches for "heart disease reversal approach of Dr._____," filling in the name of the physician you are interested in. (I have confirmed that these searches will get you to the desired information or to information about how to buy what you want.)

Why the routine below is called a "vascular cleansing routine" **(VCR).** Fortunately, my regularly doing earlier versions of the routine given below, with nearly none of the major effective supplements, actually has achieved "vascular cleansing" for me. I will repeat here very favorable results of Life Lines screenings I had done during the summer of 2017.

Carotid artery disease: left, mild; right, normal
Arterial fibrillation, normal

Abdominal aortic aneurysm, normal
Peripheral arterial disease: left, normal; right, normal
Osteoporosis, low risk

Since the numerical results regarding carotid artery disease of my right and left sides were the same, I don't understand why the left carotid artery risk was "mild."

Ideas from a highly educated, competent professional whose higher education was not in the health field. This is a quote from an email I received from him. I strongly believe that he knows much more about this than a very high percentage of MD cardiologists.

> "One of my primary research areas is reversal of atherosclerosis. To accomplish this, I take a supplement drug that dissolves the fibrin protein lattice structure on which the atherosclerotic plaques form.
>
> "The drug I take is Nattozimes substitute for Nattokinase. I also take a smaller dose of Serrapeptase, as that was the drug originally used in European clinical trials to dissolve atherosclerotic plaques. I am staggered with the lack of knowledge of American primary care docs. **I have yet to meet any primary care physician who has even a clue about using nattokinase or serrapeptase**."

Reversal of very dangerous calcification in blood vessels. Clinical nutritionist Keith Bishop reports in an article, "How to reduce blood vessel calcification," that high density intake of vitamin K2 in a major study (Beulens et al, 2009) was associated with a 20% decrease in coronary calcification. **Since vitamin K2 is a blood coagulant, any use of a K2 supplement should be accompanied by taking of sufficient anti-coagulants**.

Additional supplements to consider to reverse atherosclerosis. There have been research projects which have indicated that each of the following supplements should tend to achieve reversal of atherosclerosis.

GliSODin. This is a patented supplement which has excellent antioxidant and anti-inflammatory properties. By far the best description of research concerning use of GliSODin in reversal of atherosclerosis is an article on the Internet in *Life Extension Magazine* with the title "Reversing atherosclerosis naturally" (2007).

Nattokinase. Nattokinase is derived from a type of soy cheese. Research has indicated that it tends to dissolve blood clots. You learned above that there is a patented product, Nattozimes, which is derived from nattokinase.

Tocotrienols. There has been extensive research about heart health benefits of tocotrienols, which is a type of vitamin E. Dr. Blaylock recommends utilization of tocotrienols in prevention of heart attacks and strokes.

Pomegranate. Pomegranate can be consumed as an extract, or the juice can be drunk. The *Life Extension Magazine* article mentioned above regarding GliSODin also has detailed description of research findings about use of pomegranate juice in reversal of atherosclerosis.

Walnuts. The heart health benefits of eating walnuts are so substantial, numerous, and well researched that I think it makes sense to include eating walnuts in efforts to achieve reversal of atherosclerosis. I currently do not have scientific evidence that eating walnuts achieves this reversal.

Should you decide to implement some version of the VCR below with the supervision of a qualified medical professional, I hope that your goal will be to progressively reverse your atherosclerosis. I believe there is scientific evidence that many, if not all, of **the approaches listed above should tend to reverse atherosclerosis**.

An atherosclerosis-reversal routine (VCR). Even though this routine as given below is for women, there are very few changes needed for it to be appropriate for men. Instead of taking 25 mg of DHEA, men can take 50 mg. It is especially important for women to take folate instead of folic acid. Unless a man is experiencing troubling "senior moments," it would probably be better for him not to take folic acid.

Below is a **primary prevention VCR for women, which can be adapted by addition of some of the supplements listed above. I recommend adding pomegranate, tocotrienols, GliSODin, and nattokinase and eating some walnuts during every day.**

Primary Heart-Disease Prevention Routine (VCR) for Women

Supplements to take> > > > > Wait 30 minutes> > > > > Get 20 to 40 min. of
with large gl. water   moderate exercise.

magnesium-citrate (200–400 mg)

fish oil (1000 mg)   Another time in day,

vitamin B6 (100 mg)   take w/ lrg. glass of water

arginine (500 mg)   vitamin D3 (2000 to 5000 iu or

alpha-lipoic acid (600 mg)   as directed by MD)

coenzyme Q10 (200 mg) or, if   vitamin B12 (1000 mcg)

over 45, ubiquinol (100 mg)   DHEA (25 mg or as suggested

DHA (100 mg)   by an MD)

turmeric (500 mg)

potassium (100 mg) folate (400 mcg)

vitamin C (500 mg) turmeric (500 mg)

garlic (dose according to type) If "bad

lipids panel,"

lecithin (1300 mg) niacin (500 mg)

coconut oil (3 capsules) lecithin (1300 mg)

ginkgo biloba (60 mg) No exercise after this.

If "bad lipids profile,"

niacin (500 mg)

If not "bad lipids profile"

niacin (200 mg)

If you want to take vitamin E (tocopherols), you should not take more than 1000 mg per day. Vitamin E has significant anti-coagulant effects.

Using a major formula and additional supplements. As an alternative to taking the supplements listed above, you can take **OmegaQ Plus with resveratrol and turmeric,** which is a formula developed and marketed by prominent cardiologist, Dr. Stephen Sinatra. It includes B6, folate, B12, squid oil, DHA, EPA, turmeric, l-carnitine, coenzyme Q10, and resveratrol. Enough to take one before your VCR and one at bedtime will cost $50 per month. If I were to decide to take it, which I may decide to do, I would also take DHEA, l-arginine, garlic, lecithin, niacin, magnesium-citrate, and potassium before my exercise. At bedtime with the other capsule, I would take D3. Of course, a supervising physician would want to add or substitute supplements from the list above. **If you use OmegaQ Plus with resveratrol and turmeric in atherosclerosis-reversal efforts, you would need to add some of the supplements discussed in detail above.**

REFERENCES

Azuma, J. et al (1983). Therapy of congestive heart failure with orally administered taurine. *Clinical Thereutics*, Vol. 5, No. 4, pp. 398–408.

Baker, S.M. (1991–1992). Magnesium deficiency in primary care and preventive medicine. *Magnesium and Trace Elements*, Vol. 10, pp. 251–262.

Beulens, J.W. et al (2009). High dietary menaquinone intake is associated with reduced coronary calcification. *Atherosclerosis*, Vol. 203, Issue 2, pp. 289–93.

Crouse, John R. et al (2017). Effect of rosuvastatin on progression of carotid intim-media thickness in low-risk individuals with subclinical atherosclerosis: the METEOR Trial. *Journal of the American Medical Association*, Vol. 297, No. 12, pp. 1344–1353.

Divakaran, S. et al (2015). Use of cardiac CT and calcium scoring for detecting coronary plaque: implications for prognosis and patient management. *British Journal of Radiology*, Vol. 88, p. 1046.

Food and Drug Administration (2014). FDA warns consumers of the dangers of aspirin therapy. NBC News.

Jimenez, Guallar E. et al (2001). The association of chromium with the risk of a first myocardial infarction in men. The EURAMIC Study (abstract). *Circulation*, Vol. 103, p. 1366.

Langsjoen, Peter H. & Langsjoen, Alena M. (1999). Overview of the use of CoQ10 in cardiovascular disease. *Biofactors*, Vol. 9, Issue 2–4, pp. 273–284.

Lee, Joyce (2008). Why young adults hold the key to assessing the obesity epidemic of children. *Archives of Pediatric and Adolescent Medicine*, Vol. 162, No. 7, pp. 682–7.

Leon, Hernando et al (2008). Effect of fish oil on arrhythmias and mortality: systematic review. *British Medical Journal*, Vol. 337, p. 2931.

Mertz, W. (1993). Chromium in human nutrition: a review. *Journal of Nutrition*, Vol. 123, No. 4, pp. 626–633.

Sole, M.J. & Jeejeebhoy, K.N. (2002). Conditioned nutritional requirements: therapeutic relevance to heart failure. *Herz.*, Vol. 27, No. 2, pp. 174–178.

── CHAPTER 10 ──
Prevention, Control, and Reversal
of Type 2 Diabetes

<u>Cautionary statement</u>. Type 2 diabetes is a serious and dangerous disease. The author is not a physician or health expert. If you have type 2 diabetes or think you may have that disease, you should obtain assistance from and, if needed, medical treatment from a physician.

Prevention. If a physician has stated that you do not yet have type 2 diabetes, you may still have "pre-diabetes," which can involve constant hunger, unexplained weight loss, weight gain, high waist circumference, flu-like symptoms, blurred vision, slow healing, tingling, loss of feeling in your hands or feet, recurrent gum or skin infection, recurrent vaginal or bladder infection, and/or increased urination. If you have many of those symptoms, it will be prudent for you to talk to your physician about doing things recommended in this chapter to prevent the development of type 2 diabetes. Attempting to prevent the development of type 2 diabetes can involve weight loss, adoption of a low glycemic-index diet (including consumption of plenty of fiber), and taking carefully selected supplements, followed by moderate (not strenuous) exercise. Research has shown that, if a person with pre-diabetes loses 5% to 7% of her or his body weight and gets regular exercise, there is a 58% probability that this will prevent development of diabetes (Johns Hopkins Medicine, 2017).

Control. Obviously, if control is your goal, you have been diagnosed as having type 2 diabetes. In this chapter, you will be given some information you may decide to use to control your diabetes. I strongly recommend that you do this with medical supervision. You may be able to find an integrative or holistic MD or DO or a naturopathic doctor (ND) who will supervise your attempt to control the disease. Successful control of type 2 diabetes may involve being able to avoid taking medication and/or insulin.

Reversal. As with control, reversal should be done with medical supervision. An article on the Newsweek website (Sheridan, 2017) reports research in which nearly half of research subjects with type 2 diabetes who lost 30 lbs. during a six-month study experienced remission of diabetes.

Below I tell you about availability of three type 2 diabetes-reversal programs. Unless your physician has a particular reversal program she or he recommends, you may decide to purchase one of those documents, study it, and show it to your physician.

Elaboration. On the WebMD website, there is a March 4, 2015 article by Dennis Thompson with the title "Statin linked to raised risk of type 2 diabetes," which is about a large Finnish study (Cederberg et al, 2015). That study found nearly a 50% increase in development of type 2 diabetes in people taking a cholesterol-lowering drug. Lipids expert Dr. Ronald Goldberg was quoted in the WebMD article as saying that those researchers:

> "show evidence that statins increased insulin resistance, and that the people who developed diabetes appeared to have less ability to respond to the insulin resistance by making more insulin."

Importance of this subject. It has been reported that 40% of Americans will develop type 2 diabetes during her or his lifetime.

As discussed earlier this book, one of the worst and most preventable life sequences relating to health is, starting in your 20s or 30s and caused partly by bad diet and sedentary life style, weight gain and an increase in blood pressure. This can produce the metabolic syndrome (syndrome X), which can also involve insulin resistance. Unchecked, this can lead to development of type 2 diabetes, which can in turn lead to Alzheimer's disease. Some type of horrible death probably will follow. In chapter 1, you will find a health-motivation poster about this horrible sequence of events. This deterioration of health is easily prevented without medication. For me, the activities needed to prevent that sequence have improved my health and life experiences very greatly.

Importance of health motivation in dealing by non-medical, non-drug means with either the threat or actuality of type 2 diabetes. It is nearly certain that any person who nearly has or actually has type 2 diabetes has failed for a significant period of time to work hard enough protecting her or his health. If you have been in that situation, I encourage you to read or reread chapter one of this book. Preventing, controlling, or reversing type 2 diabetes takes strong motivation.

Relevance for young adults. Unfortunately, it is not unusual for a fairly young child to develop type 2 diabetes. I recommend that you read especially the type 2 diabetes risk factors, which are given later in this chapter.

Available information about reversal of type 2 diabetes. I have bought off of the Internet a book which appears to provide comprehensive and credible information about this subject. It is by Max Sidorov, K.N. (2017) and has the title *7 steps to health and the big diabetes lie.* It is said to have been written "in cooperation with the doctors at the International Council for Truth in Medicine." I do not have information needed to vouch for the credibility of the author or the International Council for Truth in Medicine. **If I had type 2 diabetes, I would read this 429-page book and discuss type 2 diabetes reversal with my primary physician.**

I have also bought ($39) off of the Internet a pdf document with the title "The DIABETES PROTOCOL: completely and permanently reverse both TypeI and TypeII diabetes in just 19 days."

The Health Sciences Institute (2011) has a publication, *Today's greatest alternative medicines,* which includes a chapter on reversal of diabetes.

One of the reasons I bought these three documents was that I know that "fringe" alternative-health approaches may work. For example, when I had an extremely painful kidney stone, I bought Cleanse Drops off of the Internet. I drank water containing a few drops. Within 15 minutes, the pain stopped. Within two hours, I painlessly passed the stone.

Author's relevant experience. Based on tests done in early 2018, my excellent integrative physician states that I am "pre-diabetic." My result for insulin was 105, which was vastly higher than the high risk cutoff of 12 and indicated high insulin resistance. My heart- and brain-disease risk factors have for decades indicated that I have been at risk of developing type 2 diabetes. During 2015, I started having what I thought were diabetic foot pains. I had allowed my weight to get to 222, which was far too high. To avoid development of full-blown type 2 diabetes, I lost 15–18 pounds, and the pains ended. During April of 2018, I have lost weight down to 204 and want to avoid gaining above that level. This is a minor example of what a person may be able to achieve against type 2 diabetes.

The most outrageous ad on American TV. You, like me, have probably seen many times on TV an ad for Tresiba, a diabetes medication. Accompanied by catchy, pretty, cheerful music, the ad ends by showing three or four happy, smiling adults and asking, "Are you Tresiba ready?" Learning that you need to take a diabetes medication is extremely bad news and is not a time when a rational person would look happy. A Toujeo diabetes medication ad is nearly as offensive. It shows a somewhat overweight man enjoying life very much while on Toujeo. Learning that you are Tresiba and Toujeo ready confirms that you are substantially down the road toward death from heart disease and Alzheimer's or other dementia. **No one should minimize the medical seriousness of developing type 2 diabetes.**

A wonderful triumph against type 2 diabetes. Years ago, my friend Sarah had type 2 diabetes and hypertension. She had a heart attack and later was told that she died and had to be resuscitated. After the heart attack, she was on many drugs that were not controlling her hypertension. So, she obtained excellent science-based information about controlling her various medical problems. Gradually, she was able to stop taking all of the medications. She was able to control her blood pressure by non-medical, non-drug means and was told that she no longer had type 2 diabetes. Of course, a person should try to do this only with medical supervision.

Soda consumption, weight gain and risk of diabetes in women. German researchers have reported that:

"[i]t appears that greater consumption of sugar-sweetened beverages is associated with greater weight gain and an increased risk for development of type 2 diabetes in women." (Schulze et al, 2004).

Type 2 diabetes risk factors. The source is the NIH National Institute of Diabetes and Digestive and Kidney Diseases.

Overweight or obese
45 years old or older
Family history of having type 2 diabetes
African-American or American Indian descent
High blood pressure
Low HDL (good cholesterol), high triglycerides
Not physically active
History of heart disease or stroke
Has depression

Prevention of type 2 diabetes. The NIH National Institute of Diabetes and Digestive and Kidney Diseases has on the Internet two excellent documents about prevention of type 2 diabetes. The first is for young adults. "Get real! You don't have to knock yourself out to prevent diabetes." The second is for older adults. "It's not too late to prevent type 2 diabetes."

Natural remedies for type 2 diabetes. For a person who already has type 2 diabetes, the goal may be control of the condition without taking insulin. I have looked pretty extensively on the Internet and believe that the best introduction to this in on the WebMD website, which I have found to provide high quality information about health. The article is "Natural remedies for type 2 diabetes."

Elements of prevention, control, and reversal programs.

Weight loss. To find a credible weight-loss approach, search on the Internet for "Dr. Oz and student researcher discover $5 weight loss miracle." Because of the high weight- loss rate that apparently can be achieved, I think

I should urge you to be cautious in using that approach. The weight-loss goal relating to type 2 diabetes may not be very high.

Low glycemic-index diet. There are many excellent articles about low glycemic- index diet on the Internet. A central element is elimination of high-sugar and refined- carbohydrate foods and drinks. Consumption of plenty of fiber in fruits, vegetables (various colors), and whole grains is important.

Supplements. I found two similar lists of supplements for diabetes treatment on the Internet. One was on the Healthline.com website, "Supplements that have shown promise as diabetes treatment," and "Natural remedies for diabetes" by Cathy Wong, ND. The following list combines those two lists: cinnamon, chromium, thiamine, alpha-lipoic acid, green tea, resveratrol, magnesium-citrate, zinc, bitter lemon, ginseng, aloe vera, gymnema, vanadium. I have long and positive experience with the supplements from cinnamon through zinc. Each of those supplements has a wide variety of health benefits. I have less experience using herbal supplements. Persons with pre-diabetes or type 1 or type 2 diabetes should, when taking niacin, take niacinamide, instead of nicotinic-acid.

Exercise. As I have discussed in several chapters, I recommend doing a "vascular cleansing routine (VCR)," which involves taking supplements, waiting 30 minutes, and then getting at least 20 minutes of moderate exercise. I believe that this routine provides synergy of the benefits of supplements and exercise. **I strongly recommend against strenuous or exhausting exercise**.

Reduction of stress. Several type 2 diabetes-treatment programs on the Internet include recommendation of reduction of stress. "Stressors" cause the physiological stress reaction, which, for people with diabetes, tends to increase blood-glucose levels. Chapter 14 is about dealing with anxiety and stress. You may decide to add some of the supplements listed above to the routine (VCR) in that chapter.

REFERENCES

Cederberg, H. et al (2015). Increased risk of diabetes with statin treatment is associated with impaired insulin sensitivity and insulin secretion: a 6-year follow-up study of the METSIM cohort. *Diabetologia*, the journal of the European Association for Study of Diabetes.

Johns Hopkins Medicine (2017). "Diabetes." Digestive Weight Loss Center on Internet.

Schulze, M. Et al, 2004). Sugar-sweetened beverages, weight gain, and incidence of type 2 diabetes in young and middle-aged women. *Journal of American Medical Association*, Vol. 292, pp. 927–34.

Sheridan, Kate (2017). "Type 2 diabetes reversed with weight loss: super low-calorie diet may cure the disease." Newsweek website.

Sidorov, Max (2017). *7 steps to health and THE BIG DIABETES LIE*. In cooperation with the doctors at the International Council for Truth in Medicine. http://www.TheICTM.org

SECTION 4
Brain Health and Function

CHAPTER 11
Ways to Improve Your Thinking and Memory--for Young and Healthy Persons

Cautionary statement. As indicated in the chapter title, this information is for young and healthy persons who do not have significant brain health or function problems. Chapter 4 includes information about benefits and risks of taking nutritional supplements. Several multi-ingredient supplement formulas are discussed in this chapter. The containers of those products provide cautionary information.

Importance of this subject. It can often make sense for a young person or healthy middle-age person to want to obtain a boost in quality of thinking and memory for several hours or longer. Fortunately, there are now effective and safe ways to do that.

Relevance for young adults. This is relevant for young adults for reasons in addition to getting a boost in brain performance. Richard Isaacson, MD, and Christopher Ochner, PhD, have a recently published book, *The Alzheimer's prevention & treatment diet* (2016), in which they argue strongly that prevention of Alzheimer's and other dementia should begin during early adulthood.

Very soon in this chapter, you will be told about a variety of supplement formulas that have been shown in research to improve a person's thinking, memory, attention, and focus. (I know for sure that extensive research has been done concerning specific ingredients, showing remarkable benefits. I do not know how many of the formulas have been evaluated in research.)

Author's relevant experience. The serious heart disease risk factors I reported in chapter 6 are also serious brain disease risk factors. In 2018, I had a test that showed that I have severe genetic risk factors regarding developing Alzheimer's. People in my high risk category have a 30% life time risk of developing Alzheimer's. If you have read this book to this point, you know that I started performing my own heart and brain health supplement-and-exercise routine in 1982. Starting in 1982, I worked on heart and brain health very successfully and consistently for 29 years before I first took a multi-ingredient supplement formula for brain function benefits. Instead, I took between eight and 12 of the 15 supplements listed below, waited 30 minutes, and then got moderate exercise (sometimes strenuous exercise in the early years) for at least 30 minutes.

I take numerous supplements, including a multi-ingredient supplement formula, for brain function benefits nearly every day. Before playing duplicate bridge, I take the full complement of VCR supplements, several supplements with brain function benefits, Advanced Memory Formula, and Prevagen, and, about 30 minutes later, walk very briskly at a mall for 15 to 20 minutes. Apparently, this allows my brain to use the alpha-lipoic acid and produce the very important antioxidant, glutathione, which has significant brain health and function benefits. During the late fall of 2017, my partners and I had many excellent duplicate bridge results in the very tough Columbia Bridge Club.

Update on the author's brain function. Late in October of 2017, I had a two-hour evaluation by a PhD neurologist at the Medical University of South Carolina. He reported to me that he found no evidence of abnormality concerning my brain function. My impression was that he gave me the most favorable report he had available. I continue to believe that my determined efforts to protect my brain health and function have been and will continue to be very worthwhile.

Calculated minimum cost of 15 supplements for a basic heart-and brain-health routine. If I were starting supplement use in the 25 to 45 age range, had my "bad lipids profile," and knew what I now know, I would buy and take daily (several twice daily) the following nutritional supplements. Supplements I would take twice daily would be curcumin, fish oil, lecithin, magnesium-citrate, niacin (nicotinic acid), vitamin B6, and vitamin D3. The cost totals below are based on taking all supplements once a day. Taking the indicated supplements twice a day would increase the cost by about $.30 per day.

I carefully searched for the best prices on the Internet and ended up with Puritan's Pride and Swanson supplements. Remember: I looked carefully for the best buy for the desired dosage. Obviously, your cost for "premium quality" supplements from other companies will be higher. I have mainly bought from Puritan's Pride for about 20 years, which has not kept me from achieving excellent results.

Alpha-lipoic acid, 600 mg, Swanson	$.17
Coenzyme Q10, 200 mg, Puritan's Pride	.09
Curcumin/turmeric, 800 mg, Puritan's Pride	.035
DHA, 300 mg, Puritan's Pride	.092
DHEA, 50 mg, Puritan's Pride	.064
	Women should take less, maybe 25 mg, as recommended by doctor.
Fish oil, 1000 mg, Puritan's Pride	.04
Folic acid, 400 mcg, Puritan's Pride	.014
	Men should not take unless they are having "senior moments."
L-arginine, 500 mg, Puritan's Pride	.104
Lecithin, 1200 mg, Swanson	.064
Magnesium-citrate, 200 mg, Puritan's Pride	.062
Niacin (nicotinic acid), 500 mg, Swanson	.042
Potassium-gluconate, 99 mg, Swanson	.029
Vitamin B6, 50 mg, Puritan's Pride	.03

Vitamin B12, 1000 mcg, Puritan's Pride	.02
Vitamin D3, 5000 iu, Puritan's Pride	.03
	Taking much more than the long-time recommended daily allowance is safe.
Daily cost	$.886
Monthly cost	$26.58
Yearly cost	$323.39

My recommendation to you. Instead of just taking an excellent multi-ingredient supplement formula on days when you want a boost in brain function, I recommend that you implement this routine (take supplements, wait 30 minutes, then get 30+ minutes of moderate exercise) four or five days per week.

Performing this VCR will provide many significant benefits.

(1) **Benefits of the supplements**. Please forgive me for repeating. You could write a short book just on the health and wellbeing benefits of these 15 supplements. Chapter 4 includes a section concerning benefits of and cautions relating to each of these supplements. These supplements, with good exercise and diet, can practically guarantee you a life-time of excellent heart and brain health.

(2) **Benefits of the exercise**. I have included in chapter 6 and chapter 18 a full listing of the astonishingly great benefits of exercise. Exercise improves a person's brain function in several important ways. Some young people and healthy older people have not been "into exercise." If that includes you, I greatly hope you will take advantage of this opportunity to start regularly getting these benefits.

(3) **Synergistic effects of the supplements and exercise together**. Some scientists believe that exercising not long after taking supplements will improve the body's and brain's benefits from the supplements.

If you want to be very sharp for an exam or meeting at 3:00 p.m., you could do this routine starting at 10:00 a.m. or during your lunch hour and then take a multi-ingredient supplement formula about 2:00 p.m. I think it's prudent to avoid taking a formula with many herbal ingredients at the same time as many vitamins and minerals. Though I have never had a bad interaction of various types of pills, I think it's better to be careful.

Information about supplements with cognitive functioning benefits.

Supplements which should help with brain health and/or function. The Natural Medicines Comprehensive Database lists the following supplements as probably effective in treatment of Alzheimer's: ginkgo leaf, vitamin E, huperzine A, phosphatidylserine (PS), and vinpocetine. The following are additional supplements which may have benefits regarding brain health and/or function: vitamin B12, DHEA (more for men), coenzyme Q10, alpha-lipoic acid, green tea extract, magnesium (-citrate or -glycinate), melatonin, vitamin B6, folate (for women and for men who have cognitive-function problems). Fortunately, all of this second list of supplements have established benefits regarding cardiovascular health. Research has suggested that taking turmeric and vitamin D3 together can result in some removal (regression) from the brain of beta-amyloid plaque, which is a major physical aspect of development of Alzheimer's. Acetyl-choline, which is extremely important for brain health and function, is a product of metabolism of choline found in lecithin. Taurine, which helps with heart health, is said to be an important brain antioxidant. I have read very recent expert comments to that effect that DHA, an omega-3 fatty acid, has major brain health and function benefits.

Brain function patented formulas. There are many dozens of patented supplements which are marketed to help with brain health and function. Two which appear to have excellent ingredients are Brain Ammo (a little more than $2 per day) and Advanced Memory Formula (a little more than $1 per day). NeuroHD is touted on one website as the best brain supplement of 2014. Brain Power is another brain supplement. Prevagen, which is heavily advertised on TV, is reported to have benefits regarding memory. (I take Advanced Memory Formula and Prevagen and am confident that each provides substantial benefits. I take also Elysium, an anti-aging supplement that was developed by the head of the aging research center at MIT.)

Information about a supplement formula I would recommend. Several years ago, a young man just out of college appeared on the *Shark Tank* TV show seeking investment by a shark in his company, Cerebral Success, which had developed and was marketing a multi-ingredient supplement formula for improvement of thinking, memory, attention, etc. Fortunately for him, he got the best possible investor, Barbara Corcoran. The product is SmartX, which can be found on the Internet for about $1 per capsule. For the extremely strong variety of ingredients of SmartX, I think that is a very reasonable price. I recommend against taking more than one SmartX capsule in a day.

The importance of healthful eating. Even college students and older healthy adults need to have a basically healthy diet. Chapter 3 gives information about this.

REFERENCES

Isaacson, Richard & Ochner, Christopher (2016). *The Alzheimer's prevention and treatment diet: using nutrition to combat the effects of Alzheimer's disease.* Garden City Park, NY: SquareOne Publishers.

— CHAPTER 12 —

Ways to Prevent or Attempt to Reverse
Alzheimer's Disease and other Dementia

Cautionary statement for persons who have been diagnosed as having Alzheimer's disease or other dementia. Significantly reversing Alzheimer's or serious dementia is very difficult, even if it is attempted by a top expert in the field. Experts believe that some cases of full-blown Alzheimer's simply cannot be significantly reversed.

If you or a person you are wanting to help has been diagnosed as having Alzheimer's disease or other dementia, I believe it will be important for you to have the assistance of an integrative or holistic MD or DO (osteopathic physician) or ND (naturopathic doctor) who has expertise concerning use of non-medical, non-drug approaches in attempting to reverse the Alzheimer's or other dementia. One way to start on this would be to show this chapter to your family physician. Unfortunately, in many cities, it is hard to find a physician with relevant expertise who will help with this.

The Alzheimer's Association has for decades pronounced that Alzheimer's disease cannot be prevented or reversed. This message strongly discourages individual efforts to prevent Alzheimer's and other dementias. I believe their pronouncement is based on research that has shown that there is no single drug which will prevent or reverse Alzheimer's.

Importance of this subject. The Alzheimer's Association provides the following statistics. Currently, one of nine persons over 65 has Alzheimer's or other dementia. After age 65, the likelihood of developing Alzheimer's doubles about every five years (Rosenzweig, 2018). Among persons 85 and older, 38% have Alzheimer's or other dementia. By 2050, 16 million Americans will have Alzheimer's or other dementia.

Very encouraging, successful Alzheimer's-and dementia-reversal research by Dr. Bredesen (2014) is sufficient reason to view this as a very important subject.

Relevance for young adults. Richard Isaacson, MD, and Christopher Ochner, PhD, are the authors of a recent book, *The Alzheimer's prevention & treatment diet* (2016), in which they argue strongly that prevention of Alzheimer's and other dementia should begin during early adulthood.

Author's relevant experience. As I have mentioned earlier, I have numerous severe heart and brain disease risk factors. Two of my father's sisters and two of my mother's sisters had severe dementia in their late 70s. My father and mother each had a brother who remained physically active through his 70s and did not develop Alzheimer's or dementia. A male relative has been diagnosed with Alzheimer's. In 2015, a business employee's criminal act resulted in my suffering major hearing loss in my "good ear." Hearing loss is a significant dementia risk factor.

In 2011, I noticed that I was having more "senior moments" than previously. I knew that I already was winning the heart-health fight. So, I shifted my health emphasis to prevention of Alzheimer's and other dementia. Then 67 years old, I read many articles and several books on the subject. I started taking a cognitive-function formula and now take two. Frankly, I now work hard on my brain health and function nearly every day and don't regret this effort in the slightest. If I were at the 2011 (67 years old) stage now, I would buy and read carefully *Memory rescue* by Dr. Daniel Amen.

Major reasons that I am achieving excellent brain health and function outcomes in spite of severe Alzheimer's and dementia risk factors. It is important for me to remind you that I started working very hard on my heart and brain health in 1982, when I was 38 years old. Fortunately, my consistent performance of my VCR kept me from having problems regarding hypertension (high blood pressure). Since then, I have gradually improved my VCR (supplement-and-exercise routine) by adding important supplements.

The importance of LDL regarding brain function especially in old age. Dr. Duane Graveline documents in several books possible adverse effects regarding brain function of taking a statin drug. I believe that refusing to take a statin drug has been probably the best decision of my life. Now in my middle 70s, I have nearly as much creativity relating to very difficult subjects and functions, such as music and writing, as during any other period of my life.

Explanation. **This chapter has three sections. They are concerned with (1) prevention of Alzheimer's and other dementia; (2) reversal of mild cognitive impairment; and (3) attempting to reverse Alzheimer's and other dementia.**

The information in all sections of this chapter is intended for people who do not take a statin drug for cholesterol control or BP control.

Prevention of Alzheimer's disease and other dementia.

An approach for young and healthy persons. Chapter 11 provides detailed suggestions about how to "improve your thinking and memory" and about prevention of Alzheimer's and other dementia. This section is primarily for people who are not as young or healthy.

Excellent information from three physicians. Everyone who has a strong interest in prevention of Alzheimer's and other dementia should buy an important recent book by Richard Isaacson, MD, and Christopher Ochner, PhD, *The Alzheimer's prevention & treatment diet* (2016). As mentioned above, they argue strongly that prevention of Alzheimer's and other dementia should begin during early adulthood.

Dr. Daniel Amen is a psychiatrist and an extremely capable medical expert on brain health and function. To find several excellent articles presenting his approaches concerning brain health and function, you can go to the anewdayanewme.com website and find an article, "Dr. Daniel Amen: prevent Alzheimer's. Early warning signs your brain may be in trouble." Below that article are links to additional articles describing his approaches. Dr. Amen is the author of several books regarding brain function and health, including *Change your brain: chance your life* (2015) and *Memory rescue* (2017).

Dr. Gary Small (Small & Vorgan, 2011), a psychiatrist, is the author of a book, *Alzheimer's Prevention Program*, and also the author of a regular report, *The Mind Health Report*.

A detailed, research-based article on the Internet. "15 resolutions to reduce your dementia risk in 2015," on the Alzheimers.net website

Extremely encouraging research findings. Fortunately, in recent years there has been very great improvement of available information about the prevention of Alzheimer's and other dementia. As mentioned earlier, in 2014, Dr. Dale Bredesen had an article published in which he reported research he had directed. He selected ten patients with either Alzheimer's or other severe dementia. Using measures from a document listing 25 categories of measures, he developed Alzheimer's- or other dementia-reversal programs specifically for each of the ten patients. After full implementation of those programs, nine of the patients had improved significantly, and two patients were able to return to work. **Why is this relevant to the subject of prevention of Alzheimer's and other dementia? The reason is that the prevention of a disease is virtually always much easier to do and more effectively done than reversal of the disease**. I believe it is reasonable to conclude that much of the information in Dr. Bredesen's measures can be used effectively in the prevention of Alzheimer's and other dementia. (Detailed information about Dr. Bredesen's 25 categories is in the last section of this chapter.)

Can nutritional supplements help with preventing Alzheimer's and other dementia? In his 25 categories of metabolic and body function areas, Dr. Bredesen mentions 31 nutritional supplements, many of which I already used when I discovered his 2014 article. In his recent book, *Memory Rescue* (2017), Dr. Daniel Amen mentions 53 nutritional supplements. These numbers of supplements discussed by two of the very elite brain health and function experts, both of whom are achieving extremely remarkable positive results with seriously ill patients, give us the clear answer that supplements can help.

There is scientific research suggesting that these supplements may help with prevention of Alzheimer's: Vitamin D3 taken with turmeric at bedtime, folic acid, cinnamon, vitamin E, coenzyme Q10 (ubiquinol for persons over 45), magnesium-citrate, alpha-lipoic acid followed by exercise, fish oil, DHA, acetyl-l carnitine, vitamin B12, vitamin B6, DHEA (more for men), lecithin, melatonin, and niacin. (Persons with diabetes, take niacinamide. Others take nicotinic acid.) These supplements, along with exercise and good diet, also help substantially with prevention of heart and blood vessel disease.

The importance of having good heart and blood vessel health. About 85% of persons who die from Alzheimer's and are autopsied had atherosclerosis or other "heart disease." Unfortunately, taking a statin drug can have significant **adverse** cognitive functioning effects. There are many health experts (some with information available on the Internet) who have available non-statin approaches to prevention and even reversal of heart and blood vessel disease.

Control of blood pressure in middle age. Even moderately high BP during middle age can have adverse effects on brain health and cognitive function (Reitz et al, 2007). One of the dangers is a series of small strokes, which will seriously damage your brain. Non-drug approaches for preventing or controlling hypertension are provided in chapter 7 of this book.

The importance of good diet. Research findings released in 2012 indicate that, among 6,183 women over 65 tracked for four years, consumption of saturated fat (animal fat) was associated with decline in "memory and abstract thinking," while consumption of monounsaturated fat (major source, olive oil) was associated with significantly less cognitive decline (Okereke, 2012). So, **there has been research indicating that consumption of a lot of saturated fat by older people, especially women, can result in cognitive decline**. There are specific recommendations about diet later in this chapter.

You can find the dietary approaches of Dr. David Perlmutter on the Internet. His most important recommendation emphasizes consuming good fats, such as omega-3 oils, coconut oil, and olive oil. I eat a lot of Smart Balance containing olive oil, which tastes better than real butter. An important component of brain tissue is DHA, which is found in fish oil and can be bought separately. DHA has very important brain health and function benefits.

Dr. Perlmutter also strongly recommends **against** the consumption of grains. He uses the phrase "grain brain." I love whole grain bread but think that going off of whole grain foods entirely has been a very good move for me.

The importance of exercise. Here are three statements including information you may not have. (1) All heart health programs for people who do not have very severe heart disease include regular exercise, such as brisk walking for 30 minutes four days per week. (2) The most effective way to **build** your brain power is physical exercise. (3) Among old people, the ones who think the best tend to be the ones who exercise the most.

Benefits of adopting and following a supplement-and-exercise routine (VCR). As mentioned several times in this book, my VCR routine has allowed me, at 74, to have excellent heart and brain health. You can use the VCR in chapter 11 or adapt the VCR for reversal of mild cognitive impairment, which is later in this chapter.

Internet article on Alzheimer's prevention. "Alzheimer's and dementia prevention: how to reduce your risk and protect your brain" is a helpful article on the Internet.

An important federal government resource concerning non-traditional approaches for dealing with the threat of Alzheimer's or dementia. In the National Institutes of Health, there is the National Center for Complementary and Alternative Medicine. On their website, there is a very important collection of information and resources about Alzheimer's and dementia: "Cognitive function, dementia, and Alzheimer's disease."

Reversal of mild cognitive impairment. Mild cognitive impairment (MCI) is, as the phrase suggests, an instance of compromised cognitive functioning that is significantly less severe than full-blown Alzheimer's or other dementia. Because it is less severe, reversing it is more achievable than reversal of full-blown Alzheimer's or other dementia. Below is an MCI-reversal routine.

People for whom this routine is intended. This routine is specifically for people who have been diagnosed as experiencing "mild cognitive impairment" (MCI) or for people who have strong reasons to believe they are experiencing MCI or are at risk of developing MCI. MCI involves primarily high frequency of "senior moments"—problems with memory. Having an occasional "senior moment" does not qualify as MCI. (There are excellent articles on the Internet about MCI and about recovery from MCI.)

This routine is not intended for use by people with Alzheimer's or other dementia, though their caregivers may find valuable information here.

Important Bredesen research. As mentioned above, in recent years, UCLA professor Dr. Dale Bredesen (2014) reported research in which he attempted to reverse symptoms of ten patients with Alzheimer's or other severe dementia. He used 25 different categories of measures in developing a program for each patient. (Before I found the Bredesen study, I was already doing something meaningful in 18 of his 25 areas.) Nine of the ten patients improved, and two improved enough to return to work. So, we have strong scientific evidence that cognitive-health problems can be reduced. It follows that MCI of some persons might be reversible.

The impact of cardiovascular health on brain health and function. Here is a significant quote from the Alzheimer's Association web site:

> "Some autopsy studies show that as many as 80 percent of individuals with Alzheimer's disease also have cardiovascular disease."

Research has shown that having high blood pressure (BP) can have very adverse health consequences (Chobanian, 2001). Even moderately high BP during middle age can have adverse effects on brain health and cognitive function later in life (Reitz et al, 2007). Because of these risks, it is very important for even moderately elevated BP to be controlled.

This alerts us to the most important thing to do to protect brain health: Start as early as possible in working proactively to protect, and even improve, your cardiovascular health (Isaacson & Ochner, 2016). The routine (VCR) below is intended to protect and improve heart and brain health, while providing special attention to recovering from mild cognitive impairment.

Brain-health benefits of exercise. The Alzheimer's Association frequently reports research indicating that physical exercise reduces the risk of Alzheimer's by 50%. Research shows that **physical exercise is the best way to build your brain power** (Ratey, 2008). Recent research has shown that the combination of adherence to the **Mediterranean diet** (information on the Internet) **and regular physical exercise reduces the risk of Alzheimer's by 60%** (Scarmeas et al, 2009).

Exercise can prompt growth of new brain cells in the hippocampus, which is referred to as the memory center of the brain. As reported earlier in this book, exercise has a wide variety of startlingly great heart health, brain health, and general wellbeing benefits.

Additional ways to prompt growth of new brain cells in the hippocampus. Taking DHA tends to result in growth of new brain cells. There is suggestion in research that taking phosphatidylcholine, which is found in lecithin, can result in growth of new brain cells in the hippocampus.

A brief note for people with some problems with depression. An important research project showed that, for older persons with major depression, treatment with regular exercise was as effective as treatment with an antidepressant drug after 16 weeks (Blumenthal et al, 1999). Tending to be depressed can interfere with your motivation to implement this routine. If you have some problems with minor depression, regular exercise should help you.

Adverse effects of statin drugs regarding brain health and function. Taking a statin drug can result in probably reversible dementia, which is often referred to as "brain fog." Substantial lowering of LDL can have very adverse consequences regarding brain health and function (Roberts, 2012).

Supplements which should help with brain health and/or function. The Natural Medicines Comprehensive Database lists the following supplements as probably effective in treatment of Alzheimer's: ginkgo leaf, vitamin E, huperzine A, phosphatidylserine (PS), and vinpocetine. The following are additional supplements which may have benefits regarding brain health and/or function: vitamin B12, DHEA (more for men), coenzyme Q10, alpha-lipoic acid, green tea extract, magnesium (-citrate or -glycinate), melatonin, vitamin B6, folate (for women and for men who have cognitive-function problems). Fortunately, all of this second list of supplements have established benefits regarding cardiovascular health. Research has suggested that taking turmeric and vitamin D3 together can result in some removal (regression) from the brain of beta-amyloid plaque, which is a major physical aspect of development of Alzheimer's. Acetyl-choline, which is extremely important for brain health and function, is a product of metabolism of choline found in lecithin. Taurine, which helps with heart health, is said to be an important brain antioxidant. I strongly encourage readers to make sure that DHA, an omega-3 in fish oil, is included in their brain health and function VCR.

Brain function patented formulas. There are many dozens of patented supplements which are marketed to help with brain health and function. Two which appear to have excellent ingredients are Brain Ammo (a little more than $2 per day) and Advanced Memory Formula (a little more than $1 per day). NeuroHD is touted on one website as the best brain supplement of 2014. Brain Power is another brain supplement. It is important for people with MCI to take an excellent brain-function supplement. Prevagen, which is heavily advertised on TV, is reported to have benefits regarding memory. (I take Advanced Memory Formula and Prevagen and am confident that each provides substantial benefits. I take also Elysium, an anti-aging supplement that was developed by the head of the aging research center at MIT.)

As mentioned in chapter 11, there is a multi-ingredient supplement formula, SmartX, which is made and marketed by a company in which Barbara Corcoran invested during an episode of *Shark Tank*. SmartX has excellent ingredients and a reasonable price ($1 per capsule).

I recommend that everyone performing this routine for reversal of mild cognitive impairment take Advanced Memory Formula or SmartX and Prevagen. These supplements can be taken significantly after or before taking the many supplements listed below.

Even though the routine as given below is for women, there are very few changes needed for it to be appropriate for men. Instead of taking 25 mg of DHEA, men can take 50 mg. Women can take folate or folic acid.

Routine (VCR) for Recovering from Mild Cognitive Impairment for Women
(You should alter the program below by selecting and adding supplements described above.)

Supplements to take> > > > > Wait 30 minutes> > > > > Get 20 to 40 min. of
with large gl. water   moderate exercise.

magnesium-citrate (200–400 mg)

fish oil (1000 mg)

vitamin B6 (100 mg)

cinnamon

vitamin E (2000 mg)

l-arginine (500 mg)

folate or folic acid (400 mcg)

alpha-lipoic acid (600 mg)

coenzyme Q10 (200 mg) or, if over 45, ubiquinol (100 mg)

DHA (300 mg)

potassium (100 mg)

vitamin C (500 mg)

garlic (dose according to type)

lecithin (1300 mg)

coconut oil (3 capsules)

ginkgo biloba (60 mg)

green tea extract (500 mg)

If "bad lipids profile,"

niacin (500 mg)

If not "bad lipids profile"

niacin (200 mg)

Not long before bedtime,

take w/ lrg. glass of water

vitamin D3 (2000 to 5000 iu or as directed by MD)

coconut oil (2 capsules)

vitamin B12 (1000 mcg)

vitamin B6 (100 mg)

DHEA (25 mg)
turmeric (500 mg)
If "bad lipids profile,"
niacin (500 mg)
lecithin (1300 mg)
melatonin (5 mg) (at bedtime)

Exercise as part of your routine. It is recommended that you perform the detailed routine (VCR) at least four times per week.

As discussed in previous chapters, strenuous exercise causes your blood platelets to be stickier and causes production of free radicals, which threaten cardiovascular and brain health. So, while avoiding strenuous exercise, you can do exercise in addition to your MCI-reversal routine. Getting at least 30 minutes of moderate exercise every day is a good goal.

<u>Some ideas about diet</u>. It should help to follow eating suggestions in chapter 3 of this book. Here are some very specific suggestions.

Some things to eat or drink. Coffee and other caffeinated foods and beverages (not including sugary soft drinks), dark chocolate, nuts, olive oil (including butter substitutes with olive oil as the main ingredient), fresh fruits and vegetables

Some things to avoid eating or drinking. Red meat, pizza, processed cheese, eggs Benedict, breaded chicken, sausage, Ramen noodles, sugary beverages, sugary desserts (limit consumption), refined carbohydrate foods, "white foods," including rice, potatoes, ordinary pasta, saturated fats

Research findings released in 2012 indicate that, among 6,183 women over 65 tracked for four years, consumption of saturated fat (animal fat) was associated with decline in "memory and abstract thinking," while consumption of monounsaturated fat (major source, olive oil) was associated with significantly less cognitive decline (Okereke, Olivia, 2012).

<u>Additional ways to protect and improve your brain health and function</u>. The ideas and strategies below were gleaned from a variety of books and articles on the subject. (At any given time, there is a fairly current book on the

market which is specifically about building your brain power. You may find good ideas and strategies in an Internet article written by Steve Gillman with the title "70 ways to increase your brain power.")

Don't get a flu shot. Dr. David Brownstein, MD, and Peter Doshi, PhD, Johns Hopkins, say flu shots are practically worthless and dangerous.

Mental exercise. The fact that this subject is toward the end of this chapter and is not very long should not be taken as indicating that it is not important. **Getting mental exercise, which involves strenuous cognitive activities, is extremely important to maintaining and improving cognitive functioning and brain health**. Lumosity exercises on the Internet have been shown in research to have a variety of cognitive benefits. There is an excellent article about this with the title "Brain exercise provides benefits at any age" on the Dr. Mercola web site.

Being bilingual helps with retaining strong cognitive functioning.

Playing duplicate bridge has been shown to delay the onset of Alzheimer's. I'm glad that I have played duplicate bridge regularly since 1981. I try to use duplicate bridge and studying about it as opportunities to do "brain pushups."

Research consistently shows that people who have had higher education, including graduate degrees, have more protection from cognitive decline than people who have not. Apparently what you study is not important.

Develop check lists in your work and important activities. My 39-year-old son Alex has work responsibilities in which it is extremely important for him to avoid making mistakes. He informs me that having detailed check lists helps him and that many high-level professionals have that practice.

Stay socially active. There is no doubt that social isolation is an Alzheimer's risk factor. Also, the resulting loneliness can cause depression, which also is an Alzheimer's and dementia risk factor. Loneliness is stressful, which prevents your body from healing itself.

Avoid chronic stress. Experiencing chronic stress, which involves frequently having the physiological stress reaction, during mid-life tends to result in problems with cognitive function later in life. Chronic stress is a major cause of cardiovascular disease. Fortunately, there are many good strategies for preventing the stress reaction and preventing adverse consequences of it, if it occurs. Chapter 14 is about this.

Try to solve major health problems. Uncontrolled diabetes, obesity, cardiovascular disease (CVD), and high BP (hypertension) increase the risk that a person will experience Alzheimer's or other dementia. Fortunately, performing the supplements-and-exercise routine (VCR) faithfully will help with reducing or even overcoming each of those risk factors.

Avoid heavy-metals toxicity. We need to get enough of several metals, such as cooper, chromium, iron, zinc, and manganese. Too much of even these metals can cause health problems. Other metals, such as mercury, lead, cadmium, aluminum, and thallium, apparently do not provide health benefits and cause health problems when they build up past a low level. Severe heavy-metals toxicity alone can cause dementia. People who think this might be a problem for them should check with their doctor about having one or more tests for heavy-metals toxicity. If you have this problem, there is a possibility that chelation treatment will help significantly.

Effects of prescription drugs on thinking. When people diagnosed with Alzheimer's die and an autopsy is performed, researchers have found that almost half of the individuals never had Alzheimer's at all. So what is the problem? Why were these people mentally impaired near the end of their lives? Some doctors believe it was their prescription drugs—especially statin drugs—causing memory loss, mental confusion, and even dementia. So, if you feel that you are experiencing cognitive decline, it will make sense to check carefully to see whether some of this is being caused by one or more prescription medications. It is reported in chapter 6 that experts believe that statin drugs "don't work" with people, especially women, over 65. Recent research has shown that some anti-psychotic medications tend to cause significant brain shrinkage.

Health benefits of having a good pet. Having a good pet tends to have significant heart- and brain-health benefits.

Chew gum. If you want to be as sharp as possible mentally in a particular situation, such as a bridge or poker game, **chew gum**.

(Please note that this is the end of the MCI-reversal routine.)

Ways to attempt reversal of Alzheimer's disease and other dementia. If you have a relative or friend who has Alzheimer's or other dementia, I recommend that you look at the three approaches below. Dr. Bredesen has definitely proven that a highly skilled team can achieve significant reversal of Alzheimer's and dementia symptoms with a high percentage of patients.

(1) An approach emphasizing consumption of coconut oil that should help many people with Alzheimer's or other dementia. People with Alzheimer's or other dementia probably have lost the ability to use glucose (sugar in the blood) as energy food for the brain because of severe insulin resistance. It is very amazing that, if these people eat food including a lot of coconut oil, their bodies will make "ketone bodies," which the brain can use as fuel. Physician Dr. Mary Newport has successfully used this approach with her husband, who had been diagnosed with early-onset Alzheimer's. There is a video about this on the Internet. For an article on this subject, search on the Internet for "Coconut oil and Alzheimer's: Is the misguided low-fat dietary philosophy primarily responsible for Alzheimer's disease?"

To obtain recipes of dishes that include coconut oil, you can search on the Internet for "Free coconut recipes," "Coconut oil on the ketogenic diet," or "All about ketogenic diet." There are many websites about achieving a ketogenic diet.

(2) Alzheimer's-reversal approach of Dr. Jacob Teitelbaum. If you are very concerned about yourself or a close relative or associate regarding thinking and memory, you can find on the Internet an excellent article by Dr. Jacob Teitelbaum, "Alzheimer's and senility are reversible." He provides extremely specific suggestions for physicians, concerned persons, and their relatives. Dr. Teitelbaum is listed on the Internet in "Newsmax Health's top 100 physicians who embrace integrative medicine."

(3) Important Alzheimer's reversal research by Dr. Dale Bredesen. Below are 25 areas of metabolism and body function that Dr. Bredesen used in developing detailed treatment programs for his ten research subject, all of whom had Alzheimer's or other severe dementia. As previously noted, nine of the patients improved significantly, and two were able to return to work.

LIST OF MEASURES USED IN BREDESEN DEMENTIA-REVERSAL PROTOCOL

(Based entirely on Bredesen 25 measures.
Full terms were substituted for abbreviations.)

Measure	Goal	Rational
1. Low glycemic, low inflammatory, low grain diet	Minimize simple carbohydrates, minimize inflammation	Minimize inflamm., insulin resistance
2. Fast 12 hr. each night, including 3 hr. prior to bedtime	Enhance autophagy (normal elimination of dysfunctional cells), ketogenesis (breakdown of fatty acids producing ketone bodies)	Reduce insulin levels, reduce beta-amyloid plaques
3. Yoga, meditation, and/or music	Stress reduction	Reduction of cortisol, reduction CRF (corticotropin-releasing factor)
4. 8 hr. sleep per night, melatonin, 0.5 mg, tryptophan 500 mg; exclude sleep apnea	Optimize sleep	

5. 30–60 min. exercise per day, 4–6 days/week	Multiple health and cognition benefits	
6. Brain stimulation		
7. B12, MTHF, P5P (active form of B6), TMG, if necessary	Reduction of homocysteine below 7	
8. Vitamin B12 methylcobalamin	Serum B12 over 500	B12 deficiency causes shrinking of brain.
9. Anti-inflammatory diet; curcumin with D3 at bedtime, DHA/EPA, optimize hygiene, including dental hygiene	C-reactive protein below 1.0; A/G (albumin/globulin) ratio over 1.5	Crucial role of inflammation in Alzheimer's disease
10. Diet as indicated above	Fasting insulin below 7; HgbA1c (blood sugar indicator) below 5.5	Type II diabetes-Alzheimer's relationship
11. Optimize fT3, fT4 (thyroid hormones), estradiol, testosterone, progesterone, pregnenolone, cortisol	Hormone balance	
12. Repair gastrointestinal, if needed; prebiotics, probiotics	Gastrointestinal health	Avoid inflammation, autoimmunity

13. Curcumin with D3 at bedtime, ashwagandha (herbal supp.)	Reduction of beta-amyloid plaques
14. Bacopa monneiera (herbal supp.), magnesium-threonate	Cognitive enhancement
15. Vitamin D3, K2 (coagulant)	250H-D3=50–100ng/ml (desirable level of D3)
16. H. Erinaceus (mushroom) or acetyl-L-carnitine	Increase NGF (nerve growth factor)
17. Citicoline (supp.), DHA	Provide synaptic structural components
18. Vitamin E (mixed tocopherols and tocotrienols, selelenium, blueberries, N-acetyl cysteine, ascorbate, alpha-lipoic acid (with exercise produces super antioxidant glutathione)	Optimize antioxidants
19. Depends on lab results	Optimize zinc:fCU ratio (zinc:copper ratio)

20. Exclude or treat sleep apnea; supplemental oxygen, as indicated	Ensure nocturnal oxygenation	
21. CoQ10 or ubiquinol, alpha-lipoic acid with exercise, N-acetyl cysteine, acetyl-L-carnitine, selenium, zinc, resveratrol, ascorbate, thiamine, PQQ (pyrroloquinoline quinone, an enzyme taken as supplement)	Optimize mitochondrial function	
22. Pantothenic acid	Increase focus	Acetylcholine synthesis requirement
23. Resveratrol	Increase Sir'T1 function (anti-aging gene)	
24. Evaluate heavy metal toxicity, chelate, if indicated	Exclude, eliminate heavy metal toxicity	CNS (central nervous system) effects of heavy metal
25. Coconut oil or Axona	Medium-chain triglycerides effects	

How can information about Dr. Bredesen's research be used? Unfortunately, it is very unlikely that a significant number of persons with full-blown Alzheimer's or other dementia will be able to receive treatment utilizing methods described by Dr. Bredesen. If you are very concerned about your brain health or function because of experiences of close relatives or because of having some "senior moments," I encourage you to study the 25 areas listed above more than once. Doing this very carefully will help you to acquire potentially important information about things you can do to improve your brain health and function. I take regularly or occasionally more than half of the supplements listed by Dr. Bredesen.

REFERENCES

Amen, Daniel (2017). *Memory rescue*. Carol Stream, IL: Tyndale Momentum.

Amen, Daniel (2015). *Change your brain: change your life*. NY, NY: Harmony Books.

Blumenthal, James A. et al (1999). Effects of exercise training on older patients with major depression. *Archives of Internal Medicine*, Vol. 159, No. 19, pp. 2349–2356.

Bredesen, D. (2014). Reversal of cognitive decline: a novel therapeutic program. *Aging, 6*, 707–717.

Isaacson, Richard & Ochner, Christopher (2016). *The Alzheimer's prevention and treatment diet: using nutrition to combat the effects of Alzheimer's disease*. Garden City Park, NY: SquareOne Publishers.

Okereke, Olivia et al (2012). Dietary fat types and 4-year cognitive change in community-dwelling older women. *Annals of Neurology*, Vol. 72, No. 1, pp. 124–34.

Ratey, John J. with Hagerman, Eric (2008). *Spark: the revolutionary new science of exercise and the brain*. NY, NY: Little, Brown and Company.

Reitz, C. et al (2007). Hypertension and the risk of mild cognitive impairment. *Arch Neurol.*, Vol 64 (No. 12), pp. 1734–40.

Roberts, B. (2012). *The truth about statins: risks and alternatives to cholesterol-lowering drugs*. NY, NY: Pocket Books.

Rosenzweig, Andrew, MD (2018). How important is age as an Alzheimer's risk factor? Verywellhealth.com website.

Scarmeas, Nikolaos et al (2009). Physical activity, diet, and risk of Alzheimer's disease. *Journal of the American Medical Association*, Vol. 302, No. 6, pp. 627–637.

Small, Gary & Vorgan, Gigi (2011). *The Alzheimer's prevention program: keep your brain healthy for the rest of your life.* NY, NY: Workman Publishing.

─── CHAPTER 13 ───
Anti-Aging Approaches

Elaboration. Here's the cover verbiage of a book (1998) by Dr. Timothy Smith.

Renewal
THE ANTI-AGING REVOLUTION
THE BREAKTHROUGH PROGRAM
REVERSE HEART DISEASE
DESTROY CANCER CELLS
FEEL MORE ENERGETIC WITH EVERY DECADE
BOOST YOUR BRAINPOWER
ATTACK AGING AT THE CELLULAR LEVEL
EXTEND YOUR LIFE SPAN

Most Americans would think that the writer of a book with this cover language is a "snake oil salesman." Dr. Smith expected to have additional editions of the book, which did not occur. Nearly 20 years after that book's publication, there is additional scientific support for all of the claims on his book cover. I am trying to improve my health and functioning in each of those areas and believe that I'm making good or excellent progress in all of them. If this is a very interesting subject for you, you can buy one of Dr. Smith's books on the Internet.

Subjects not included in this chapter. Anti-wrinkling creams, hair coloring, hair restoration, breast augmentation, face lifts, cosmetic surgery.

If you have seen a picture of me, age 74, in this book, you may have noticed that my hair is fairly light brown. I have never used hair coloring. Since the early 1980s, I've taken vitamin B12 once or twice a day. A benefit of B12 is that it tends to prevent your hair from turning white.

Author's relevant experience. As you may have already read, I have had to work determinedly to overcome several types of health problems, nearly all of which I did not create for myself. I could have been a premature casualty of several of those problems.

Recently, a cousin who knows me very well said to me, "John, I think you are better positioned to enjoy living in your 90s than any other person I know." Of course, I was delighted to hear those words as I was approaching 74.

When I was 26, a person asked me if a brother who is eight years older than me was my twin brother. From that time through probably my late 60s, everyone who guessed how old I was guessed that I was older than I was. Since I turned 73, people have consistently guessed that I'm younger than I am, sometimes significantly younger. Maybe my substantial anti-aging efforts are paying off. (I do a high percentage of the things recommended in the VCR below.)

I am not exaggerating in saying that usually I feel as good as I did in my 30s. It is possible that a supplement I take, Elysium (discussed later), helps with this.

Importance of this subject. In an article ("What is the role of genetics compared to environment in aging?") on the sharecare.com website, Dr. Michael Roizen, MD, states that genetics account for 25% a person's aging. So, ordinarily, a person can, over time, greatly influence her or his own aging and longevity.

Nearly all humans want to live as long as possible with good health. It's obvious, therefore, that many people will be interested in learning highly credible information about things to do to slow and maybe, in some cases, reverse aging.

Persons who are especially interested in this subject may benefit from knowing that the following two organizations exist: Buck Institute for Healthy Aging and the American Federation for Aging Research.

Relevance for young adults. Research has shown that cardiovascular disease can start to develop in the bodies of children. As I have mentioned earlier, Dr. Richard Isaacson and Christopher Ochner, PhD, have recently had a book published (Isaacson & Ochner, 2016) about prevention of Alzheimer's disease and other dementia. They emphasize that the earliest evidence of development of Alzheimer's disease appears in the bodies of humans during early adulthood.

If a person genuinely wants to live a long, healthy, and happy life, there is no question that the person should start to learn and implement anti-aging approaches as early as possible during adulthood.

The importance of joint health. The supplement-and-exercise routine (vascular cleansing routine (VCR)) below is primarily concerned with heart and brain health. I want to mention now the unfortunate truth that having problems concerning the health and comfort of your joints, especially your knees and hips, tends to make a person look and feel old. In chapter 5, I tell some about approaches (mainly taking chondroitin-sulfate for many years) that I have used to maintain, and sometimes restore, my joint health and comfort. During the summer of 2017, I experienced significant hip pain and discomfort. Frankly, I was afraid that I was headed for hip replacement. I purchased a supplement formula, LunarFlex PM. The formula is said to help with sleep (which is occurring for me) and with health and comfort of joints, which is also occurring. I want to provide full disclosure here. I expect that I will protect my right hip from unnecessary exertion and strain for the rest of my life. That is much better than needing to have hip-replacement surgery.

The anti-aging benefits of working hard to maintain competence in difficult activities. Decades ago, I decided to try to play golf reasonably well through my 70s because I had two uncles (one on each side) who played tennis or golf quite well through their 70s. Each lived to his 90s and did not fall prey to dementia, even though each had two sisters who did. Now 74, I am sure that this is an excellent goal for me. Incredibly, I in the spring and summer of 2018 experienced substantial improvement of my golf game. Though I am a decent golfer now, I knew a Pinehurst golfer in his middle 70s and two Hendersonville, NC, golfers in their middle 70s who have been significantly better golfers than me in that age range. All three of them work or worked consistently on physical strength for golf.

As you may know by now, I work very hard also on remaining competitive in bridge. As a "night owl," nearly every night at 1:00 a.m., I study two free Internet websites (Bridgeclues2 and Frank Stewart bridge) about bridge. Because duplicate bridge is a very difficult activity, I have had to experiment to discover the best things to do to prepare to play well.

Two additional books about anti-aging approaches. If this topic appeals to you, you may want to buy one or both of following books.

> de Grey, Aubrey (2008). *Ending aging: the rejuvenation breakthroughs that could reverse human aging in our life time.* NY, NY: St. Martin's Press.

> Null, Gary (2003). *Power aging: the revolutionary program to control the symptoms of aging naturally.* Stamford, CT: Bottom Line Books.

The importance of CVD (cardiovascular disease) prevention. The information in this chapter has primary goals of preventing CVD (cardiovascular disease) and brain disease and even improving heart and brain health and brain function. A combination of cardiovascular disease and deterioration of brain health can cause a person to look and seem older than she is. So, if you succeed in improving your heart and brain health, you will be slowing your aging in important ways. Of course, this chapter includes extensive information about preventing or retarding other aspects of aging.

Supplements which help against aging. In chapter 4 of this book, you read about selected supplements which can, especially along with exercise, improve some aspect of your health and functioning, which will have an anti-aging effect. Here are some examples:

Ubiquinol. At some time in one's 40s, the human body becomes much less able to convert ordinary coenzyme Q10 (ubiquinone) into the form which "does the work," ubiquinol. The ubiquinol supplement is worth the price.

Supplements which promote production of nitric oxide. L-arginine supplementation causes production of nitric oxide. There is evidence that around the age of 40 our bodies become less able to allow arginine to produce nitric oxide, which is extremely important for health. I recently started having excellent heart beat slowing effects of taking, instead of l-arginine, l-arginine/citrulline. You can take an expensive supplement, CircO2, which is "guaranteed" to achieve production of nitric oxide. The cost is about $1.25 per day. Another approach is to buy l-citrulline powder and consume it with a beverage.

Alpha-lipoic acid. Glutathione is produced in the body after the consumption of alpha-lipoic acid or an expensive cold-processed whey protein, followed by exercise. Research suggests that glutathione, Dr. Oz's "superhero of the antioxidants," has a wide variety of positive functions in the human body. I think this should be a crucial aspect of anti-aging efforts.

DMG. DMG is close in composition to the B vitamins. I have only recently learned that Balch & Balch, the authors of an influential book about supplements, **recommend DMG for 48 different health conditions**.

As a person ages, her or his body gradually loses the ability to produce DMG. So, it would not be irresponsible for you to consider taking DMG regularly.

Nattokinase. Nattokinase is derived from a type of soy cheese. It has a powerful ability to dissolve blood clots. As we age, the potential for blood clots causing a heart attack, stroke, deep vein thrombosis, or pulmonary embolism increases. Especially when you expect to be sitting for a long stretch of hours, it will make sense to take nattokinase.

Tocotrienols. Telomeres are extensions from some cells that shorten as we age. Byron J. Richards, board certified clinical nutritionist, has an article on his website with the title, "Tocotrienols extend telomeres and turn back the clock," dated February 2013. He describes research that showed that, in addition to extending telomeres, tocotrienols have other anti-aging benefits. For example, tocotrienols help with reversal of atherosclerosis.

Turmeric and vitamin D3. Taking curcumin/turmeric and vitamin D3 together at bedtime apparently can help the brain in its nightly process of clearing out beta-amyloid plaques in the brain. That is the plaque found in the brains of persons with Alzheimer's. People in India, where there is nearly no Alzheimer's or other dementia, consume a lot of turmeric in curry.

Resveratrol. Several years ago, there was a terrific amount of interest in the telomeres of our cells. As mentioned above, the shorter a telomere is, the closer the cell is to death. I have purchased from a highly reputable physician a book in which he claims that taking resveratrol, a powerful antioxidant found in red wine and grape juice, can prompt the production of telomerase, which is supposed to cause actual lengthening of telomeres. I recently came across a study which found that consuming resveratrol does not have the expected benefits. My reading suggests to me that there is still a possibility of significant benefits of resveratrol. Especially because it is important for heart and brain health to have enough antioxidants, I continue to take reservatrol about every other day.

Folate. I have recently become aware of potential health problems for men when they get too much folic acid from diet and supplements. Folate is vitamin B9 and is found especially in foods like greens, broccoli, and Brussels sprouts. Folic acid is a synthesized product which is not nearly as easily digested and metabolized in the human body as folate is. There is strong evidence that folate has cardiovascular health benefits for women. Unless a man is challenged regarding brain function, he shouldn't take folic acid.

DHA. DHA is an omega-3 found in fish oil. A high percentage of the human brain is DHA.

<u>"Pricey" supplements and supplement formulas you may decide to include in your routine.</u> It may help you to know about several supplements and supplement formulas, including cost.

Telovite. Research suggests that an enzyme, telomerase, can slow or even reverse shortening of telomeres.

Telovite is a patented supplement formula including 14 ingredients which are said to produce telomerase. Telovite can be taken as a substitute for a multivitamin. A bottle provides capsules for a month, and four bottles can be bought for $49.95 each. So, the cost can be about $1.70 per day.

GliSODin. GliSODin is a patented antioxidant with important anti-inflammatory effects. The formula is derived partly from cantaloupes. A substantial amount of scientific research has been done regarding health effects and benefits of GliSODin. If I wanted to achieve some regression of atherosclerosis (I don't need to, having done so decades ago.), I would very seriously consider this product. GliSODin is said to reduce problems regarding oxidative stress. Below is a quote from the evercare BrilliantBrightBrain website:

> "Oxidative stress is known to significantly contribute to the process of inflammation, which underpins conditions like rheumatoid arthritis, metabolic syndrome, and diabetes, as well as to neurodegenerative diseases like Alzheimer's."

The cost is about $.55 per day. To purchase, you can simply search for "buy GliSODin" on the Internet. If a person is concerned about having some hardening of the arteries and about potential brain health and function problems, buying and taking GliSODin is, I think, a "no-brainer".

OmegaKrill 5X. This is a patented and heavily promoted omega-3 oil formula from BioTrust. It includes more DHA than ordinary fish oil and includes krill oil, which contains astaxanthin, a powerful antioxidant. There are several apparently costly steps in the manufacturing which are said to produce a substantially superior product with better health benefits. The cost is a little less than $1 per day.

Kyolic Garlic Extract Cardiovascular Formula #100. The cardiovascular-health benefits of garlic are so numerous and great that it makes sense to invest in an excellent garlic supplement, which this appears to be. The cost is about $.30 per day.

Elysium. This is an anti-aging supplement that was developed by the head of the anti-aging center at MIT. I believe in Elysium as much as I believe in alpha-lipoic acid and the glutathione it produces.

L-carnosine. (500 mg) When you have many sugar molecules in your system, they "glom" onto fats and proteins in a process known as glycation. This forms advanced glycation end products (AGEs), which causes protein fibers to become stiff and malformed. Research has indicated that l-carnosine prevents glycation. L-carnosine is a dipeptide that is ordinarily produced in sufficient amounts in the bodies of young people. As with ubiquinol, not enough l-carnosine is produced in the bodies of elderly people. By preventing glycation, l-carnosine tends to retard an aspect of aging. Dr. Oz has called l-carnosine "the miracle pill to stop aging." The cost per day should be $.60 or less. You can take l-alanine, which is less expensive, and your body may produce l-carnosine.

Phosphatidylserine. This product is derived from lecithin. The primary intended benefit is the improvement of cognitive functioning. I have recently learned about a great deal of research showing impressive cognitive functioning benefits of phosphatidylserine. The supplement companies have so much confidence in it that it is included in several expensive cognitive functioning supplements. Several companies sell phosphatidylserine with a cost of about $2 per day.

Brain Ammo. Life Essentials sells this product. While Procera AVH and Cognizin have been shown in research to have cognitive functioning benefits, I believe that Brain Ammo has better ingredients, based on recent research. Those ingredients are phosphatidylserine (most important), gingko biloba, acetyl-carnitine, St. John's wort, l-glutamine, DMAE, bacopin, and vinpocetin. The cost per day is slightly less than $2. Anyone with the slightest concern about cognitive function (e.g., memory, alertness, etc.) should take one of these cognitive functioning supplement formulas.

Procera AVH. This is a cognitive-functioning patented formula which was tested through clinical trials. So, there is scientific evidence that it works.

Cognizin IQ 150. I know less about this patented cognitive functioning formula.

Advanced Memory Formula. Advanced Bionutritionals sells this product. This formula contains eight well selected ingredients. For a six-month supply, the cost is a little more than $1 per day. I have been taking this product for about three years and am happy with the apparent benefits.

Cresceo. This patented cognitive-functioning formula was developed by or for Dr. Daniel Amen, noted psychiatrist, who has become an important neuroscientist.

Blood Pressure Essentials. This BP formula is from Optimal Naturals. The cost per day of this product should be less than $.60 per day. If you have troublesome elevation of BP, I suggest that you read chapter 7.

Ways to increase normal production of human growth hormone (HGH) in the body. There could be a full chapter about human growth hormone. I strongly believe that working to increase my natural production of HGH for several decades has been worthwhile for me. The following actions increase production of HGH: taking glutamine; taking melatonin,; possibly consuming lecithin; taking l-lysine; taking l-arginine, waiting a while, and then exercising; taking goji-berry supplement, eating goji berries; physical exercise; avoiding high glycemic-index carbohydrates; and weight lifting with high repetitions. While I would never take HGH injections or HGH in pill form, my impression is that increasing your HGH by these natural means can have a wide variety of benefits. Research which involved HGH injections for the experimental group but not for the control group resulted in more lean muscle mass, less fat tissue, and thicker skin for the experimental group (Rudman et al, 1990). I have not found good scientific evidence about effects of production of HGH by natural means and have no research evidence that this has heart-or brain-health benefits. Natural production of HGH may help with the improvement of sexual enjoyment, athletic performance, and stamina/energy/strength.

An anti-aging routine for women. Obviously, you may decide to add some of the supplements described above to the routine (VCR) below or take them separately.

Even though this routine as given below is for women, there are very few changes needed for it to be appropriate for men. Instead of taking 25 mg of DHEA, men can take 50 mg. It is especially important for women to take folate instead of folic acid. Unless a man is experiencing troubling "senior moments," it would probably be better for him not to take folic acid.

Anti-Aging Vascular Cleansing Routine (VCR) for Women
(I encourage you to study the supplement information above and select additional supplements to take, possibly at a different time in the day.)

Supplements to take> > > > > Wait 30 minutes> > > > > Get 20 to 40 min. of
with large gl. water   moderate exercise.
magnesium-citrate (200–400 mg)
fish oil (1000 mg)
vitamin B6 (100 mg)
l-arginine (500 mg)
alpha-lipoic acid (600 mg)
coenzyme Q10 (200 mg) or, if
over 45, ubiquinol (100 mg)
DHA (300 mg)
potassium (100 mg)
vitamin C (500 mg)
garlic (dose according to type)
lecithin (1300 mg)
coconut oil (3 capsules)
ginkgo biloba (60 mg)
green tea extract (500 mg)
If "bad lipids profile,"
niacin (500 mg)
If not "bad lipids profile"
niacin (200 mg)

At another time in the day,
take w/ lrg. glass of water
vitamin D3 (2000 to 5000 iu or
as directed by MD)
vitamin B12 (1000 mcg)
coconut oil (2 capsules)
folate (400 mcg)
DHEA (25 mg or as directed
by an MD)
turmeric (500 mg)
chromium picolinate (200 mcg)
If "bad lipids profile,"
niacin (500 mg)
lecithin (1300 mg)

Exercise as part of your program. It is recommended that you perform the detailed program above at least four times, maybe more, per week.

As mentioned previously, strenuous exercise actually makes your blood platelets stickier, and moderate exercise makes your blood platelets less sticky (Wang et al, 1994). While avoiding strenuous exercise, you can do exercise in addition to a supplement-and-exercise routine (VCR). Getting at least 30 minutes of moderate exercise per day is a good goal. I have walked about 22,000 miles while playing golf and have no doubt that doing so has been very helpful regarding my heart and brain health. As discussed previously, EWOT (exercise with oxygen therapy) involves setting an oxygen concentrator gauge between 5 and 10 and getting meaningful exercise for 15 minutes. EWOT has so many health benefits that, for a person wanting to do potentially helpful anti-aging activities, there are strong arguments for doing it nearly every day. During EWOT, I use all of my ankle and wrist weights to increase the demands of walking very briskly in my house.

Increasing your stamina by gradually increasing the intensity of your exercise. One way to do this is to buy adjustable wrist and/or ankle weights (You can buy Gold's Gym adjustable weights at Walmart.) and gradually increase the amount of weight you use while walking or jogging. Now, instead of doing that, I walk as briskly as I can.

Benefits of exercise against aging. There is a detailed list of benefits of exercise in chapters 1 and 6 of this book. Nearly all of those benefits will help with slowing aging. The Alzheimer's Foundation states that exercise reduces the risk of Alzheimer's by 50%. There is a tendency for older people who exercise a lot to have good or excellent brain function.

You probably see evidence of benefits of exercise among your acquaintances.

Some experimentation by you. Since people vary in many important ways, it may help you to experiment to see which supplements and how much of what types of exercise seem to work best for you.

Foods which help against aging.
Fresh fruits and vegetables, especially greens
Cruciferous vegetables (e.g., broccoli, Brussels sprouts, etc.)
Other fruits, especially blueberries and other berries, and vegetables
Enough protein, including omega-3 rich fish
Whole-grain foods, whole-grain pasta (complex carbohydrate food)
Brown rice
Watermelon
Red wine (women, one glass; men, 1.5 or 2 glasses)
Nuts
Dark chocolate
Avocado
Garlic
Ginger
Some soy foods (for women, not men)
Water (Sufficient hydration is very important. Dehydration can result in brain shrinkage.)

Behaviors which tend to increase longevity.

Avoidance of obesity. How many obese very old people do you know?
Maintenance of social connections. Church, family, bridge clubs, tennis group, friends, and many other types of affiliation help.

"Stress busting". If you have a major source of stress in your life, try to figure out how to solve the problem(s) or at least reduce the stress.

Volunteering

Being married. Married people tend to live longer.

Having an active sex life

Keeping your cool. Fortunately, we have some control over how often we get made and even how mad we get.

Getting enough sleep

Taking a multivitamin

Flossing every day. I carefully pick all of my teeth several times every day.

Having a pet

Belonging to a spiritual community

Having a medical checkup regularly

Being optimistic is better for longevity than being pessimistic.

REFERENCES

de Grey, Aubrey (2008). *Ending aging: the rejuvenation breakthroughs that could reverse human aging in our life time*. NY, NY: St. Martin's Press.

Isaacson, Richard & Ochner, Christopher (2016). *The Alzheimer's prevention and treatment diet: using nutrition to combat the effects of Alzheimer's disease*. Garden City Park, NY: SquareOne Publishers.

Null, Gary (2003). *Power aging: the revolutionary program to control the symptoms of aging naturally*. Stamford, CT: Bottom Line Books.

Smith, Timothy (1998). *Renewal: the anti-aging revolution*. Emmaus, PA: Rodale Press.

— SECTION 5 —
Mental Health

— CHAPTER 14 —
Ways to Prevent or Deal with Anxiety and Stress

Importance of this subject. "One third of Americans are living with extreme stress" is a quote from an article, "Stress a major problem in the U.S.," on the website of the American Psychological Association.

Having significant problems with anxiety is a type of mental illness. A *Newsweek* article (Bekiempis, 2014) reported that about one in five Americans suffer from mental illness each year. Mental illness can lead to engaging in many types of self-destructive behavior and, for some people, failure to do what is needed to protect and improve health.

Very current event showing the effects of "stress" on human behavior. In the Master's golf tournament in early April of 2018, Jordan Spieth was, as his Sunday round began, so far behind that he felt no stress. Late in the round, he was 9 under par for the day and tied for the lead. Rory McIlroy started three strokes behind the leader, Patrick Reed, and knew that a win in the Master's would move him up substantially in the hierarchy of golf greatness. McIlroy entirely failed to meet the challenges of his very difficult situation and played two over par for the day. (This obviously shows connections between this chapter and chapter 36 about high-risk activities and decision making.)

<u>Elaboration.</u>

Clarification of definitions. In the medical literature, "stressors" are things that cause "stress", which is the physiological stress reaction (also called the "fight-or-flight" reaction).

Great significance of "stress" as a cause of cardiovascular disease. In an important book Scottish physician Dr. Malcolm Kendrick (2008) argues persuasively that the physiological stress reaction is by far the most important cause of cardiovascular disease (CVD). He compares CVD rates in several countries during several periods in history and makes a strong case that, in every case, high CVD rates were associated with unusually high rates of "stress" experienced by the residents before and during those high-CVD periods.

Tendency of physiological stress reaction to cause increase of blood sugar. Anxiety and emotional stressors can cause the body to experience the physiological stress reaction. This causes increase of blood sugar, which will increase danger of developing type 2 diabetes.

<u>Relevance for young adults.</u> Young adults encounter many types of stressful challenges, including the need to complete education and pay higher-education debt, find and succeed in a job, be financially self-sufficient, and more. Unquestionably, early adulthood tends to be very stressful.

<u>Author's expertise and experience.</u> Though I am not now an expert concerning "stress" or even "work-related stress," my doctoral dissertation in criminology at Florida State University concerned work-related stress and had the title "Work-related stress of state criminal trial court judges" (Memory, 1981).

When I practiced law briefly after law school, before going on active duty in the Army, I discovered that ordinary civilian practice of law was too stressful for me. So, I have more than a scholarly interest in "stress." Years ago, I happened upon the statistic that about one of eight practicing lawyers is giving some thought to committing suicide. When I was a JAG captain in the 82nd Airborne Division (1971–73), we had PT (physical training) about three days a week at 7:00 a.m. That exercise helped me to deal successfully with the potential for stress and anxiety as an active duty Army lawyer.

During 2015, after moving from the NC mountains to a house I owned in South Carolina, I tried very hard to get my house in the NC mountains sold. As my fund of available cash was being depleted by having two mortgages to pay, I developed continuing, chronic anxiety that was harmful to my health and wellbeing. One result was occasional tachycardia (my pulse going to 180 bpm and staying there), which resulted in several visits to the emergency room. So, I know what chronic serious anxiety feels like.

Goals of this chapter. This chapter is for people who especially want help in dealing with stress and anxiety, in addition to help in preventing heart and brain disease. As you will shortly see, when you deal better with stress, you will tend to improve your cardiovascular health. Then, as you improve your cardiovascular health, you will greatly improve your prospects regarding brain health and function.

Distinguishing anxiety and stress. When you are anxious, you are worrying about the possibility that something bad will happen. You may be anxious about the possibility that you or your actions will prove to be inadequate in some way. When you experience stress, you generally are feeling inadequate in some way. You tend to feel stressed when you are experiencing the physiological stress reaction.

Related research. Salmon (2001) has concluded, based on review of relevant research, that exercise training helps a person to cope with stress.

Two Harvard scientists (Kubzansky & Kawachi, 2000) have reviewed research concerning the contribution of emotions to the development of CVD (cardiovascular disease). They found that there is strong evidence that anxiety results in cardiovascular disease but that the evidence relating to anger and depression is not strong. This may be because anxiety is much more likely to involve occurrence of the physiological stress reaction than anger or depression.

Researchers who reviewed research concerning the effects of life stress and social support on development of coronary heart disease (CHD) (Greenwood et al, 1996) found that psychosocial stress tended to be associated with development of CHD and that social support tended to inhibit the development of CHD.

Some definitions. "Stressors" are the things that cause a person to experience the physiological stress reaction, and "stress" is that physiological reaction. (Contributing to misunderstandings, the stress reaction is also called the "fight-or-flight reaction" and, especially in medical literature, the "general adaptation syndrome.") A very wide variety of things can be stressors, such as feeling somehow inadequate in a situation, danger, threat, talking or singing in public, doing a difficult and important function in work (qualitative stress), having too much work to do (quantitative stress), having to take care of an unappreciative, uncooperative relative, trying to do something difficult and important in sports, loneliness, feeling very angry, and many more things.

Stress causes the body to secrete "stress hormones," cortisol and epinephrine (adrenaline).

Supplements which should help regarding stress. Supplements that should help you with stress coping include lecithin (1200 mg), fish oil (1000 mg), niacin (250 to 500 mg), melatonin (5 mg) (at bedtime), alpha-lipoic acid (600 mg) (before exercise), and magnesium (400 mg). For more omega-3 fatty acids, you can eat some walnuts. Eating almonds may help. Later in this chapter, there is a recommended routine, which includes these supplements and exercise. Research has indicated that GliSODin has benefits regarding avoidance of adverse effects of stress (GliSODin technical publication, 2012). The cost of GliSODin is about $.55 per day. Research has shown that phosphatidylserine helps significantly with brain function. While phosphatidylserine alone can cost $2 per day, you can obtain it along with seven other well selected ingredients in the patented formula, Advanced Memory Formula, for a little over $1 per day.

Irwin Naturals markets a supplement formula with the following language on the bottle: "Stress-Defy. Balanced-Relaxed-Calm. Stressful Day Neutralizer."

The importance of good brain function in "dealing with stress." If your brain is working well, you should have good ability to solve problems which have potential to make your life stressful. If your brain is working well, you should have good ability to think and otherwise perform in "stressful situations." So, it makes sense to consider taking a cognitive-function supplement formula to help in coping with stress. Chapters 11 and 12 provide information about this.

Some experimentation by you. Since people vary in many important ways, it may help you to experiment to see which supplements and how much of what types of exercise help you the most in dealing with stress and anxiety.

Important books about dealing with "stress." I strongly recommend that persons who feel they have major "stress" problems in their lives obtain Dr. Lisa Rankin's book (2013), *Mind over Medicine*. She emphasizes that self-sabotaging thought, negative thoughts generally, helplessness, and loneliness are stressful and increase adverse health effects of the stress reaction. Ways to get rid of the stress reaction and allow natural self-repair in our bodies include meditation, relaxation, dancing, exercising, and laughing. Of course, relationships help us to overcome loneliness.

Wayne Froggatt is a counselor and very successful writer on subjects relating to psychology and psychotherapy who lives in New Zealand. He is the author of a book, *Taking Control* (2006), which is primarily intended to help people with problems concerning stress management.

Ideas from the "guru" of scientific study of and dealing with stress. Hans Selye, the aforementioned guru, recommended an approach to stress, which he described as "living wisely in accordance with natural laws." In his classic book *The Stress of Life* (1978), he discussed the following as important dimensions of living wisely:

Adopting an attitude of gratitude toward life, rather than seeking revenge for injuries or slights.

Acting toward others from altruistic, rather than self-centered motives.

Retaining a capacity for wonder and delight in the genuinely good and beautiful things in life.

Finding a purpose for one's life and expressing one's individuality in fulfilling that purpose.

Keeping a healthy sense of modesty about one's goals or achievements.

The author's thinking about a synergistic spiraling upward of health, wellbeing, and happiness. To help you to understand what synergy is, I will give an example. If parents relate to a child with love but not reasonable discipline (expectation of moral behavior), there is a substantial chance there will be problems with the child. If the parents relate to the child with reasonable discipline but not with love, there is a substantial chance there will be problems with the child. Fortunately, if the parents relate to the child with love **and** reasonable discipline, there is an excellent chance that there will not be problems with the child. There can be positive synergy of the love with the reasonable discipline, with each supporting the other.

There is giant potential for positive synergy relating to stress coping, heart health, and brain health. Here is a model about that. The arrows indicate that the process which sends out the arrows tends to promote achievement of the thing that the arrows point to.

Efforts to avoid, reduce and cope with stress in >>>> healthy ways	Efforts to improve cardiovascular >>>> health	Efforts to improve brain health and function
^		v
^		v
^		v
Efforts to increase happiness and <<<<<<<<<<< avoid depression	Efforts to perform well to reduce <<<<< stress	Efforts to solve problems to reduce problems with stress and improve your well being

We often hear of a "spiraling down" of a person's health. This model depicts the exact opposite—a spiraling upward relating to a person's health, wellbeing, and happiness. Every time you make progress in one of these six efforts, you tend to promote achievement of the other efforts. Fortunately for me, those types of favorable things have occurred in my life.

Synergy regarding nutrition (including supplements) and exercise. Happily, all of the supplements which are suggested in this chapter to help with stress also help with cardiovascular and brain health. Exercise helps in achieving all six of the efforts above. Very significantly, there is substantial positive synergy of good nutrition and moderate exercise.

"Stress busting." Solving problems which result in experiencing stress is part of the model above. Americans seem to be attracted to the idea of energetically "going at" stress and problems and situations which cause stress. Stress generally involves some sort of at least perceived inadequacy. Problems continue as a result of inadequacy in solving the problem, and the problem itself can involve some type of inadequacy. The obvious point is that problems and "stress" tend to be very closely connected in our lives.

Deep breathing in stressful situations. Some basketball players take a deep breath before shooting a free throw. Partly because I have a problem regarding level of dissolved oxygen in my blood, I take deep breaths often while playing duplicate bridge and playing golf. A deep breath tends to oxygenate your brain and can help you to relax and think and perform well.

Stress-related benefits of relaxation and meditation. Though relaxation and meditation have not been important in mental health promotion for me, there is an extensive body of literature that documents that both relaxation and meditation have benefits against problematic potential to experience the physiological stress reaction (to become over-stressed).

Using relaxation against stress and anxiety. For some people, regular relaxation is very important against stress and anxiety. You can do a search for "use of relaxation against stress and/or anxiety" and select an approach that appeals to you.

Using meditation against stress and anxiety. Similarly, for some people, using a carefully selected meditation routine can help greatly against stress and anxiety. You can do a search for "meditation routine against stress and anxiety" and select an approach that appeals to you.

A suggested supplement-and-exercise routine (VCR). Even though the routine as given below is for women, there are very few changes needed for it to be appropriate for men. Instead of taking 25 mg of DHEA, men can take 50 mg. It is especially important for women to take folate instead of folic acid. Unless a man is experiencing troubling "senior moments," it would probably be better for him not to take folic acid.

A Routine (VCR) for Women about Reduction of and Coping with Stress
(You should select and add some supplements described above.)

Supplements to take> > > > > Wait 30 minutes> > > > Get 20 to 40 min. of
with large gl. water   moderate exercise.
magnesium-citrate (200–400 mg)
fish oil (1000 mg)
vitamin B6 (100 mg)
l-arginine (500 mg) or, if over 45, l-arginine/citrulline
alpha-lipoic acid (600 mg)
coenzyme Q10 (200 mg) or, if
over 45, ubiquinol (100 mg)
DHA (300 mg)
potassium (100 mg)
vitamin C (500 mg)
garlic (dose according to type)
lecithin (1300 mg)
coconut oil (3 capsules)
ginkgo biloba (60 mg)
green tea extract (500 mg)
If "bad lipids profile,"
niacin (500 mg)
If not "bad lipids profile"
niacin (200 mg)

At another time in the day,
take w/ lrg. glass of water
vitamin D3 (2000 to 5000 iu or as directed by MD)
vitamin B12 (1000 mcg)
folate (400 mcg)
DHEA (25 mg or as directed by an MD)
turmeric (500 mg)
chromium picolinate (200 mcg)
If "bad lipids profile,"
niacin (500 mg)
lecithin (1300 mg)
melatonin (5 mg) (at bedtime)

Exercise as part of your program. It is recommended that you perform the VCR above at least four times, maybe more, per week.

Strenuous exercise actually makes your blood platelets stickier, and moderate exercise makes your blood platelets less sticky (Wang et al, 1994). If you decide to do strenuous exercise, it will be especially important for you to take before that exercise supplements that have enough anti-coagulant and antioxidant effects. Nattokinase is an effective anti-coagulant. Obviously, **a person wanting to prevent a stroke or deep vein thrombosis (DVT) must avoid strenuous exercise**.

While avoiding strenuous exercise, you can do exercise in addition to a supplements-and-exercise routine. Getting at least 30 minutes of moderate exercise every day is a good goal. I have walked more than 22,000 miles while playing golf. Since learning that EWOT (exercise with oxygen therapy) is a recognized anti-cancer treatment, I have been doing EWOT nearly every day. It involves setting an oxygen concentrator gauge between 5 and 10 and then getting meaningful exercise for exactly 15 minutes—no more, no less. To make my walking in my house more demanding, I use ankle and wrist weights.

Increasing your stamina by gradually increasing the intensity of your exercise. One way to do this is to buy adjustable wrist and ankle weights (You can buy Gold's Gym adjustable weights at Walmart.) and gradually increase the amount of weight you use while walking or jogging. Now, my main exercise is walking as briskly as I can, pumping my arms along with my leg movements.

Some experimentation by you. Since people vary in many important ways, it may help you to experiment to see which supplements and how much of what types of exercise seem to work best for you.

Ideas about dealing specifically with anxiety.

Anxiety remedies. You can search on the Anxiety Remedies website for "2016 Looking for a natural anxiety remedy that actually works." You may find helpful information there.

Taking anti-anxiety medication when needed. There can be times when, for some people, everything in this chapter will not totally "get the job done" in dealing with stress and anxiety. For example, anxiety resulting from stressful life situations and the stress reaction can be one of the triggers of tachycardia, which is elevated pulse which can be as high as 200 beats per minute. For some people, this type of tachycardia can be life-threatening by causing a heart attack or stroke. One type of help in dealing with chronic anxiety can be anti-anxiety medication prescribed by a psychiatrist or other physician.

Talking therapy. It may help to have "talking therapy" with a qualified practitioner, such as a PhD clinical psychologist or a psychiatrist. This talking therapy can involve developing good strategies for dealing healthfully with stressors, stress and anxiety. Unfortunately, many psychologists don't know much about psychological and health benefits of supplements and exercise.

Some ideas about diet. It should help to follow eating suggestions in chapter 3 of this book. Here are a few very specific suggestions.

Some recommended things to eat or drink. Dark chocolate, nuts, coconut oil, olive oil (including butter substitute with olive oil as the main ingredient), fresh fruits and vegetables. Consume only a small amount of coffee and other caffeinated beverages and foods.

Some things to avoid eating or drinking. Sugary beverages, sugary desserts (limit consumption), refined carbohydrate foods, "white foods" (including rice, potatoes, ordinary pasta), saturated fats. (Though coconut oil is saturated, consuming it is health-enhancing in several ways.)

Research findings released in 2012 indicate that, among 6,183 women over 65 tracked for four years, consumption of saturated fat (animal fat) was associated with decline in "memory and abstract thinking," while consumption of monounsaturated fat (primarily olive oil) was associated with significantly less cognitive decline (Okereke, Olivia, 2012).

Information specifically about anti-stress diet. The Stress Management Society has an excellent document on the Internet with the title "Combating stress with a balanced nutritional diet." Dr. Oz has on the internet information with the title "Cortisol-reduction grocery list."

Stress management. There is a very detailed and helpful article about stress management, "Stress management," December 2011, by Melinda Smith, M.A. and Robert Segal, M.A. on the helpguide.org website.

Try to always be and act as a good, decent, and honest person. We've all heard the "folk wisdom" that "Honesty is the best policy." A "good and decent" person is not just honest. One way to communicate this fairly well is that she or he probably tries to abide by the Golden Rule, "Do unto others as you would have them do unto you."

If you do this, you may be able to avoid many types of events that can create more life stress for you and make having good mental health more difficult.

Value of humor. Be alert to notice if you encounter something that is funny and enjoy it.

REFERENCES

Bekiempis, V. (2014). Nearly 1 in 5 Americans suffers from mental illness each year. *Newsweek*. February 28, 2014.

Foggatt, Wayne (2006). *Taking control*. Auckland, NZ: Harper Collins.

Greenwood, D.C. et al (1996). Coronary heart disease: a review of the role of psychosocial stress and social support. *Journal of Public Health*, Vol. 18, No. 2, pp. 221–31.

Kubzansky, L.D. & Kawachi, I. (2000). Going to the heart of the matter: do negative emotions cause coronary heart disease? *Journal of Psychosomatic Research*, Vol. 48, Issue 4, pp. 323–37.

McKendrick, Malcolm (2008). *The great cholesterol con*. London: John Blake Publishing, Ltd.

Okereke, Olivia et al (2012). Dietary fat types and 4-year cognitive change in community-dwelling older women. *Annals of Neurology*, Vol. 72, No. 1, pp. 124–34.

Rankin, L. (2013). *Mind over medicine*. Carlsbad, CA: Hay House, Inc.

Salmon, P. (2001). Effects of physical exercise on anxiety, depression, and sensitivity to stress: a unifying theory. *Clinical Psychology Review*, Vol. 21, Issue 1, pp. 33–61.

Selye, Hans (1978). *The stress of life*. Columbus, OH: McGraw-Hill Education.

Wang, J.S. et al (1994). Different effects of strenuous exercise and moderate exercise on platelet function in men. *Circulation*, Vol. 90, pp. 2877–2885.

— CHAPTER 15 —
Ways to Prevent, Control, and Reduce Depression

Cautionary statement. Depression is a serious and dangerous mental illness. It can "trick" a person into thinking that she or he cannot have hope for the future. This is proven by the fact that many people who fail in a suicide attempt go on to live enjoyable and fulfilling lives.

This chapter is not primarily intended for people who are experiencing serious "clinical" depression, including people who are having recurring thoughts of suicide. Those persons should as soon as possible obtain treatment by a fully qualified psychiatrist (MD) or psychologist (PhD). Because psychologists and psychiatrists don't always provide helpful information about benefits of exercise and supplements, even people with "clinical" depression may benefit from reading this chapter.

Helpful resources on the Internet. If you would like to read an excellent short article on the Internet about preventing depression, I suggest that you find "Depression prevention—how to prevent depression." Another very well produced resource is on the wikihow.com web site. The title is "WikiHow to prevent depression." In my opinion, both of these articles can be much more helpful than a comparable article on the Mayo Clinic website.

Author's relevant experience. Tragically, more than one of my relatives have committed suicide. So, I am confident that I have inherited vulnerability to becoming depressed. Also, I have low thyroid function (hypothyroidism), which can increase my tendency to become depressed. As any psychiatrist would predict, I have experienced troublesome depression several times. Fortunately, I decided in 1969 to make dealing with my vulnerability to experiencing depression a priority for me. I've learned valuable things about this, such as the depression-reduction benefits of exercise and of taking fish oil. I will, for the rest of my life, take an **extremely** low-dose antidepressant drug and an **extremely** low-dose anti-anxiety drug.

If I had not worked very hard on my physical health, heart health, brain health, and mental health for many decades, I would now, if I were alive, be very much more vulnerable to being depressed than I am.

Importance of this subject. There is on the Health.com website an article with the title "CDC: Nearly 1 in 10 U.S. adults depressed." (September 30, 2010). I have read a credible report that one of eight practicing attorneys is giving some thought to committing suicide. This undoubtably is related to the fact that working in some lawyer specialties is extremely stressful. A *Newsweek* article in 2014 reported that about one in five Americans suffers from mental illness each year (Bekiempis, 2014). Having significant problems with depression is a type of mental illness.

Statistics about suicides and suicide attempts in the U.S. in 2013. In 2013, there were 41,149 suicides in the U.S. The rate was 12.6 per 100,000 population. Males commit suicide at four times as high a rate as females. Among students in grades 9–12, 17% seriously considered committing suicide (22.4%, female; 11.6%, male). **In grades 9–12, 8% of students (10.6%, female; 5.4%, male) attempted suicide one or more times in the previous year.** ("Suicide: facts at a glance in 2013," Centers for Disease Control (CDC))

Relevance for young adults. It is not uncommon for a young adult to experience depression. It is important for young adults to make important decisions, such as decisions about education, career, dating, marriage, children, etc., which will not be likely to result in problems regarding mental health. For example, when I practiced law for six months in NC in 1968–69, I realized that ordinary practice of law was too stressful for me. That was a realistic perception and decision which has helped me to make good decisions about my working career.

Supplements which may help with depression prevention and control. Over many years, I have been impressed with the quality of information on the WebMD web site. For that reason, I am providing here information from that website (Vitamins and Supplements search concerning depression) regarding supplements that help regarding depression. Those supplements and likely effectiveness based on user reviews are: zinc (possibly effective), 5-HTP (possibly effective), DHA (possibily ineffective), DHEA (possibly effective), EPA in fish oil (possibly effective), folic acid (possibly effective), Saffron (possibly effective), SAM-e (likely effective), St. John's Wort (likely effective). There are many other supplements, some of which I think are worth taking, concerning which there is said to be "insufficient evidence" of effectiveness. You can experiment with including these supplements in a supplement-and- exercise routine (VCR), which is provided below.

Benefits of fish oil against depression. Daniel K. Hall-Flavin, MD, is the author of an article on the Mayo Clinic website, "Fish oil supplements: Can they treat depression?" He writes, "Fish oil supplements may help ease symptoms of depression in some people."

A multi-ingredient supplement formula. Irwin Naturals markets a supplement formula with the following language on the bottle: "Sunny Mood. Feel Good, Feel Balanced." This product is intended to help with problems relating to depression.

Talking therapy. For some people with vulnerability to developing depression, having continuing therapy with a qualified and capable therapist (psychiatrist or psychologist) can be extremely helpful. Research has shown that continuing therapy can actually change the structure of the brain.

Taking an anti-depressant drug. If your psychiatrist recommends one or more psychotropic medications, you should take that advice very seriously. At any given time, many millions of Americans are refusing or failing to take prescribed, potentially helpful psychotropic drugs.

Benefits of exercise against depression. In major research, exercise was found to be as effective for old patients as taking an anti-depressant drug in dealing with depression (Blumenthal et al, 1999).

The importance of having hope for the future. Very few feelings and beliefs of humans are as important as hope, which I believe is a combination of a feeling and a belief. Hope (or absence of hope) is crucial concerning many important things, including health motivation, violent crime, self-destructive behavior, retrieving something good from failure, and dealing with anxiety, stress, and depression.

I greatly value the Christian morality I learned as a child. One of the most revered verses of the Bible is 1 Corinthians 13:13. "And now these three remain: faith, hope and love. But the greatest of these is love." I have developed my own adaptation of 1 Corinthians 13:13:

> "And now abideth frugality, problem
> solving, and work; these three;
> but the greatest of these is work."

So, what do I think humans should try to gain or improve through working persistently on solving problems? If you solve or significantly reduce a problem you have, you probably achieve some improvement of your quality of life. Even a fairly small improvement in your quality of life can result in some increase in hope for the future. Improvement in hope reduces vulnerability to becoming depressed.

As a result of trying to live according to this saying, I have been able to put more time and energy into recreation and creativity than most people.

Examples of adverse health consequences of depression and troublesome emotions. A 1998 article (Sesso et al) reports research that showed that depression tends to increase the risk of cardiovascular disease. Other researchers have reported that anger can contribute to later development by the individual of cardiovascular disease (Chang et al, 2002) and to occurrence of myocardial infarction (Mittleman et al, 1995).

Solving problems relating to emotions. Maybe because I inherited a vulnerability to becoming depressed and vulnerability to becoming stressed (experiencing the physiological- stress reaction), I have sometimes experienced negative emotions that have been troubling in number and/or strength. So, I developed many years ago my own strategy for dealing with troubling emotions.

I write on a sheet the date and then some of these questions:

> Troubling emotions exercise   December 14, 2017
>
> What am I depressed about?
> Comment by Elaine
> What am I mad about?
> No response to my email about Forum topic   Email Jim
>
> What am I worried (anxious) about?
> Results of biopsy
>
> What is stressing me?
> Need to pay property tax   Borrow $1850
>
> What am I sad about?
> Rosalie's death   Call Henry

I leave under each question enough space to write a few answers.

I then brainstorm answers to those questions and write the answers under the questions, as shown above. Next, I brainstorm actions I can take to reduce the troubling emotions and write the actions to the right of the troubling emotion I think it can help with, as shown above. **I think it is important to be very careful about actions to take.** It can help to "sleep on" what you have written down for several days. Then, usually for at least a week, I work on carrying out the actions I have listed. When I feel I have carried out an action, I cross it off. Doing this exercise occasionally over many years has helped me significantly.

Relevant information about "stress." People who are depressed often are having problems concerning stress. The same life situation, such as feeling inadequate to deal with a significant problem, can cause depression and "stress." It is important to know that experiencing the physiological stress reaction too much can result in depression and in cardiovascular disease. In his important book (2008) Scottish physician Dr. Malcolm Kendrick argues persuasively that the physiological stress reaction is by far the most important cause of cardiovascular disease. He compares CVD rates in different countries at different periods in history and makes a strong case that, in every case, high CVD rates were associated with unusually high rates of "stress" experienced by the residents before and during those high CVD periods.

Some definitions. Because of the potential for troublesome "stress" to result in depression, some definitions relating to stress are given here.

"Stressors" are the things which cause a person to experience the physiological stress reaction, and "stress" is that physiological reaction. (Contributing to misunderstandings, the stress reaction is also called the fight-or-flight reaction and, especially in medical literature, the "general adaptation syndrome.") An incredibly wide variety of things can be stressors, such as feeling somehow inadequate in a situation, danger, threat, doing a difficult and important function in work (qualitative stress), having too much work to do (quantitative stress), having to take care of an unappreciative, uncooperative relative, trying to do something difficult and important in sports, loneliness, feeling very angry, and many more things.

Stress causes the body to secrete of the "stress hormones," cortisol and epinephrine (adrenaline).

If you think you are experiencing problems concerning stress and/or anxiety, you can get more information and suggestions in chapter 14.

Potential for positive synergy and spiraling upward relating to health and wellbeing. To help you understand what synergy is, I will give an example. If parents relate to a child with love but not reasonable discipline (expectation of moral behavior), there is a big chance there will be problems with the child. If the parents relate to the child with reasonable discipline but not with love, there is a big chance there will be problems with the child. Fortunately, if the parents relate to the child with love and reasonable discipline, there is an excellent chance that there will not be problems with the child. There can be positive synergy of love with reasonable discipline, with each supporting the other. If synergy occurs, the positive effects of the two together are greater than the sum of the positive effects of the two separately.

There is giant potential for positive synergy and spiraling upward relating to coping with stress and depression, heart health, and brain health. Here is a model about that. The arrows indicate that the process which sends out the arrows tends to promote achieving the thing that the arrows point to. Though I developed this model to deal with stress, the model can be adapted to deal with depression. The point is that, if you continue to work on reducing an emotional problem, such as stress or depression, there is a good chance that your life will gradually improve.

Efforts to avoid, reduce and cope with depression in healthy ways	>>	Efforts to improve cardiovascular health	>>>	Efforts to improve brain health and function
^				v
^				v
^				v
Efforts to increase happiness and avoid depression	<<<<<<<<<<<<	Efforts to perform well to reduce depression	<<<	Efforts to solve problems to reduce problems with depression and improve your well being

We often hear of a "spiraling down" of a person's health and wellbeing. This is exactly the opposite—a spiraling upward regarding a person's health, wellbeing, and happiness. Every time you make progress in one of these six efforts, you tend to promote achievement of the other efforts. Those types of things have happened fairly often in my life.

A suggested supplement-and-exercise routine (VCR). I suggest that you experiment regarding taking Saffron, SAM-e, and St. John's Wort. It might be better to take one or more of those supplements at some time in the day other than with the supplements listed below.

Even though this routine as given below is for women, there are very few changes needed for it to be appropriate for men. Instead of taking 25 mg of

DHEA, men can take 50 mg. It is especially important for women to take folate instead of folic acid. Unless a man is experiencing troubling "senior moments," it would probably be better for him not to take folic acid. You can add supplements described above to the following VCR.

ROUTINE (VCR) FOR WOMEN TO PREVENT, CONTROL, OR REDUCE DEPRESSION

Supplements to take> > > > > Wait 30 minutes> > > > > Get 20 to 40 min. of
with large gl. water   moderate exercise.
magnesium-citrate (200–400 mg)
fish oil (1000 mg)
5-HTP
Folic acid
DHEA
Zinc
vitamin B6 (100 mg)
l-arginine (500 mg); if over 45,
l-arginine/citrulline
alpha-lipoic acid (600 mg)
coenzyme Q10 (200 mg) or, if
over 45, ubiquinol (100 mg)
DHA (300 mg)
potassium (100 mg)
vitamin C (500 mg)
garlic (dose according to type)
lecithin (1300 mg)
coconut oil (3 capsules)
ginkgo biloba (60 mg)
green tea extract (500 mg)
If "bad lipids profile,"
niacin (500 mg)
If not "bad lipids profile"
niacin (200 mg)

<u>At another time in the day,</u>
<u>take w/ lrg. glass of water</u>
vitamin D3 (2000 to 5000 iu or
as directed by MD)
vitamin B12 (1000 mcg)
folate (400 mcg)
DHEA (25 mg or as directed
by an MD)
turmeric (500 mg)
chromium picolinate (200 mcg)
If "bad lipids profile,"
niacin (500 mg)
lecithin (1300 mg)
melatonin (5 mg) (at bedtime)

    <u>Exercise as part of your program.</u> I recommend that you perform a routine (VCR) at least four times, maybe more, per week.

    Strenuous exercise actually makes your blood platelets stickier, and moderate exercise makes your blood platelets less sticky (Wang et al, 1994). Obviously, **a person wanting to prevent a stroke or other dangerous blood clot must avoid strenuous exercise**. While avoiding strenuous exercise, you can do exercise in addition to this routine's exercise. Getting at least 30 minutes of moderate exercise every day is a good goal. I have walked more than 22,000 miles while playing golf and have no doubt that doing so has been very helpful regarding my heart and brain health and in dealing healthfully with vulnerability to experiencing depression. In recent years, I would occasionally walk 18 holes of golf in Hendersonville, NC, when I felt somewhat depressed. I could sense **down to the minute** when my walking overcame the depression. Since learning that EWOT (exercise with oxygen therapy) is an accepted anti-cancer treatment, I have been doing it nearly every day. EWOT involves turning the gauge on an oxygen concentrator between 5 and 10 and then getting meaningful exercise for 15 minutes—no more, no less. I believe that EWOT has significant anti-depression effect.

    Increasing your stamina by gradually increasing the intensity of your exercise. One way to do this is to buy adjustable wrist and ankle weights

(You can buy Gold's Gym adjustable weights at Walmart.) and gradually increase the amount of weight you use while walking or jogging. Obviously, you can take as long as you wish in increasing amount of weight. Now, instead of using weights, I walk as briskly as I can, which appears to be sufficiently strenuous for me.

Stress-related benefits of relaxation and meditation. Though relaxation and meditation have not been important in mental health promotion for me, there is an extensive body of literature that documents that both relaxation and meditation have benefits against the problematic potential to experience depression.

Using relaxation against depression. For some people, regular relaxation is very important defense against depression. You can do a search for "use of relaxation against depression" and can select an approach that appeals to you.

Using meditation against depression. Similarly, for some people, using a carefully selected meditation routine can help greatly against depression. You can do a search for "meditation routine against depression" and can select an approach that appeals to you.

Some ideas about diet. It should help to follow eating suggestions in chapter 3 of this book. Here are a few very specific suggestions.

Some things to eat or drink. Dark chocolate, nuts, coconut oil, olive oil (including butter substitute with olive oil as the main ingredient), fresh fruits and vegetables, a limited amount of coffee and other caffeinated foods and beverages

Some things to avoid eating or drinking. Sugary beverages, sugary desserts (limit consumption), refined carbohydrate foods, "white foods" (including rice, potatoes, ordinary pasta), saturated fats

Finding activities that are fun, inexpensive, and brief. I think it can help against a tendency to become depressed to weave into your life schedule activities that are fun, inexpensive, and brief. For me, that includes drinking exactly two glasses of red wine every day, a very hot tub bath (especially in cold weather), eating a nutritious and healthful cereal that includes lots of chocolate, scratching my back with a stiff brush with a long handle, and watching and enjoying a winning sports team. In 2018, I'm enjoying the excellent Atlanta Braves. I believe that, in life, small things can matter.

REFERENCES

Bekiempis, V. (2014). Nearly 1 in 5 Americans suffers from mental illness each year. *Newsweek*. February 28, 2014.

Blumenthal, J.A. et al (1999). Effects of exercise training on older patients with major depression. *Archives of Internal Medicine*, Vol. 159, pp. 2349–2356.

Chang, P.P. et al (2002). Anger in young men and subsequent premature cardiovascular disease: the precursors study. *Archives of Internal Medicine*, Vol. 162, p. 901.

McKendrick, Malcolm (2008). *The great cholesterol con*. London: John Blake Publishing, Ltd.

Mittleman, M.A. et al (1995). Triggering of acute myocardial infarction by episodes of anger. Determinants of Myocardial Infarction Onset Study Investigators. *Circulation*, Vol. 92, p. 1720.

Okereke, Olivia et al (2012). Dietary fat types and 4-year cognitive change in community-dwelling older women. *Annals of Neurology*, Vol. 72, No. 1, pp. 124–34.

Sesso, H.D. et al (1998). Depression and the risk of coronary heart disease in the Normative Aging Study. *American Journal of Cardiology*, Vol. 82, No. 7, p. 851.

Wang, J.S. et al (1994). Different effects of strenuous exercise and moderate exercise on platelet function in men. *Circulation*, Vol. 90, pp. 2877–2885.

—— CHAPTER 16 ——
Self-Destructive and Dangerous Behavior

Acknowledgment. I want to acknowledge that I do not have strong understanding of the types of behaviors that fit in this category. Also, I want to apologize in advance if some sections I have written fail to exhibit compassion for people who, no doubt, are or have been in challenging circumstances in important ways.

Elaboration. Smoking, alcoholism, excessive consumption of alcoholic beverages, abuse of legal drugs, use of illicit drugs, obesity, sedentary lifestyle, and engaging in unreasonably dangerous activities are examples of self-destructive or dangerous behaviors. Of course, suicide and suicide attempts are part of this giant national problem. Addiction-driven gambling usually has adverse effects.

Annual deaths relating to drug use, including tobacco. Tobacco, 480,000; alcohol, 31,000; overdose of illicit drug(s), 22,000 (Internet article based on Centers for Disease Control data: "How many people die each year from drug use"). Opioid overdoses increased from 2500 in 2013 to 20,146 in 2016. The reported drug overdose total in 2016 was 64,070. It was reported on TV that the number of opioid deaths in 2016 was 42,000. As an experienced social scientist, I will state that this is the most startling health-related trend I know of. The end of this trend is not in sight. I believe this phenomenon tells us that there are giant underlying human problems in the U.S. Those problems may be related to economic disparities. During the Trump Presidential campaign in 2015 and 2016, the gap between the wealth and quality of life of the very wealthy and of the poor were more visible than ever in the U.S.

Statistics about suicides and suicide attempts in the U.S. in 2013. In 2013, there were 41,149 suicides in the U.S. The rate was 12.6 per 100,000 population. Men commit suicide at four times as high a rate as women. Among students in grades 9–12, 17% seriously considered committing suicide (22.4%, female; 11.6%, male). **In grades 9–12, 8% of students (10.6%, female; 5.4%, male) attempted suicide one or more times in the previous year** ("Suicide: facts at a glance in 2013," Centers for Disease Control (CDC)). For helpful additional information about suicide in the U.S., go to "Suicide prevention" on the American Foundation for Suicide Prevention website. From 1999 to 2014, suicide in the U.S. increased by 24% (Curtin, et al, 2016).

Connection of self-destructive deaths and academic performance. Students reporting many D's and F's have much higher adverse outcomes from the above causes than students with higher academic performance (Internet article: "CDC releases new data on the connection between health and academics.")

Connection of this topic and the topic of chapter one, health motivation. People who engage in self-destructive behavior probably do not have enough health motivation. They are not sufficiently motivated to avoid behavior that can seriously damage their health. If you fit that description, I would like for you to read chapter one with an open mind. (Heck, read it twice. I need repetition to learn important things.) Maybe this will help you to get onto a safer and more rewarding life path.

I do not know why so much self-destructive behavior occurs in the U.S. For instance, virtually everyone knows that smoking is very hazardous to your health. Still, smoking is a major cause of 480,000 deaths annually in the U.S. If someone asked me, a PhD criminologist, to explain the high rate of self-destructive behavior that violates the criminal law in the U.S., I would answer, "I believe it has something to do with inadequacy of hope for the future." I, however, am not an expert on any type of self-destructive behavior, except for juvenile suicides in secure detention facilities.

Sexual enjoyment and performance benefits of taking supplements, waiting 30 minutes, and then getting nearly strenuous exercise. I hope a significant number of people who are at risk for doing self-destructive activity will learn and remember that taking healthful supplements, waiting 30 minutes, and then getting 30 to 45 minutes of nearly strenuous exercise is very likely to significantly improve your sexual enjoyment and performance. That is discussed in detail early in chapter one.

Author's relevant expertise and experiences. I wrote and had published in a refereed health journal an article (Memory, 1989) about suicide of juveniles in adult jails and was a consulting editor of a refereed health journal, *Suicide and Life-Threatening Behavior,* for two years. As a lawyer and Criminal Justice professor, I was sometimes concerned with self-destructive behavior.

Unfortunately, more than one member of my extended family have committed suicide. As a result of my father's tragic death when I was five, I developed a strong fear of death. Over decades, that fear "morphed" into very strong enjoyment of living. These emotions have motivated me to stay away from self-destructive activities.

Since the early 1970s, I have drunk nearly exactly two glasses of red wine on at least 95% of days. If I drink more than two glasses during a day, I get a bad headache. This "problem" has guaranteed that I will not become an alcoholic or "a problem drinker." I am very aware that many people with more talent and human potential than me have become victims of their own self-destructive behavior.

Living successfully is a difficult activity. Doing self-destructive activities can strongly tend to reduce a person's ability to perform difficult activities well, such as living successfully.

Importance of this subject. The statistics above indicate that there is in the U.S. an alarmingly high rate of several types of self-destructive behavior. Currently, our country is experiencing an epidemic of opioid addiction and overdoses. Several demographic groups in the U.S. are experiencing elevation of suicide rate. These are just the most vivid indicators of the importance of learning about and preventing self-destructive behavior.

It is important for readers and others to understand and remember that the adverse consequences of smoking, excessive drinking of alcoholic beverages, taking dangerous illicit drugs, obesity, and engaging in irresponsibly dangerous activities, such as drunk driving or extremely fast and/or reckless driving, have significant probabilities of occurring and can be very severe. Several decades ago, two Duke University Basketball All-Americans, Bobby Hurley and Jay Williams (who did not play on the same team) shortly after signing extremely lucrative NBA basketball contracts were, in different incidents, injured in a vehicular accident, resulting in the loss of their ability to compete in the NBA. Another example involves the very severe adverse consequences of obesity.

Relevance for young adults. Many knowledgeable people have said something to the effect, "If you aren't moving ahead, you are falling behind." I believe, consistent with this, that, if a young person is not attempting to have a healthful lifestyle, she or he is probably lapsing toward some type of unhealthful lifestyle.

Self-destructive and dangerous behavior is rampant on university and college campuses. That includes excessive and dangerous consumption of alcoholic beverages, use of illicit drugs, high-speed, reckless, and drunk driving, persons putting themselves into physically and sexually vulnerable situations, having unprotected sex, and a variety of other high-risk behaviors young people are likely to engage in. For some, obesity is already a problem. Many suicide attempts occur and may succeed. Though I enjoyed being a member of Sigma Chi fraternity at Wake Forest College, I believe now that fraternities and sororities are actually contributing to the problem of self-destructive behavior on campuses.

A tragic story of self-destructive behavior. I told you earlier about a young man I knew in the 1960s. He enjoyed relationships with women and had no trouble succeeding in that area. He took up golf during college. During his 30s, he won an amateur golf tournament, which was an astonishing athletic achievement. After college, he completed graduate education and received a doctorate in a health specialty. "The world was his oyster!" While working in his specialty, he drank heavily, became an alcoholic, became severely overweight, probably developed the metabolic syndrome, became a type 2 diabetic, lost the ability to work in his profession, and had his house foreclosed on. At the age of 70, he had a fall that caused fatal injuries.

He could have prevented the following: alcoholism, obesity, metabolic syndrome, and type 2 diabetes. Walking more carefully might have prevented his fatal fall.

A short pep talk about our wonderful human species. **Being very healthy is not very hard to achieve, and living that way is great!**

Nearly all humans have countless ancestors who flourished in challenging environments. I believe that a very high percentage of humans have the talents and personality to be self-supporting and self-reliant. A person does not need fabulous talents and capabilities to achieve at least modest success in life.

I have joked with my son about wanting to live in retirement in a used mobile home on the southwest side of a small mountain in the Shenandoah Valley, growing a big garden and listening to bluegrass music. That could provide enjoyable living and wouldn't require much money. The point, affirmed in chapter 20 about frugal living, is that an enjoyable quality of life doesn't have to cost very much.

Participation in high-risk activities by people without sufficient skill. Chapter 36 is about high-risk activities. For me, trying to ride a skateboard or doing more than very easy rock climbing without safety ropes would qualify more as a self-destructive activity than as a high-risk activity. So, there is some overlap of these two chapters.

Suicide. I must mention the recent tragic suicide of Anthony Bourdain. Though I have never watched an entire Bourdain TV show, I years ago concluded that Bourdain had the best job "on the planet." I wish I had something wise and helpful to say about his death. His death does remind us that suicide may threaten many more people than we would assume it threatens.

Suicide, of course, is the most severe form of self-destructive behavior. Because of this severity, I've decided to share some information and impressions.

(1) Most people who commit suicide are in the grips of depression, which is a powerful form of mental illness. When a person is depressed, it is very likely that she or he will **substantially overestimate the difficulties**

she or he is confronting and **substantially underestimate the adaptive resources** that are readily available to use in dealing with difficulties. So, depression can trick a person into thinking her or his situation is hopeless.

(2) A high percentage of people who unsuccessfully attempt to commit suicide go on to have long, happy, and productive lives.

(3) I believe that many people who are considering suicide **incorrectly** think, "They will be better off without me."

(4) As a surviving relative of several people who committed suicide, I will sadly report that having a close relative commit suicide can be very traumatic for surviving relatives.

(5) I believe that nearly everyone who commits suicide believes that she or he did not have hope for the future in one or more important aspects of her or his life. Maybe a first step in increasing hope could be reaching out for emotional support and advice from a loved one or friend or calling one of the phone lines devoted to helping potentially suicidal people. Getting professional treatment for depression is probably needed. Then, the person may want to work determinedly on solving problems that stand in the way of feeling hopeful about the future. Chapter 15 of this book is specifically about dealing with depression.

Avoiding behavior that can be self-destructive or otherwise very harmful for the individual.

Try to think rationally about possible bad consequences of the behavior you are considering. Here's an example from my life. During graduation from Wake Forest College in 1965, I was commissioned as an Army second lieutenant. Three months later, I started the three-year program of studies of the Wake Forest University School of Law. That was when recreational illicit drugs were rapidly increasing in popularity in the U.S.

I was keenly aware that, if I should be convicted for possession and/or use of an illegal drug, I could lose the opportunity to take the NC bar exam and become a licensed attorney. Conviction could also result in my being dishonorably discharged from the Army. I strongly believed that being a licensed lawyer and being a commissioned Army officer could be extremely valuable to me. Therefore, **I never considered using an illicit drug**.

Many types of potentially self-destructive or dangerous behaviors can result in a serious injury for that person or some other person. A disabling injury can keep a person from enjoying many wonderful aspects of living.

When about to behave in a self-destructive way, get some exercise. You could go on a brisk walk or jog, play an active sport, or do some weight lifting. In chapter 15, there is a supplement-and-exercise routine (VCR) for dealing with depression. In chapter 14, there is another routine, which is about dealing with anxiety and stress. There is plenty of scientific evidence that the listed supplements and exercise tend to fairly quickly help you concerning depression, stress, and anxiety.

Talk with someone you trust. This can be a loved one, friend, or some other person or service you think could help you.

Possibility that performance of a supplement-and-exercise routine (VCR) might help persons with problems regarding self-destructive behavior. Having done a VCR many thousands of times since 1982, I know for sure that doing that can make you feel good and function well.

A suggested approach. There is a supplement formula, San Dr. Feel Good, that is intended to help a person to feel good. Irwin Naturals markets a supplement, Sunny Mood. Below that is the following language: "feel good, feel balanced."

(1) Take one of those supplements, alpha-lipoic acid, fish oil, coenzyme Q10, and curcumin with a very large glass of water.

(2) After waiting 30 minutes, get 30 minutes of moderate exercise, such as very brisk walking.

It would be terrific if a qualified person would do some experimentation about this.

REFERENCES

Curtin, Sally C. et al (2016). Increase in suicide in the U.S. 1999-2014. National Center for Health Statistics, Centers for Disease Control and Prevention.

Memory, J.M. (1981). *Work-related stress of state criminal trial court judges.* Unpublished doctoral dissertation, Florida State University, Tallahassee, FL.

— SECTION 6 —
Recreation

— CHAPTER 17 —
Importance of Health- and Vitality-Enhancing Recreation

Elaboration. Because of limited health benefits, non-active, non-demanding recreational activities that you do by yourself are not emphasized in this chapter. Instead, the focus is on types of recreation that clearly enhance a person's health and vitality, such as walking golf, music (making, not just listening), dancing, playing chess or bridge, square dancing, and hiking. Of course, there are many other wonderful and helpful types of recreation.

Proposal of a course. While I realize that many colleges and universities have one-hour courses introducing recreational activities, I believe there is a need for a two-hour course that is about describing a wide variety of available recreational activities and discussing their benefits. Chapter 1 of this book is about bolstering your health motivation. It is very important to know that the best way to bolster your health (e.g., exercise, diet) motivation is to "over-learn" the benefits of healthful activities.

Trend toward addiction to playing with a smart phone. I learned recently that especially teenagers are now at risk of becoming addicted to playing with a smart phone. Since I'm an old guy who wouldn't take a smart phone if it were offered to me, I will admit that I probably couldn't provide good suggestions for dealing with this problem, which I view as very significant and likely to cause major adverse effects. An undergraduate course about benefits of recreation should include a discussion of this problem.

Importance of this subject. "All work and no play makes Jack a dull boy" is a saying that nearly everyone agrees with. While I believe it is very desirable for young and middle-age adults to enjoy regular recreation, I think it is especially important for retired persons to have recreational activities and enjoy them regularly.

One of the best examples in U.S. history of enjoyment of healthful recreation was my **very** distant cousin, George Washington. He valued many recreational activities in which he was remarkably accomplished, including horse riding, fox hunting, dancing, and bowling.

It's interesting that, very often when we learn about the life of a famous person, we learn that she or he enjoys or enjoyed one or more types of recreation. Bill Gates and Warren Buffet are avid duplicate bridge players. I was interested to learn decades ago that nearly all of the members of the U.S. Supreme Court at the time enjoyed growing roses. Go figure! All of our three most recent former Presidents, Bill Clinton, George W. Bush, and Barack Obama, are avid golfers. I assume that, unfortunately, all three nearly always ride in a golf cart.

Since mechanization, automation, computerization, robotics, and AI (artificial intelligence) are continuing to eliminate many jobs annually in the U.S., it may in the future be very important for unemployed adults to have several types of inexpensive, time-consuming, and healthful recreation.

Relevance for young adults. I believe that, for young adults, it is very desirable to choose and participate in enjoyable, healthful recreational activities.

Many recreational activities are best learned when you are young. Golf is so difficult that only very talented athletes can successfully take up golf "later in life." People usually learn whether they have aptitude for music fairly early in life. If you discover a musical skill you can acquire and enjoy, you can enjoy it for the rest of your life. While people with aptitude can successfully take up bridge "later in life," it does not work to take up duplicate bridge at an older age if you are having too many "senior moments." So, these three recreational activities, with which I am very familiar, clearly are better learned earlier rather than later.

Making good decisions about recreation you will enjoy regularly. This can be especially challenging if you have limitations concerning availability of time and/or money. Traditionally, golfers have played 18 holes, which will take at least five hours out of your day, counting time spent driving, getting your clubs out of your car, etc. The U.S. Golf Association is urging Americans to be willing to play nine holes, which has been my practice for years. Here's a suggestion for a father or mother with children. Try **walking** nine holes with one or more family members late on Saturday or Sunday afternoon at an inexpensive public course. This can be very enjoyable, inexpensive, excellent exercise, good development of sport skills, and high quality family time.

Important tradeoffs. Undoubtedly, many parents are concerned that, if they pursue recreational activities, that will reduce their "quality time" with their spouse and children.

A friend of mine was a varsity golfer in the Big10 decades ago. During several decades when his business and children were growing, he got away from golf. He now has a great marriage, great children, wonderful grandchildren, great finances, a very beautiful home, and, given his background, a pretty good golf game. He made much better decisions than the guys who desert their wife and children for many hours on Saturdays and/or Sundays to ride 18 holes of golf, followed by beers in the clubhouse.

Significance of cost. Since I know golf well, I will describe the extremes. The cost to play Pinehurst #2 during the fall or spring (the prime seasons) **one time** is at least $450. You can walk nine holes at many public courses for $10 or a little more. If I went back to live in Pinehurst, it would cost me probably $400 per month in club dues and at least $350 per month for the cart fee. When I lived in Hendersonville, NC, I was a member the Crooked Creek Golf Club, which is known as the most walkable golf course in the mountains, and had unlimited walking golf for $67 per month. While I could play any of six courses as a Pinehurst member, I never got bored playing nearly all of my golf at Crooked Creek. I expect that there are fairly big variations in cost of some other types of recreation, such as sailing.

A "stripped down" version of recreation: walking in a VCR group. Problems regarding availability of time and money in having good, frequent recreation were discussed above. I want to applaud the probably millions of American women (Men aren't that smart.) who regularly walk briskly with one or more friends. In my opinion, **walking briskly, while your brain is working great, you feel great, and you can talk with one or more good friends, actually constitutes recreation**. I suggest that you consider referring to your walking group as a "VCR (vascular cleansing routine) group," if you regularly take healthful supplements, wait 30 minutes, and then walk. You'll find a detailed supplement-and-exercise routine, a VCR, in many of the early chapters of this book. We're told, "If it sounds too good to be true, it probably isn't true," which does not apply here. In this case, just taking the right supplements, waiting 30 minutes, and then enjoying walking briskly with your friends will put yourself on the path to great health and improved enjoyment of life.

Dealing with a very tight time schedule. If a person has an extremely tight schedule, it might make sense to do what was described in the previous paragraph—getting 20 to 30 minutes of very brisk walking that is in some way(s) recreational four or five days per week. The obvious point is that this would meet important needs for recreation and exercise.

High quality TV watching. If there is a family of two busy, smart, and intellectually curious parents and their two busy, smart, and intellectually curious children (13 and 16), I think it could be high quality family recreation for them to watch Jeopardy together every day.

Author's relevant experience. From the age of five through graduation from high school, I lived in Riverton, North Carolina, a rural area, which was (and is) owned nearly entirely by my relatives. Many families of relatives migrated there during summers to enjoy a wide variety of safe recreational activities. Having lived from the age of 5 through 17 in a rural area that offered many types of enjoyable, free, and healthful recreation may partly explain the strong emphasis I have given to recreation in my life.

More information than you want to get about my recreational activities. I'm sharing this to let you know how important I think recreation has been in my life and how I obtained information about many types of recreation.

I learned tennis in Riverton and played varsity tennis at Wake Forest. During law school I made the shift from tennis to golf, virtually always walking. I've walked about 22,000 miles playing golf. I've enjoyed making several types of music from childhood to the present. My mother taught bridge to me and my twin brother when we were 11. In 2016, I earned the bridge rank of Golf Life Master, which is four levels above Life Master. During my teens, I learned how to dance several dance steps, including "the shag." Like many of the other male and female members of my large extended family, I am an accomplished canoeist.

For several years after retiring in 2004, I would go thrift shopping as a type of recreational activity. Fortunately, I have recently reduced the amount of time I spend in thrift shopping. While I strongly believe that thrift shopping can be an important part of frugal living, I don't think it has health or functioning benefits. (Buying the beautiful $50 coffee mug for $1.75 at Goodwill recently was, however, quite gratifying.)

A question you may have. "Since no responsible person who works and has a family will engage in lots of types of recreation, why does the author even tell about his recreation?" I respect that question and point of view. To answer that question, I will tell some about benefits of recreation for me.

Benefits I have obtained from recreation. As I mention in chapters 14 and 15, I inherited some vulnerability concerning anxiety, stress and experiencing depression. Also, I have very severe heart- and brain-disease risk factors. Recreation has helped me to deal healthfully with those potential problems. Now, as I approach 75, I feel sure I've been right about that.

In the following section, I give detailed information about the benefits of physical exercise, which I have enjoyed obtaining many thousands of times. In chapter 36, I list many benefits of playing duplicate bridge. I think recreation has helped me in overcoming boredom, depression, stress, and loneliness; in bolstering my self-esteem (For example, having been one of the best male handball players in my WFC freshman class, which included countless male all-conference and all-state athletes, bolstered my self-esteem concerning the physical challenges of manhood.); bolstering my intellectual self-esteem (Success in bridge helped with this.); in developing friendships; and in having fun.

An apparent contradiction. I made this request to two success-ful male professionals who are enjoying retirement in Hendersonville, NC, "Finish the sentence, 'Life is _____.'" One said, "A bowl of cherries." The other said, "Great!" I finish the sentence, "Life is work." I think that nearly always when I am participating in recreation, I am working to achieve one or more of the important benefits I discussed in the previous paragraph. I've known four men who have worked as hard as or harder than me preparing to play golf. I've never known anyone who works nearly as hard as I do preparing to play duplicate bridge.

I do not resent that I have had to work hard, sometimes even in rec-reation, on physical health, mental health, heart health, and brain health. Instead, I feel extremely fortunate that my efforts have been successful and, very often, enjoyable.

A confession. Since some time in my 20s, I have watched too much TV. I have tried to watch "high quality TV." For the last three years, I have very often studied old *Bridge Bulletin* magazines while watching TV.

Benefits of recreation. To obtain an excellent document about benefits of parks and recreation, find on the National Recreation and Park Association website "Relevant research for practice 2017: focus on conservation and re-siliency" by Teresa L. Penbrooke, PhD. To look at a model that suggests the relationship of recreation and parks to many other things, go to page 9 of that document.

Benefits of playing bridge frequently and seriously. If you would like to read my long list of benefits of playing duplicate bridge, you can turn to chapter 18. Since two pairs of bridge players sit at a square table, bridge doesn't involve physical exercise.

Benefits of physical exercise. This is the most amazing information I have ever read on any subject. The points listed below come from a variety of sources. In some cases, I am able to provide a research article reference. Based on extensive reading over many years, I have a high degree of confidence concerning the accuracy of this information.

Deterrence of cardiovascular disease and related conditions hypertension, type 2 diabetes, obesity, and problems with endothelial function (function of blood vessels) (Taka-aki Okabe et al, 2006)

Strengthening of the heart

Improvement of blood circulation (Thompson et al, 2003)

Most effective way to build brain power (Ratey, 2008)

Combined with Mediterranean diet, reduces Alzheimer's risk by 60% (Scarmeas et al, 2009)

For older persons with serious depression, as effective as taking an anti-depressant drug in depression control (Blumenthal et al, 1999)

Reverses detrimental effects of the physiological stress reaction (Salmon,2001).

Helps with troublesome anxiety.

Moderate exercise produces growth of new brain cells in the hippocampus.

Improvement of brain function

Promotion of production of DHEA

Improvement of sex life

Help with achieving healthful sleep

Production of human growth hormone (HGH)

Production of glutathione after taking alpha-lipoic acid

Helps with delivery of nutrients and oxygen to body tissues

Promotion of production of serotonin and dopamine

Promotion of release of endorphins

Reduction of risk of coronary artery disease, type 2 diabetes, osteoporosis, obesity, depression, and cancer of breast and colon (Thompson et al, 2003)

Also, exercise contributes to fitness. There is a positive association between fitness and career success ("The link between fitness and career success," briancalkins.com website). Especially during the 1990s, when I was trying to develop excellent ideas to use in scholarly research and writing projects, I often had a good idea "pop into my brain" when I was walking golf. That would not have happened if I had sat in my office all afternoon staring at my computer screen and drinking coffee.

Benefits of dancing for senior citizens. In 2009, it was reported in a scientific research article (Hui, E. et al, 2009) that regular dancing has significant physical and psychological well-being benefits for older people. Since the early 1980s, I have often attended a ballroom dance on a Friday or Saturday night and have danced nearly every dance, including fast-tempo dances, for more than two hours. You have to be "in good shape" to do that. Maybe because of my low dissolved oxygen, I have never had above-average running speed for any distance. It is peculiar that, even at 74, I can dance a swing dance on tempo probably as fast or very nearly as fast as any other dancer of any age at most ballroom dances.

A very important benefit of recreation during your working career is that it can help in prevention of "burnout" from long-term experiencing of work-related stress. Though my doctoral dissertation was on work-related stress of state criminal trial court judges (Memory, 1981), I am not now an expert on work-related stress.

Fortunately, nearly everyone can find one or more types of recreation the person can perform well. Consequently, a significant percentage of people can achieve some self-esteem benefits from their recreation.

Some new retirees have so much additional free time on their hands that they experience troublesome boredom. During a short hiatus in my working career in the early 1990s, I experienced very disconcerting boredom nearly every afternoon between 1:00 and 4:00 p.m. Recreation can healthfully oc-cupy free time and prevent boredom.

Some possible criteria for personal recreational activities.

Should unequivocally be fun

Should at least sometimes provide rejuvenation

Should enhance several aspects of the person's wellbeing, such as health

Very positive for it to enhance mental health

Very positive for it to enhance brain health and function

Should not be costly, unless this is not an important criterion for the person

Should not take a lot of time, unless you want it to

Very positive for it to enhance family and friendship relationships. Of course, very negative for it to adversely affect family relationships.

Examples of types of recreation which probably don't have significant health and wellbeing benefits. Shopping, collecting clothes, shoes, or jewelry, playing on your iPhone, riding a jet ski, fishing in a powerful motorboat, sunbathing, watching sitcoms on TV, watching old movies, listening to popular music, watching FoxNews, CNN, or MSNBC (select one), riding golf carts, enjoying too many drinks at your favorite bar, bowling (very limited exercise), stamp or coin collecting, standing in a hunting stand or sitting in a hunting blind for countless hours. Though I have enjoyed doubles tennis, I don't think it generally allows players to get even moderate exercise. Playing singles tennis may provide moderate exercise.

I think that these listed activities won't come close to providing the benefits of many other recreational activities.

It is important for me to acknowledge that some of the recreational activities listed above may have types of valuable benefits that are not apparent to me. For example, a friend especially enjoys watching old movies. He may be receiving benefits that I'm not aware of.

A few examples of high quality recreation.

Very brisk walking. Of course, you need to add some aspect, maybe talking to a friend, that will make it recreational.

Jogging. For most people, jogging should not be strenuous enough to cause problems. (Strenuous exercise makes your blood platelets stickier and causes release of free radicals—two things you don't want to have happen.) Again, you need to add enjoyable aspects. I occasionally see a couple jogging together as one is pushing a baby carriage. They always appear to be having fun.

Square dancing. I have two friendly couples in the NC mountains who enjoy square dancing. All four of them are unusually active and young looking for their age. Square dancing provides exercise and demands recollection of intricate dancing routines.

Gardening and cooking. Growing a lot of vegetables, harvesting them, delivering some to neighbors' houses, cooking them at your home, and enjoying them with family and friends is great, healthful recreation.

Walking nine holes of golf. While many women are smart enough to walk briskly with friends during weekday lunch hours, men can walk nine holes of golf with buddies. I live on a golf course and know that some women walk golf with female friends. Of course, you can do this with one or more family members.

Hiking. Hiking with family and friends in beautiful state and national parks

Swimming. During the 1990s, my main exercise for four months of the year was swimming an easy backstroke (adapted breast stroke, upside down) against the current of the beautiful Lumber (or Lumbee) River in south-central NC. This was so pleasant that it constituted recreation for me.

Bicycle riding. While I am fairly well coordinated, I make too many mistakes to ride a bicycle or motorcycle regularly.

Hiking, biking, or canoeing in beautiful nature taking photographs.

Writing can be an enjoyable recreational activity. Having last worked (as a Criminal Justice associate professor) in 2004, I have during retirement put in many hundreds of hours trying to do the best job I can writing a wide variety of documents. This is, in effect, "play work" I do for various benefits. For "senior citizens," learning new things helps in prevention of Alzheimer's and other dementia.

For women (and a few men) who spend many hours preparing family meals, dining out can be important recreation.

The future of recreation in the U.S. Golf is losing 3 million golfers annually. Many other recreational activities are losing participants, including square dancing, chess, duplicate bridge, and, I think, bowling.

I hope the "wave of the future" in recreation is not sitting, playing with your iPhone.

Exercise to improve golf performance. I have known well three men in their 70s and one man in his 80s who played golf very well. All four of them regularly did exercise that enhanced their ability to play golf. I started exercising to bolster my golf performance in the 1970s. (As a member of Pinehurst G&CC, I never broke 80 on courses #2 or #4. So, I can't credibly share tips about playing golf.) Here are golf exercise approaches that have worked for me.

Hands. I use a V-shaped hand exercise device. It is desirable for your hands to have equal strength.

Wrists. Wrist curls with as much weight as possible. For a right-handed golfer, right wrist does regular curls, left wrist does reverse curls.

Arms. Pushups

Core. I have strong elastic bands, which I anchor at the bottom of a door. Then I pull the bands with both hands moving how I would move in a golf swing.

Legs. I hold a 36-pound barbell in each hand and go up and down bending my knees. **Optional or occasional**

Arms and shoulders in downward motion. You anchor the elastic bands at the top of a door, stand either facing the door or with your back to the door, and, with a handle in each hand, push toward the floor. It is easy for a person to lose the strength needed for this exercise. When you lose it, you're vulnerable to rotator cuff problems. **Optional or occasional**

I know a man who was an elite golfer during high school and is now about 75. His best score on a very difficult course when he was 18 would have been 73. Unfortunately, he has lost so much ability to hit a golf ball with power and consistency that playing golf is extremely frustrating for him. I'm sure that, if he had done strength work for golf consistently for decades, he could have prevented these problems.

REFERENCES

Blumenthal, J. A. et al (1999). Effects of exercise training on older patients with major depression. *Archives of Internal Medicine*, Vol. 159, No. 19, pp. 2349–2356.

Hui, E. et al (2009). Effects of dance on physical and psychological well-being in older persons. Archives of Gerontology & Geriatrics, Vol. 49, Issue 1, pp. e45–e50.

Memory, J. M. (1981). *Work-related stress of state criminal trial court judges.* Unpublished doctoral dissertation, Florida State University, Tallahassee.

Ratey, John J. with Hagerman, Eric (2008). *Spark: the revolutionary new science of exercise and the brain.* NY, NY: Little, Brown and Company.

Salmon, Peter (2001). Effects of physical exercise on anxiety, depression, and sensitivity to stress: a unifying theory. *Clinical Psychology Review*, Vol. 21, Issue 1, pp. 33–61.

Scarmeas, Nikolaos et al (2009). Physical activity, diet, and risk of Alzheimer's disease. *Journal of the American Medical Association*, Vol. 302, No. 6, pp. 627–637.

Taka-aki Okabe, B.M. et al (2006). Effects of exercise on the development of atherosclerosis in apolipoprotein E-deficient mice. *Experimental Clinical Cardiology*, Vol. 11, No. 4, pp. 276–279.

Thompson, Paul D. et al (2003). American Heart Association scientific statement: exercise and physical activity in the prevention and treatment of atherosclerotic cardiovascular disease. *Arteriosclerosis, Thrombosis, and Vascular Biology*, Vol. 23, pp. e42–49.

AN ESSAY ABOUT EXCEPTIONAL, MEMORABLE EXPERIENCES IN RECREATION

Looking back over many years, I'm struck that engaging in recreation has helped me substantially in acquiring friends and having great experiences.

Playing Golf below Mount Mitchell

For about six years (2006–2015) while I lived in Hendersonville, NC, I played golf with my friends Jim and Dave nearly every Monday afternoon. Since they were both much better golfers and younger than me, I had incentive to work during weekends preparing for the tough golf match on Monday. Though they would have happily "given me strokes" to make the contest fair for me, I never asked for them.

While I have practiced short golf shots (chips and pitches) for many hundreds of hours, Dave has never practiced them: He is so talented that he hasn't needed to. Jim is a religious agnostic and a Republican. Some liberal readers may think, "Oops, sounds like bad morals to me." Wrong! I haven't known a more moral and unselfish person than Jim. Though he had played varsity golf for the Michigan Wolverines, he "let golf slide" during the crucial years of parenting two great children and "growing" his printing business.

In 2012 one of us suggested that we, on a Monday in mid-October, drive 40 miles to play golf at the Mount Mitchell Golf Course. Fortunately, we hit the most beautiful fall day of that year. While walking the rolling fairways, we saw breath-taking panoramas of hills and mountains covered by bright yellow, gold, orange, and red leaves. You may be thinking, "Why didn't he mention the beautiful leaves on Mount Mitchell itself?" Mount Mitchell, which is visible from many spots on the course, is so tall that beautiful oak, red maple, tupelo, river birch, sweet gum, and hickory trees don't grow on the high elevations, which have a slightly surreal dark gray or black color.

I don't remember who won. I probably lost about $2.50 to Dave and $3.25 to Jim. That's a small price to pay for challenging and enjoyable (and healthful) golf in an exquisite natural setting.

Floating the Lumbee with Alex

In 1991, my son Alex (then 12) and I spent an April weekend at the log cabin in which I grew up (1949–61) in the rural Riverton community in Scotland County, NC. We decided that on Saturday afternoon we would canoe about four miles down the meandering, tea-colored Lumbee River (Lumber River on the map).

During every season of the year, the river is beautiful. For about two weeks in April, it is so exquisite that my grasp of the English language does not allow me to communicate well in words the nature, power, and complexity of the beauty. But I will try.

During those two weeks, the oak, red maple, river birch, tupelo, and hickory trees have early leaves with sometimes dazzling, sometimes subtle colors—dark red, pink, gold, orange, very light green, and darker green. As we floated, the bright afternoon sunshine glistened on the swirling river current. Much of the time, we heard a chorus of songs of bird species that were in early breeding season in the deep swamp.

After about an hour of floating, we came to a challenging stretch of the river that required that we paddle close to the bank on the right and then turn sharply to the left and shoot with a strong current through a narrow opening in the logs, branches, and vines. As we emerged safely from that maneuver, we entered a long corridor with red-, pink-, gold-, orange-, and green-colored trees of many shapes and sizes standing by or drooping over the river. I hope I will see that again.

Singing with Lorraine

When I was married and living in Pinehurst, NC, from 1999–2003, I was fortunate to have the first of four wonderful female singing partners,

Lorraine. She had sung professionally many years earlier in the DC area, as I had. Her fairly low voice allowed me to sing harmony comfortably on "the old songs." I accompanied us on my electric guitar. Lorraine and I never argued, except for when she wanted me to sing a solo, and I insisted that she sing it. We had fun practicing and performing, often for seniors in some type of residential facility. The audience would sometimes light up as they sang with us one of their favorite songs from the late 1920s or 1930s.

The 2001 Pinehurst Country Club Christmas formal dance in the beautifully decorated main ballroom was on a Saturday evening in December, about three months after 9/11. During the band break, we sang a short program of Christmas music, and it went well. As we were ending, I asked those successful, accomplished, decent, golf-loving Pinehurst folks in their elegant formal attire to stand for us to sing together "God Bless America." The couples from Pennsylvania and New Jersey, Ohio and upstate New York, who were living a wonderful version of the American dream, stood and sang their hearts out, leaving no doubt that they really did love America.

CHAPTER 18
Bridge (the card game)

<u>Elaboration</u>. As an unregulated social activity, bridge is referred to as social bridge or contract bridge. As a highly regulated recreational activity with local clubs and tournaments, it's known as duplicate bridge. In the 1930s, 60 million Americans played bridge. Now, the organization regulating duplicate bridge, the American Contract Bridge League (ACBL), has 165,000 members.

ACBL has not done a good job of capitalizing on the fact that the two richest people in the U.S. for several decades, Bill Gates and Warren Buffet, are very avid duplicate bridge players.

Many duplicate-playing couples enjoy mini-vacations attending bridge tournaments. You may be surprised to learn that a significant percentage of couples who enjoy duplicate bridge have concluded that it's better not to play together.

<u>A way to learn to play bridge</u>. Teaching readers to play bridge is not a goal of this chapter. Fortunately, you can go to the ACBL website and click on "LEARN." You will be directed to two different ways to learn to play bridge.

<u>Opportunities to play duplicate bridge online</u>. Because I especially value opportunities to interact in person with other people in bridge club games and tournaments, I have never played bridge online. If that appeals to you, you can do searches and find several opportunities. I know a good player in western SC who earned 600 masterpoints online in not much more than a

year. (Earning Life Master previously took only 300 masterpoints. Now, it takes 500 masterpoints of several types.)

Ways to improve your abilities as a bridge player online. For at least the last ten years, on a high percentage of nights I have gotten on my computer at 1:00 a.m. to study superb—and free—instructional bridge hands on the Bridge Clues website, which in spring of 2018 was improved. To find it, search for "bridgeclues2.com" on the Internet.

As previously discussed, I did research in the 1980s about ways judges can improve their knowledge of search and seizure law. Clearly, **the most effective method was regular self-study**, which is what Bridge Clues offers. Shortly before 1:00 a.m., I study the day's Frank Stewart bridge column, which also is excellent, free, and on the Internet.

A warning. Duplicate bridge is a difficult, challenging activity. For example, I know well two **extremely intelligent, well-educated** (both with a doctoral degree) men in their 60s who played a lot of social bridge earlier in their lives. In spite of their determined efforts during retirement, their average duplicate bridge score has been far below average. I still can't figure that out.

Many of the few college students who learn and continue to play duplicate bridge are math, science, computer engineering/science, or engineering majors.

It can be difficult to find one or more bridge partners with whom you are compatible and with whom you (and that partner) can improve in bridge. The best situation is to find an excellent mentor who is willing to play with you regularly. During the 1990s, I fortunately was able to play nearly every Friday night with one of the top two players in the Pinehurst, NC area.

Relevant experience of the author. In about 1954, my math-teacher mother started teaching bridge to me and my twin brother, David. While David could have been an excellent duplicate player, he hasn't had the slightest interest. I have played organized duplicate bridge often since 1981 and in 2016 achieved the rank of Gold Life Master, which is four levels above ordinary Life Master.

When I was a Criminal Justice professor, I presented a lengthy paper

(2003) comparing a specific form of bridge with two-officer patrol policing at the annual meeting of the Academy of Criminal Justice Sciences. I have written an unpublished 78-page book (Memory, 2017) about bridge, concerning which a highly ranked duplicate player has provided a very positive endorsement. I think my best bridge results were in 2015. Unfortunately, I believe that father time and my genetic vulnerability to developing brain disease have reduced my maximum performance level. Fortunately, preparing determinedly to play still allows me and my fine partners to often get a score we're very happy with.

Importance of this subject. I strongly believe that playing duplicate bridge seriously and frequently has a wide variety of benefits, which are listed below. Also, bridge is analogous to several types of "real world" high-risk activities. Poker, on the other hand, is not analogous to types of situations and activities that are often encountered in life.

A proposal. I believe that, because bridge is an exceptionally fine recreational activity, there is justification for colleges and universities to offer a one- or two-hour for-credit course about bridge. It is common for colleges and universities to offer one-hour courses about recreational activities that involve physical exercise. As discussed in this chapter, bridge can provide benefits that are at least as valuable as those of types of recreation that involve physical exercise.

Relevance for young adults. It helps to learn to play bridge seriously sooner rather than later. For example, if a person in his or her 70s is experiencing many "senior moments," it will be too late to learn and genuinely compete in duplicate bridge. If two young adults meet on the Internet and then play duplicate bridge as partners, they will learn more about each other than in any other activity I know of (except, maybe, robbing a bank).

Some information about methods to use in duplicate bridge. Most readers of this book would be astonished to learn how extremely complex the methods used by many duplicate bridge players are. In the *Bridge Bulletin* in 2009 Larry Cohen, who is a very well respected bridge player and teacher, said,

"On any level, players should cut back on the methods, conventions and 'science' and concentrate on basic bridge logic and not making mistakes. Many new players clog their brains with so much memorization that they don't have any brain power left for the beauty of the game."

I entirely agree with Larry. Research was done comparing fairly simple bridge methods with "super-scientific" methods. The "super-scientific" methods barely won.

In my bridge book, I emphasize using low-complexity, high-power methods. Though only duplicate players will understand this, I'll report that in 2015 and 2016 I played for only four days in regional tournaments with an excellent female player from California. Fortunately for me, she agreed to play my methods, which are much less complex than her preferred methods. During the four afternoon games and the four evening games, we won a total of 60 gold masterpoints. During my early years in bridge, you needed to win 25 gold points to make Life Master.

Duplicate bridge rules. The rules governing duplicate bridge are very complex and are changed some occasionally. The zero-tolerance policy requires courteous player behavior. If a player is careful to be honest, fair, and courteous, she or he will probably be able to play without violating rules. The directors, who supervise games, try to help new players to be comfortable.

Professions and vocations that are common among duplicate-bridge players. It's not uncommon for a strong female player to be or have been a math teacher or professor. Though I am a social scientist, I haven't found any other persons with that career among strong players. There are about equal numbers of doctors and lawyers, and they're about equally good.

In chapter 36 of this book, "High-risk activities and decision making," bridge is included as a recreational activity in which there is simulation of risks of very adverse outcomes as players compete to win valuable rewards. For example, in a certain type of bridge scoring, you can make a serious mistake on one of 24 hands and, as a result, nearly certainly lose the 24-hand, three-hour contest.

Bridge is somewhat like two hunter-gather men in Africa 100,000 years ago hunting and confronting many types of dangers that could cause serious injury or death. As I discuss in chapter 33, I think that a high percentage of these men were so highly skilled in hunting and dealing with serious risks that their possibility of death or serious injury was very low. Bridge is different in that even the best players occasionally suffer a devastating defeat on a hand. To succeed in bridge, you must be willing to take substantial risks.

Similarity of duplicate bridge to working as an engineer. In bridge, players go into a situation, try to learn about risks and problems there, about possibly available rewards, about resources they can use in preventing adverse outcomes and in attempting to achieve a favorable outcome. The players have strong knowledge of many agreed-upon methods and problem solutions that they may need to use in a given situation. Like engineers, bridge players nearly never make up a new method or problem solution on the spot. Based on obtained information, the players utilize their vast array of proven methods in developing an action plan. During the play of the hand, the action plan is implemented. If difficulties are encountered, the action plan can be changed and a revised plan developed and implemented. I believe that this is similar to what engineers do in their professional lives. It would make sense for university colleges of engineering to sponsor duplicate bridge games for students, faculty members, and alumni.

Benefits of playing bridge seriously. Here are what I think are likely benefits of playing duplicate bridge seriously for a significant percentage of players. (An excellent article about this is on the AARP website, "A bridge to brainpower?") Of course, not everyone will receive all of these benefits.

Improvement of thinking and memory and building of brain power
Help with preventing or delaying Alzheimer's and other dementia
Bolstering immune system
Provision of a regularly available fun activity
Avoidance of boredom or a low-quality activity (e.g., couch potato)
Very low cost for high quality recreation
Production of more enjoyment of life (including depression prevention and reduction)
Provision of exquisitely challenging pair v. pair game (not important to everyone)

Provision of an excellent activity for some couples

Improved functioning in a partnership and in teamwork

Increase in friendships (with partners and opponents)

Development of a support net (maybe)

Affirmation of the importance of hard work learning methods and
using them

Improvement of problem solving using proven solutions

Practice in taking great care to avoid mistakes (important in work
and life generally)

Practice in extremely well simulated high-risk decision making

Practice in making good decisions, exercising good judgment in
stressful circumstances

Affirmation of the importance of acting honestly, ethically, and according to rules

Self-esteem enhancement (for some)

Provision of close social interaction, which is important to health
in several ways

A preliminary study at UC-Berkeley by Dr. Marian Diamond has suggested that playing bridge causes the body to produce more white blood
cells that attack viruses and other threats to health. Research has indicated
that playing bridge prevents or delays the onset of problems regarding brain
health and function.

I told a female player in her 70s about my thinking concerning benefits
of playing duplicate bridge. She immediately said, **"Bridge saved my life!"**

For many years in my early adulthood, I did not think that I had notably
good memory. When I turned 70, after 32 years of frequent duplicate bridge
play, my Lumosity memory percentile was 99.3. Since I take heart- and brain-
healthy supplements and exercise before nearly every duplicate game, bridge
strongly supports my overall health program.

One of the most important benefits of bridge is that it provides usually
amicable contact with other people. This type of social contact is very important to maintenance of mental health and prevention of deterioration of
brain functioning.

Playing bridge can possibly help you to perform in various types of
partnerships better. Types of partnerships that are to a significant extent

analogous to bridge partnership include marriage, romantic relationships, two-officer police teams, some types of business partnerships, hunters, law partners, cooperating physicians, co-facilitators of therapy and discussion groups, and mechanics cooperating in car repair.

Superiority of bridge to poker as a recreational activity. Probably the most important difference of bridge and poker is that luck in drawing cards is vastly more important in poker than in duplicate bridge. The importance of luck in the drawing of cards in poker was vividly shown in the final table of the 2017 World Series of Poker main event. When the eventual winner was slightly ahead of the other remaining player, the eventual winner got much better cards on ten straight hands, which allowed him to gain an insurmountable lead. During 2017-18, a poker player, Justin Bonomo, won several consecutive poker tournaments, which seriously challenges my statement that luck is much more important in poker than in bridge.

Though you may not believe this, I will assure you that, in duplicate bridge, you have an equal chance to win against your competitors on every hand, no matter how bad your cards are. This is because the most important aspect of competition in duplicate is against people who play the same cards that you play. You and your partner are trying to get better results than those other pairs. Bridge involves partnership with another player, which can be rewarding and enjoyable, while in poker you are competing against all of the other players.

What is the future of duplicate bridge in the U.S.? This may be the most important section of this chapter. As mentioned earlier, there were 60 million bridge players in the U.S. in the 1930s. The ACBL membership, recently about 165,000, continues to decline. Turnouts for many tournaments have been down recently. I encourage interested individuals to find one or more duplicate games in which they can play. Because some intelligent people readily conclude that duplicate bridge is an excellent activity, I predict dwindling survival for the indefinite future.

Being a good partner. Playing bridge can give a person an opportunity to figure out how to be a good partner generally. Below is the last page of my bridge book.

I LEARNED ABOUT PARTNERSHIP AT THE BRIDGE TABLE

Have a partner you can trust, and then trust your partner.

Have a partner you can respect, and then treat your partner with respect and courtesy.

Try to avoid putting your partner in unnecessarily risky or uncomfortable situations.

Do everything you can to keep partner from feeling uncomfortable or uneasy in potentially difficult situations.

Don't hesitate to compliment your partner.

If your partner makes a mistake, there's nothing to be gained by criticizing him or her.

If you feel disappointed with your partner around others, express your concern when you two are alone.

Don't hesitate to acknowledge it if a bad outcome was your fault.

Make sure you and your partner know how you can communicate with each other about lots of things and in lots of ways.

It helps to talk about how to work together effectively and enjoyably.

Teach only if you know your partner wants to be taught.

Both of you should be able to take the lead if the circumstances suggest it.

Know each other's strengths and weaknesses, and use that information to get good outcomes and avoid bad outcomes.

If you communicate and work together well, you can capitalize on good opportunities and avoid or reduce bad outcomes.

You owe it to your partner to be well prepared to do important things well.

If you try to help your partner to have fun, most likely you will both have fun.

REFERENCES

Memory, J. M. (2017). *Low-complexity, high power duplicate bridge methods.* Unpublished. Available free as pdf file.

Memory, J. M. (2003). "Application of the theory of Chicago-scoring partnership bridge to two-officer patrol policing." Presented at annual meeting of the Academy of Criminal Justice Sciences in Boston, MA.

— SECTION 7 —
Ideas about Successful Family Living

An Essay about Teaching Moral Behavior to Children

Since human pre-history, religion has had a significant role in teaching morality to children and in behavior control. At a time when a substantial decrease in affiliation of Americans with churches is occurring (Pew Research Center, 2015), this is a very important subject. Also, our national leaders often aren't good role models concerning moral behavior.

I don't think parents will need to read a book about this. At the end of this essay, there are citations to excellent, fairly short, and helpful articles on this subject that are available on the Internet.

Information and ideas I have about this come mainly from: (1) having received a wonderful moral education in a small-town Baptist church (1949–61) (Note: I have been an agnostic since about 1960.); (2) being the father of a highly moral and successful 39-year-old son; (3) having, as a holder of a PhD in criminology, continuing strong interest in morality of individuals and within groups.

I believe it's especially important to teach children the following: **Behaving in good ways helps you to have a happy life and have fun, to get along well with other people, to do good things, and to keep from having troubles and worries in your life.** Also, your good behavior will help other people in your life. For example, it will make being a parent easier for your parent(s). If members of many types of groups, including families, businesses, military units, and schools, behave well, their group probably will be successful.

It is sometimes recommended that parents wait for bad behavior by a child, in order to have a "teachable moment." Instead, I recommend that you and your child(ren) have happy conversations about good ways to behave, which is what my extremely well behaved son and I did.

The information below would need to be customized to be appropriate for the level of vocabulary and understanding of a particular child or children. I know from experience that it is possible for children who are quite young to understand this information.

Obviously, it's important for parents to "live by" the ideas about moral behavior they are trying to teach to their children. "Do as I say, not as I do" probably won't work. It would probably work for the parent to occasionally tell about a mistake she or he made in behavior during childhood or maybe even as an adult.

While I am leaving much of the "how to" thinking to the authors of the articles listed below, I will share my belief that the ideas in *Games people play* by Berne (1964) and *I'm OK, you're OK* by Harris (2004) should be helpful. (You can find a Wikipedia article about transactional analysis.) These books argue that every person has a "parent", "adult", and "child" aspect of his or her thinking and feeling. I think it isn't desirable for a parent to teach from his "parent" directed toward the child's "child." When Alex was three years old, I tried to teach things "adult" to "adult." I was trying to communicate from my rational capacity to his rational capacity.

<u>A list of desirable ways for a child (or even an adult) to behave</u>. Instead of being a list of things to believe, this is a list of words that hopefully will describe good ways for a child to be and behave. So, this list strongly emphasizes teaching the children good ways to behave, rather than bad ways not to behave.

One danger is that children will think that this subject is too big, hard, and complicated. As several authors mentioned in the article list below suggest, it is good to talk with a child about one thing (or maybe a few related things) at a time.

Loving (able to love other people). What is love? It is very normal and good for a person to like and care about herself or himself very much. You love someone when you like and care about that person as much as you like and care about yourself.

Loving other people and having them love you helps you to have a good and happy life. You can't force people to love you. Instead, you can be a good and nice person and hope for the best.

"Love your neighbor as yourself" is a very old and good idea from the Bible about how to live and behave. This idea about loving your neighbors assumes that it is good for you to love yourself. "Neighbors" (people you should love) can include your family, friends, real neighbors, and maybe other students in your school.

"Do unto others as you would have them do unto you." (The Golden Rule from the Bible) "Others" doesn't include just your family and friends. This rule encourages being kind and helpful with other people, including people of other races and religions. Doing this helps us to live happily in a peaceful world.

Caring (compassionate). For example, you learn that a student you don't know very well is sick. It is good for you to sincerely care about that student and hope she or he will get well soon. If you really do care about other people, you probably aren't self-centered, which is caring mainly about yourself and what's good for you.

Kind (not mean). I had an uncle who was big and strong. He could have been a mean bully. Instead, he was a caring and kind person who enjoyed helping other people. He had more happiness and fun in his life than any other person I have known.

Helpful. It's good to help other people, not just family, teachers, and friends. For example, your next-door neighbor, who is an old lady, can't find her cat. It's good and maybe even important for you to catch the cat and return it to your neighbor.

Generous (giving). We know that most children don't have much money and property (such as toys). So, instead of being generous by giving away money or toys, a child can be generous by helping people who need their help. If you're generous, you're probably not selfish (always wanting to get and keep things for yourself).

Joyful (able to be happy). Having enough happiness and fun is good and important. Of course, it's desirable also to do good things. Doing good and maybe even important things may make you happy.

Dependable (trustworthy). People who don't do what they say they will do have troubles finding real friends and people who love them. As adults, they often aren't able to get good jobs.

Obedient. It's important to do what a parent, teacher, police officer, and other adults tell you to do. Refusing to do this can lead to having troubles and worries in your life.

Honest. "Honesty is the best policy." Honesty helps a person to be happy, successful, and not bothered by problems and worries that you cause for yourself. It is dishonest (not honest) to tell a lie, which is saying something that you know is not true.

Friendly. You know what it means to be friendly. It's good also to be courteous, which means you are careful not to be rude to other people.

Respectful. Being respectful is sort of like being courteous. Being respectful is not just for kids. Adults need to treat children with respect.

Not "anger-prone." Anger-prone means getting mad very often.

Peaceful. It's very bad for people to start fighting and violence when it's possible to avoid it. It's important to avoid hurting other people on purpose or accidentally.

Thrifty. This means being careful to avoid spending too much money. Being thrifty doesn't keep you from having a lot of fun. Remember the old saying: "The best things in life are free."

Fair (just). It's important to try to treat people fairly. For example, there are five pieces of candy for three kids. It's not fair if one kid takes and eats three of the pieces of candy.

Self-disciplined (showing self-control). Some people can't keep from doing bad things. That is a bad way to live. For example, your mom doesn't want you to eat candy before supper. You're not showing self-discipline or self-control if, not long before supper, you eat two candy bars you had in your room.

Able and willing to work hard. It's possible to need to work hard in many parts of life. If you have chores at home, it's important to be willing to work hard doing them. Working hard on not eating too much, on exercising, and on being healthy is good for people of all ages and will really pay off. People who are willing to work hard are not lazy.

Persevering. Sometimes, we need to not give up in doing something important, even if continuing is difficult. Thomas Edison, the famous inventor, persevered and ended up inventing more wonderful things than anybody else in human history. People can persevere concerning many types of difficult situations.

Tough. People who persevere probably are tough. If a mean or nasty person treats you in a bad way, it will be good for you to be tough, without getting into a fight. You can ask your parent(s) for advice about dealing with mean and nasty people.

Brave. People need to be brave (and careful) about physical danger. Sometimes, a situation in life is difficult and scary. We need to be brave when that happens and try to do the right things.

Able to apologize (admit you were wrong or made a mistake). "Everybody makes mistakes." It's not the end of the world if you make a mistake. Sometimes, it's good to say to somebody, "I'm sorry I made that mistake." People who can't do that will cause worries and troubles for themselves.

Able to forgive other people when they say they're sorry. Why not answer, "Thank you. I accept your apology"? Some people forgive other people even if the other person hasn't said, "I'm sorry I did that." Is that a good idea? I'm not sure.

Not bragging or being arrogant. It's OK to believe you are a good person with talents and abilities. It's not good to brag and act like you believe you are better than other people.

Grateful (appreciative). People who have been fortunate (have had good things happen) in life should feel grateful and honestly tell other people that they feel grateful. If someone does something nice for you, it's good for you to say, "Thank you very much."

Cooperative. It's good, for example, to cooperate with other students in working on a class project at school.

Willing to try to have friends who behave in good ways. Some children who behave in bad ways can influence other children, causing trouble for the other children. It's good for you to make decisions that will help you to have nice friends and avoid "getting into trouble."

Willing to tell your parents when you feel disappointed or upset. You are an important person. It's OK for a parent to tell a child that the parent feels disappointed or upset about something the child has done or said. Also, it's OK for a child to tell a parent or parents that she or he is disappointed or upset about something. For example, it's OK for a child to say in a respectful way to his parent or parents, "I'm disappointed that you won't let me have Jimmy sleep over at our house this Saturday night. I would like for us to talk about that."

Helpful articles on the Internet.

Adadoni, Laura (no date given). "How to teach morals to children." Howtoadult.com website

Grant, Adam (2014). "Raising a moral child." NewYorkTimes.com website

Jennings, David (2012). "7 ways to teach morals to children." childrensministry.com website

Sweat, Becky (2008). "10 practical ways to teach your children right values." Beyondtoday.com website

Weissbourd, Richard (2009). "Why teaching values isn't enough." PsychologyToday.com website

REFERENCES

Berne, Eric (1964). *Games people play*. NY, NY: Grove Press.

Harris, Thomas (2014). *I'm OK, you're OK*. NY, NY: Galahad Books.

Pew Research Center (2015). America's changing religious landscape. Pew Research Center Religion and Public Life website (May 12, 2015).

—— CHAPTER 19 ——
Parenting

Elaboration. Research on parenting has not clearly shown that parenting makes much difference regarding outcomes for children. Having conducted a fair amount of statistical research and having been a parent for 39 years, I suspect that there are serious flaws in research that is interpreted as indicating that parenting doesn't make any difference.

If you would like to read a short, sensible introduction to that subject, search on the Internet for "Does good parenting make any difference?" by Thomas Kidd.

Importance of this subject. In spite of conclusions often reached in research concerning effects of parenting, I, like many other parents of fine and capable children, intuitively feel and think that parenting can make a significant positive or negative difference in life outcomes for children.

I have recently realized that society tends to treat this as involving a one-way (unilateral) human interaction, with parents "parenting" their children. Especially since I wrote the essay about teaching moral behavior to children, I think that it is better to remain aware that this is actually a bi-lateral human interaction.

Sharing an opinion that I have. Since sometime early in my life, I have thought that young children are the most important humans. It follows that I believe that how adults treat and parent children is extremely important.

A proposal. I suggest that colleges and universities offer a one- or two-hour for-credit course about parenting. Except, possibly, in institutions with religious affiliation, it would be undesirable for the instructor to teach approaches based on a particular religious tradition.

A course could cover examples in history and literature of especially important parenting. It would make sense to identify and discuss issues relating to parenting concerning which "reasonable people can disagree." I am confident that an instructor with relevant expertise (e.g., psychology PhD and experience) could develop and teach an excellent course.

Some ideas about course content. I was a very experienced and, I think, capable Criminal Justice generalist. My favorite course was the CJ major "capstone" course. There was no text. I wrote the best issues about criminal justice I could write, one or more for each class. While this probably wouldn't be the best way to structure a course about parenting, covering important issues relating to parenting would be crucial. I'll list a few. "How important is it for parents to treat their children equally?" "What are examples of circumstances that would justify deviating from equal treatment of children?" "Can use of corporal punishment with children be justified?" "Through what age do children tend to need their parents?" I've heard age 35. "Given that 'bad peers' definitely can have very bad effects on teenagers, are there potentially effective ways parents can steer their child away from one or more 'bad peers'?" "What are examples of situations in which it would be OK or not OK for parent(s) to make suggestions to their children?" (Suggestions might include "constructive criticism.") "How important is age of the child concerning this?" "What is a good 'rule of thumb' concerning whether parents will pay for a child's higher education v. the child developing significant higher-education debt?" "Is it a significant problem that progressively more children are returning to live in their parents' homes?" "What are safe ways for a parent or child to attempt to move into discussion of an important, potentially difficult subject with a child or parent?" "If a parent has such a busy schedule that she or he can't find time to get the minimum amount of healthful exercise, would it be acceptable for a child or children to be asked to do chores that will make that minimum amount of time available to the parent?" Of course, the most important set of issues would concern findings of research about parenting. Each of the Internet articles listed below could provide content for a class or part of a class.

Relevance for young adults. This is obviously an important subject for young adults who are or will soon become parents.

A way to access excellent books about parenting. Go to textbooks,com "Parenting Textbooks." Though the list may not include many textbooks on the subject, it includes many interesting books.

Articles about research relating to parenting. Here are titles of articles about parenting I recently found on the Internet. (Searching for "what the research says about parenting" seems to produce helpful results.)

"Parenting that works" by Amy Novotney

"Parenting styles: what they are and why they matter"

"Learning to read: what research says parents can do to help their children"

Authoritarian parenting: What happens to the kids?

"The case against spanking." American Psychological Association

"A call to commitment: fathers' involvement in children's learning"

"What the research says on parenting after divorce"

What does research say about marriage and child wellbeing?

"Kids and screen time: what does the research say?"

Author's relevant experience. Several years ago, I had the epiphany that having my mother, who was a school principal, church deacon, and a North Carolina Mother of the Year, was the most important thing that happened to me in the early decades of my life. She took four sons to live in our family's one bedroom "summer cabin" after my father died tragically in 1949. My experience with parenting has been very much less demanding than hers was.

A high percentage of parents have more experience living with their young children than I have had. I enjoyed living with my son Alex during his crucial first two years. His mother and I separated when he was 2 years old, and he later lived with her.

Being Alex's father has very greatly enhanced the quality of my life experience since his birth in 1978. Because of my limited experience as a parent, my discussion in this chapter is very limited in scope. As mentioned below, there are many excellent books available about parenting.

Teaching morals to children. I hope you read the essay that preceded this chapter. Of course, I tried to do a good job of teaching moral behavior to Alex. It was fun. Actually, nearly all activities with Alex have been fun.

My ideas about being a live-in father during my son's first two years.

(a) **Try to be realistic about your preparation and capabilities to be the parent of a very young baby**. Partly because I grew up without a father from the age of five, I did not believe or feel that I knew how to be a good and effective parent during my young adulthood.

(b) **Buy and read an excellent book about parenting from birth through the first six months**. When my wife was pregnant in 1978, I bought for us a popular book about parenting in the first six months of a baby's life. You can search for "top 10 best-selling parenting books for newborns." When Alex was a young baby, I went to the Michigan State library and found and read articles reporting research concerning the parenting of infants and toddlers.

(c) **Have lots of close, loving, stimulating contact with your young baby.** One article reported that **having frequent loving contact with a baby, including talking to the baby, tends to result in the child progressing on a higher intellectual trajectory.** I enjoyed carrying baby Alex out onto our back deck during the beautiful fall season and talking to him about the beautiful hickory and maple leaves we could reach out and touch and the creek we could barely see at the bottom of the ravine. Since early childhood, Alex has progressed on a very high trajectory intellectually. Now 39, he will soon earn a PhD in computer science at a major U.S. university.

So, my experience is that studying high quality information about parenting can have positive payoffs. I believe also that the first two years of child's life are so important that it can be a big mistake for the parents or parent to fail to interact very extensively and lovingly with the child during those years.

(d) **Before the end of the first six months, buy and read an excellent book about parenting during the first two years.** When Alex was about six months old, I bought and read a popular book about parenting during the first two years. You can do a search for "parenting books that have stood the test of time."

My ideas about being a good long-distance father after the first two years. As I mentioned earlier, Alex's mother and I separated when Alex was about 2 years old. From then until going to college, Alex lived with his mother. It appears to me that she did a very good job. I'll share some of my ideas about being a long-distance father.

(a) **Try to be a consistently interested, loving, and supportive presence in your child's life.** Even when Alex was a toddler, I called him and talked with him on the phone about once a week. I am very glad that I was able to spend nearly all of my vacation days with Alex through about his 16th birthday.

(b) **Try to never say a negative word about the other parent.** If you can do so sincerely, try to make positive comments about her or him.

(c) **Demonstrate healthful lifestyle during your visits with your child**. Every day during visits, Alex and I shared some type of exercise, mainly walking. We ate healthfully and inexpensively.

(d) **Develop fun traditions with your child**. From his age of two through about the age of 14, Alex and I had a "candle time" tradition. Near bedtime, we would turn off the TV and all of the lights and light a candle or lamp. Then, we would talk about lots of (I hoped) fun and interesting things about our day and about various aspects of living. For example, by the age of 2½, Alex knew some about the benefits of physical exercise. Maybe as a result, starting about age 20, he has exercised before school or work on four to five days per week. Happily, Alex has great healthful lifestyle and is healthy in all ways I know about. Though he has not been "into" sports, I felt sure that, if he had wanted to, he could have played and started in football at his big high school. Physical exercise is the best way to build your brain power. I feel sure that his regular exercise has built his brain power.

I think it's very important for parents to have fun with their children. Having fun and being happy is important to successful living.

(e) **Try to be responsible about having other children**. I realized that I was terrifically fortunate to have a happy, healthy, talented son. I decided that it would be good to avoid being the father of one or more additional children.

Possible reasons why colleges seldom offer a for-credit course on parenting. So, what are possible reasons that few colleges and universities have an undergraduate course on parenting? My guess is that there may be four primary reasons. First, many college students probably feel no urgency to prepare for parenting. Second, many students, some incorrectly, probably feel that they know enough about parenting. Third, some undergraduate students may fear that they will offend their parents if they take a course on parenting. Fourth, university and college administrations probably think that, since research has not clearly shown that parenting practices make any difference in life outcomes for children, there is not an appropriate literature to draw on in teaching such a course.

AN ESSAY MAINLY FOR YOUNG ADULTS: SOME COMMON SAYINGS WITH QUESTIONABLE VALIDITY

For decades it has seemed to me that many of our society's well accepted sayings don't provide correct information or good guidance. Here are some of those sayings.

"To succeed in life, you must conform." Actually, many people succeed and flourish with non-conforming (but still legal) approaches and behaviors. Many successful innovations were initially viewed as unconventional.

"Live for today, for tomorrow you may die." (This is taught in an often seen gin commercial on TV.) Actually, people who achieve much in life tend to have the ability to "delay gratification," instead of "living for today."

"You can do anything you really want to do." I realize that there are some very exceptional people for whom this is nearly true. For the rest of us, there are many careers and skills for which we do not have the required talent and/ or personality. A "success" book I read years ago had as its main idea that a high percentage of successful people do work that other people don't want to do.

"Go for the gold!" Sometimes, "going for the gold" involves trying to earn work promotions. The Peter Principle says, "In hierarchical organizations, people tend to rise to a level at which they are incompetent." When I was an Army Reserve JAG LTC, I was fortunate to have a job I knew well and could perform well. When the first Iraq war occurred, the Army needed to install an Army Reserve JAG LTC or colonel as the Staff Judge Advocate (top Army lawyer) at Fort Bragg, NC. I knew well that, should I be tapped for that job, I would have moved significantly past my level of competence and comfort.

"It's more important to work smart than hard." Edison said that genius is 5% inspiration and 95% perspiration. I think Edison came closer to giving sound advice. In writing, I need to work very hard.

"Only the strong survive." Being strong helps, but so do being smart, wise, creative, cooperative, determined, and well connected.

"Things will work out for the best in the end." Unfortunately, I no longer have this as a "working assumption" about how something important will work out.

"In the long run, people get what they deserve." Again, this is not proven true in the lives of many people.

Abolitionist Theodore Parker said, "Even though the arc of the moral universe is long, it bends toward justice." I think this is metaphysical gibberish. Unfortunately, the prospects for justice in many countries around the globe, including the U.S., are dismal. Those of us who support justice need to work "smart and hard."

"Variety is the spice of life." I think that, for many people, this is not the best approach to selection of work to do. Being a specialist is a good strategy in many sectors of the work world. I think I paid some price in my career for being a generalist.

"People appreciate constructive criticism." I actually believed that many decades ago. In most life situations, volunteering "constructive criticism" is best avoided. Even in bridge, in which I am a fairly high status player, I am very careful to ask a player if I can make a suggestion about how to best deal with a particular bridge situation.

"Do what your doctor says." Research shows that patients who insist on being involved in decision making about their health live longer than very compliant, unquestioning patients. Ornery patients have above-average survival prospects, also.

"It's important to age gracefully." While young adults aren't very concerned with this subject, I'll share that I think that fighting many aspects of aging is a better goal and strategy than aging gracefully.

"If you use good commonsense, you'll be OK." A similar sentiment is, "The only things I've needed to know I learned in kindergarten." I believe that a significant percentage of the situations we encounter in life require knowledge and judgment that are not at all commonplace or obvious.

"It is important to be assertive." Many experts have in recent decades conveyed this message. Recently, I have detected a less articulated suggestion: "In making decisions **about** being assertive, be very careful."

"I don't get mad: I get even." "Forgive and forget." "If someone slaps you on your right cheek, turn to him the other also." (Matthew 5:39) I don't support any of these maxims.

"Friendship is forever." Like other fraternity and sorority members, I was told and believed that friendships in a Greek organization would remain strong for the rest of your life. Of course, this actually does occur for some people, but I know it does not always occur. Maybe 15 years ago a popular book taught readers skill in getting rid of old friends.

"In the long run, the only thing that matters is how much you were loved." In life, there are many great things to achieve in addition to being loved. Some of these achievements contribute to self-actualization, which was Maslow's highest level of human need.

"A human life is over in the blinking of an eye." As I approach 75 years old, I believe that one of the many great things about living as a human being is that you may live for a genuinely long time.

"Enjoy celebrating Christmas!" On the Internet we find an estimate that the average person gains from three to seven pounds from Thanksgiving to New Year's Day. One expert estimated that the average continuing increase in weight during the holidays is one pound. Though that doesn't sound like very much, it's 15 pounds in 15 years. I think, also, that Christmas overspending contributes a lot to the financial woes of many people.

"No pain, no gain." A similar saying is, "The more strenuous your exercise is, the more you benefit." You probably don't know that very strenuous exercise makes your blood platelets stickier (bad!) and causes release of free radicals (bad). Moderate exercise makes your blood platelets less sticky (good!). I've settled on very brisk walking.

"Don't ever give up." People who've lived a long time with many activities probably tend to disagree. I actually do try very hard to avoid giving up my integrity and my hope for the future.

"It's only natural for men to 'wear the pants.'" Hunter-gatherer bands have been by far the most successful and continuing type of human social group. In them, band decision is egalitarian, which involved women participating fairly equally with men in group decision making.

"Nice guys finish last." This is a very thought-provoking saying that could easily be the subject of a book chapter or short book. Many self-described sexy and attractive women and men assume that this saying concerns only a man's success in gaining sexual access to attractive women. I think that broader interpretation makes the subject much more interesting and important. I assume that being "nice" includes being decent and moral.

Theresa E. DiDonato, PhD, has an article on the PsychologyToday.com website, "Do nice guys really finish last?" Based on her study of several research reports on the subject, she answers that, regarding acceptance by desirable women, nice guys don't finish last.

Please think for a second about whether the following men finished last: Will Rogers, Jimmy Carter, Arnold Palmer, John McCain, Gerald Ford, Billy Graham, Walter Cronkite, and Colin Powell. I enjoy thinking about nice guys I have known who finished far from last. Unfortunately, in nearly every professional/vocational field, some people use indecent and immoral behavior to "succeed." (So, not-nice guys don't necessarily finish last.)

An old man's short speech that you may decide to skip. Sometimes young adults get guidance from a type of unconventional society which urges them to do things like dangerous behavior, drinking too much, reckless sexual behavior, illegal behavior, cheating in school, bullying, taking illicit drugs, etc. As we all know but sometimes forget, each of these behaviors can have unexpected, bad results that may never go away. As mentioned in an earlier chapter, soon after winning lucrative NBA player contracts several years apart, Duke all-American players Bobby Hurley and Jay Williams both suffered career-ending vehicular accidents.

── CHAPTER 20 ──
Joys of Frugal Living

Importance of this subject. You cannot over-emphasize that one of the greatest joys of frugal living is avoidance or minimization of money worries, which can be caused by overspending. I will readily bet that the happiest people tend to be those who consistently "live within their means."

"The best things in life are free." The fact that many types of wonderful things and activities are free or nearly free is probably the main reason that there really are great joys of frugal living. One of the best aspects of my childhood was being taught several types of very enjoyable, healthful recreation that were free or nearly free.

Societal promotion of maximum purchasing and borrowing. I believe it is accurate to say that the total mercantile, industrial, and financial complex in the U.S. operates to promote and achieve maximum purchasing and borrowing by Americans. Persons, including young adults, who respond to this marketing and advertising pressure by overspending and/ or over-borrowing tend to get into financial trouble very quickly. The information in the next section suggests that, at any given time, many millions of Americans have overspent and/or over-borrowed or simply are earning too little.

Information about financial circumstances of Americans. Available information about the economic circumstances of Americans suggests that a high percentage of Americans need to have a frugal lifestyle.

In an article on the CNBC website (12/13/16), Jessica Dickler quotes NerdWallet as reporting the following average levels of debt of U.S. families that have a particular type of debt: credit cards—$16,061; mortgages—$172,806; auto loans—$28,535; student loans—$49,042; and "any debt"—$132,529. The average credit card interest rate is reported as 18.76%.

There is on the DQYDJ website an article with the title, "Net worth in the U.S." Zooming in the top centiles," dated August 22, 2017. The article reports average net worth of families in particular centiles, as follows:

99.9%—$30,644,280
99.5%—$11,898,128
99%—$7,869,549
95%—$1,868,640
90%—$943,656
80%—$428,540
70%—$247,026
60%—$147,732
50%—$81,456
40%—$38,322
30%—$14,840
20%—$4,314
10%—$2,066

Results of a survey by CareerBuilder.com are reported on the CBSPhilly website, August, 24, 2017. It was found that 78% of workers say that they are living from paycheck to paycheck to make ends meet. This percentage is increasing because cost of living is increasing faster than wages are increasing.

All of these financial findings strongly support a conclusion that a very high percentage of U.S. families need to have a frugal lifestyle.

Author's relevant experience. In the middle 1960s, a close male relative had a very expensive lifestyle (e.g., new Buick, yacht, expensive clothes, etc.). Unfortunately, he completely fell apart psychiatrically and has never come back. After that happened, I resolved that I would do whatever was necessary to live within a realistic monthly budget, which has often necessitated being frugal in many ways. That was one of the best decisions of my life. I'll assure you that being reasonably frugal does not keep you from having an excellent lifestyle and life.

As my twin brother David and I grew up, literally, in a log cabin on a dirt road, our mother did not have money for expensive trips, toys, and treats. So, we learned recreation that was free (e.g., basketball, singing, bridge, canoeing, tennis, and looking for interesting things as we explored the swamp and pine forest). Free, healthful recreation can be an important part of joyful frugal living.

Though tens of millions of Americans within five years of my age have earned more money during their working careers than I have (often very much more), my frugal lifestyle has allowed me to now be financially ahead of millions of those people.

Having paid off my debts in 2015, I enjoy several inexpensive splurges. For example, I have bought about 100 terrific, previously expensive shirts at thrift stores and greatly enjoy wearing them. My favorite shirt had a tear on the cuff. I got out my sewing box and repaired the tear in ten minutes.

Relevance for young adults. Early in your working career can be a good time to learn how to be frugal and to actually start being frugal. You can learn early that it doesn't hurt.

Comparison of examples of affluent and frugal living.

	Affluent option	Frugal option
Housing	Expensive new construction	Fixer-upper with "sweat equity"; a "tiny house," as featured on HGTV
Transportation	Expensive new car	I bought excellent Volvo for $2700, drove it for 100,000 miles (no breakdowns), and sold it for $1700.
Vacation trips	DisneyWorld	Camping at state and national parks
Vacation housing	Expensive hotel, resort	Buy beach or mountain condo, rent it, stay there two weeks per year, plus some weekends.

	Time share (very expensive)	Share ownership of condo with 5-to-10 other families. Cost is a small fraction of time share cost. Later, you can sell your share for a profit.
Vacation vehicle	Expensive RV	Camper trailer
Movies	Expensive trips to movie theater	Rent movie, watch in home video room.
Water recreation	Expensive, fast, loud water transportation, such as jet skis	Buy canoe, enjoy wonderful canoe floats. Canoeing can provide meaningful exercise.
Golf	Expensive country club, always riding 18 holes	Walk 9 holes at inexpensive public course.
Dining	Expensive restaurants	Enjoy inventive grilling with family and friends. Excellent Marie Callender's frozen dinners cost less than $2.75.
Wardrobe	Expensive purchases	Identify great thrift and consignment shops; make excellent purchases.
Entertainment	Expensive concerts, sometimes with travel expenses	Museums, zoos, concerts on TV
Haircuts	Expensive female or male cuts	Cut your own hair. This saved me $10,000 in 30 years and $10,000 worth of my time.
Internet shopping	Shopping on expensive sites	Subscribe to a discount catalog, such as HeartlandAmerica.com.

Over about 30 years, I have received the free HeartlandAmerica catalog and have been able to shop also on their website. I've made many excellent, cost-saving purchases. Currently, you can buy beautiful wing-tip men's shoes for between $24 and $28. Recently, I bought a $340 retail watch for $33 and a $160 electric shaver for $40.

If a family or individual adopts an affluent lifestyle, moderate income is inadequate, and low income is disastrous. If a family adopts a frugal lifestyle, low income is survivable, and moderate income is more than adequate.

I think the families who opt for the frugal options can have as much fun as the affluent lifestyle folks and will not be worried by drains on family budget. Research has shown that, up to some annual income ($75,000 in one study), additional income is associated with an increase in happiness. Past that income level, there is no predictable increase in happiness as income increases.

Tips about thrift store shopping from a 40-year veteran. (1) Many people contribute potentially valuable items in December, which is at the end of the tax year, in order to qualify for a tax deduction in that year. That is a good time to check out thrift stores that sometimes offer high value items. (2) For a town or city area to have thrift stores with many excellent items, the surrounding area needs to have an excess of affluent people and a shortage of poor people. The Pinehurst area (especially Southern Pines) in North Carolina meets those criteria. (3) I suspect that the management of a big Goodwill store near me is allowing persons to purchase the best items before they are put on display in the store.

Healthy eating on a budget. On the Money Crashers website, there is an article with the title "How to eat healthy on a budget." I fully realize I should have been doing those things for many years. Unfortunately, in our society bad food costs less than good food.

Influential writing about frugal living. For some number of years before 2000, there was an important regular publication about frugal living, *The Tightwad Gazette.* You can buy *The Complete Tightwad Gazette* (1998) by Amy Dacyczn.

A website about "living large on a small budget". If this appeals to you, you can go to the Wisebread website. That website and the information it provides appear to be a contemporary attempt to meet the needs *The Tightwad Gazette* previously sought to meet.

Tips about spending less and enjoying more. Search for that phrase, and you will find several potentially helpful articles. For example, on the *Psychology Today* website, there is an article by Heidi Grant Halvorson, PhD, with the title "5 easy tips for spending less." That article focuses on dealing with a problematic tendency to spend too much.

Article about starting to save money. On the MyFINANCE website, there is an article with the title "Easy ways to start saving money." (I've elected not to provide other information about what appeared to be a rip-off scam about achieving excellent income with virtually no effort. If it appears too good to be true, it probably isn't true.)

REFERENCES

Dacyczn, Amy (1998). *The Complete tightwad Gazette*. NY, NY: Villard Publishing.

—— CHAPTER 21 ——
How to Retrieve Some Good from a Failure

Elaboration. Nearly everyone eventually experiences what they believe and feel is a significant failure. People differ in how they respond to failure. The main idea of this chapter is that, after surviving the failure, which can be a significant challenge, a person who has failed in some way may be able to figure out how to benefit in some significant way from the experience of failure. While doing that, one can remember two well accepted sayings: "Anything that doesn't kill you makes you stronger" and "Try to turn lemons into lemonade."

Thomas Edison said, "I haven't failed. I've found 10,000 ways that don't work." After serving as Arkansas governor for a term, Bill Clinton was defeated in his reelection run. Instead of giving up, he and Hillary learned from this failure. He was later elected as the Arkansas governor and served for ten additional years.

The framers of the Articles of Confederation (adopted 1781) failed to create the structure for continuing and successful government in the area that became the original 13 states of the U.S. That failed attempt provided information and insights needed to write the current U.S. Constitution, which has provided the framework for by far the longest lasting constitutional government in world history.

Bankruptcy law is based on the assumption that financial failures happen and that it is good to give people who have experienced serious financial failure a chance to become financially viable and successful persons again. There are countless examples of individuals and companies that have gone through bankruptcy and have later become extremely successful.

In many work activities, to achieve major success, you must risk failure. It is likely that nearly all very successful doctors, lawyers, and investors have failed some.

Post-traumatic growth. Failure is often traumatic. Stephen Joseph has an article, "What doesn't kill us: post-traumatic growth," May 12, 2013, on the Huffington Post website. He states,

> "Post-traumatic growth refers to how adversity can often be a springboard to a new and more meaningful life in which people reevaluate their priorities, deepen their relation-ships, and find new understandings of who they are."

Author's relevant experience. An understanding (and maybe sympa-thetic) person who knows me well might say, "John has had more success in scholarly research and writing than in university teaching and more suc-cess in parenting than in marriage." I may have experienced more than my "fair share" of failure. A female professor once told me, "If you were black or female, you could teach anywhere you wanted to teach." Never being con-sidered for academic tenure, even though I believed I met the criteria, was a significant failure for me.

Whether you view an outcome in your life as a failure is very important. Imagine a couple who get a divorce, and each of them and their child or chil-dren are fine and are looking forward to the future. Instead of focusing on the failure, the ex-husband and ex-wife can remember that they were substantially unscathed when they went through a difficult transition (divorce) in which horrible damage to personalities, finances, and life prospects can occur.

A suggestion based on decades of experience. For decades, I thought that self-deprecating humor is the best type. While I'm proud of how I have lived my life, I've decided in recent years that nothing good is gained by making yourself the butt of jokes referring to your actual life experiences.

Importance of this subject. We all know that it is possible for a person to experience a failure as very devastating. Some people who marry and later separate and divorce are deeply wounded by that experience and never recover. Just as bankruptcy allows a person who has experienced financial failure a chance to get a fresh start, I believe it is important for people encountering many types of failure to realize that "some clouds have a silver lining."

Relevance for young adults. Failure is probably most likely to occur during a person's young adult years.

An excellent book exactly on this subject. Dr. Tim Harford is the author of *Adapt: Why success always starts with failure* (2011), which does an excellent job of communicating the main message of this chapter. You can find a review which communicates many of the points of the book on the 99u website and another review on the *Guardian* website.

Examples of possible failure and benefits that might be derived from the failure.

(1) Failure of an excellent young athlete in his or her favorite sport. For every basketball player in the U.S. who makes a living playing basketball, there are undoubtedly thousands of "wanta be's" who have spent many thousands of hours trying to get good enough to succeed in professional basketball. Such a person's failure can allow him or her to concentrate on realistic career pursuits.

(2) Failure in a marriage. The "spurned" partner can learn many types of important life lessons. Obviously, having that type of marriage with that type of spouse probably won't work in the future. Maybe a "spurned" male who got married before having a solid situation regarding career and finances can realize that, prior to a second marriage, those things should be more solid.

(3) Failure of an innovated product or service. As Dr. Herford argues, every successful innovation is preceded by some number of unsuccessful versions of that innovation. So, the innovator can learn from the failure and improve the innovation.

(4) A young lawyer discovers that general practice of law is too stressful for her or him. (It has been reported that one of eight practicing lawyers is giving some thought to committing suicide, probably because of the stress.) Learning this lesson can prompt the lawyer to find a low-stress legal specialty, such as patent law.

(5) Failure of a young singer-songwriter who had moved to Nashville. A town the size of Columbia, SC, needs about 3,000 lawyers. It doesn't need any singer-songwriters. Maybe this is a dose of reality that will motivate this musician to pursue another type of work, which may be connected with music.

(6) Failure of a university physics major to make sufficiently good grades in physics to be accepted in a physics master's degree program. This student needs to grasp that a student with enough talent and drive to make mainly Bs and Cs in college physics has the talent and drive to succeed in many other subjects and careers.

(7) An excellent student who has earned an MBA (master of business administration) gets a high paying job in business, gets married, buys an expensive house, buys a new car, and joins an expensive country club. He loses the job and has no prospects of making that much money again. He and his wife can discover the joys of frugal living, lower their blood pressure, and maybe improve activities in their home's master bedroom.

(8) A newly graduated physician gets a job in an expensive suburb of Philadelphia. For whatever reason, she or he is not able to get enough paying patients in this highly competitive medical services environment. Maybe moving to a much smaller city/town that needs a doctor with that specialty is the right move.

I can give literally hundreds of hypothetical situations of this sort. In life, the important question often is not whether a person will be "put on his butt" (knocked down). The most important question is, "Will she or he get up?"

Do you tend to be over-optimistic (over-confident) or pessimistic (possibly under-confident?). I think that this is an important question for nearly everyone. (Socrates said, "Know thyself.") I have tended to be over-optimistic and over-confident. This has led to some disappointments. A person who tends to be over-confident may tend toward being somewhat grandiose. Experiencing a failure can help you to gain valuable self-knowledge.

A relevant maxim from poker. In poker, strong players agree, "If you are never called when you bluff, you aren't bluffing enough." There is a similar maxim in duplicate bridge. The point is: **In some life activities, it can be very important to be willing to take risks that you will experience failure to some extent. If you are unwilling to do that, your ability to succeed meaningfully will be decreased.**

The importance of trying to figure out how to benefit from adversity. For many decades, I have tried to be alert to do this and think I have often succeeded. I will give you a current example in my life. I believe my right hip is vulnerable to injury. So, when walking upstairs, I grab the stairs rail with my right hand and use my right arm to reduce exertion/strain of my right hip. I have been hoping that this will strengthen my right arm and improve my golf game. As of June of 2018, my golf play had improved substantially, probably because of this strengthening of my right hand, wrist, and arm.

Possible benefits of minor neuroses.

Depression. The tendency to experience depression is so common among humans that it is possible that having that vulnerability had survival value in the evolution of man.

When a person experiences depression, it is likely that the person has very recently experienced some type of failure or even defeat. It's possible that she or he has experienced severe stress, resulting in the physiological stress reaction. In that type of situation, "continuing the fight" is probably not a good option. Being depressed can force the person to retreat and, probably, be less active. That can provide helpful rest and physical and/or emotional healing. This break can give the person an opportunity to think carefully about what has happened and about how she or he can avoid that outcome in the future. Maybe more importantly, this gives the individual ample time to discover or develop opportunities and consider them.

Anxiety. I believe that experiencing anxiety can have survival value, as when a person awakens in the middle of the night and can't go back to sleep because of anxiety (worrying) about something. While awake, the person can do some possibly helpful "brainstorming" about the problematic situation. After feeling less anxious allows him to eventually go back to sleep, his brain can continue to "work on" the difficult situation. As we have often heard, it can help to "sleep on it."

Paranoia. *Shark Tank* regular, Robert Herjavec, said during a recent show, "In my business, only the paranoid survive." I will share, however, that, because my oldest brother became a totally disabled paranoid-schizophrenic 50 years ago, I have always consciously tried to avoid engaging in paranoid thinking.

REFERENCES

Harford, T. (2011). *Adapt: Why success always starts with failure*. NY, NY: Farrar, Straus and Giroux.

CHAPTER 22
Sources of Supplementary Individual Income

Elaboration. This chapter concerns ways that a person with a primary job can either earn or otherwise lawfully acquire additional money. Of course, these approaches can be used by a stay-at-home mom or dad, a retiree, or a person who is "between jobs."

A way to find side gigs. I think that the best way to find a side gig (part-time job) is to go to Craig's List and click on "gigs."

Information on financial circumstances of Americans. In an article on the CNBC website (12/13/16), Jessica Dickler quotes NerdWallet as reporting the following average levels of debt of U.S. families that have a particular type of debt: credit cards—$16,061; mortgages—$172,806; auto loans—$28,535; student loans—$49,042; and "any debt"—$132,529. The reported average credit card interest rate is 18.76%.

There is on the DQYDJ website an article with the title, "Net worth in the U.S. zooming in the top centiles," dated August 22, 2017. The article's report of average net worth of families in particular centiles follows:

99.9%—$30,644,280
99.5%—$11,898,128
99%—$7,869,549
95%—$1,868,640
90%—$943,656
80%—$428,540

70%—$247,026
60%—$147,732
50%—$81,456
40%—$38,322
30%—$14,840
20%—$4,314
10%—$2,066

Results of a survey by CareerBuilder.com are reported on the CBSPhilly website, August, 24, 2017. It was found that 78% of workers say that they are living from paycheck to paycheck to make ends meet. This percentage is increasing because cost of living is increasing faster than wages.

Obviously, this information suggests that many people, probably especially young adults, could benefit from developing one or more sources of supplementary income.

Relevant experience of the author. My main source of supplementary income was staying in the Army Reserve for 17 years after five years of Army active duty (1969–74). Actually, pay for my monthly weekend drills and the summer two-week stints of Army Reserve duty provided a reasonable level of compensation for my time and work. The modest retirement and medical coverage (Tricare) I acquired at age 60 are quite helpful. With Tricare, I don't need to have a health insurance policy that would be secondary to Medicare. Given my various health challenges, such a policy for me would be very expensive.

My other source of supplementary income was real estate ownership. For example, I bought a house on a 15-year mortgage in 2004. I rented it from 2006 until 2015 and did not have to pay income tax on the rent because of house depreciation. My renter paid nearly 2/3 of the entire mortgage.

Since retiring in 2004, I have often had the opportunity to direct duplicate bridge games, which takes nearly five hours and pays $40 to $50. Making no more per hour than a high school dropout or illegal immigrant doesn't appeal to me. Obviously, people prefer side gigs with meaningful monetary payoff.

Importance of this subject. Years ago, the average job of a professional person lasted 24 years. Now the average is about 4.5 years. It is not unreasonable for some people who change jobs several times to want to make or acquire some extra money, especially between jobs.

For some people, a supplementary income activity eventually becomes the primary source of income. Fortunately, a side gig can be recreational, which, as discussed in chapter 17, can produce various types of non-monetary benefits.

Relevance for young adults. Obviously, this subject can be of special interest to recent college graduates who have a main job that doesn't pay well and college debts to pay off.

One advantage of having a for-credit course about this is that students may obtain information that will allow them to take one or more courses to prepare themselves to acquire supplementary income. Students who wanted to prepare income tax returns during "tax season" could take a course about taxes.

To find information about this on the Internet, I suggest that you search for "ways to earn extra money." You will find several lists of ways to earn extra money. There is a good article about side gigs on the Daily Worth website, "The best ways to make extra money freelancing, telecommuting, or starting a side job." Also, there are excellent books about good side gigs.

Information about new careers. On the MyLifeStyleCareer website, there is an article that may provide valuable information about sources of supplementary income: "100 great second-act career resources."

Real estate investment and ownership. In the U.S., a high percentage of wealthy people, including a U.S. President, became wealthy through real estate investment and improvement.

I am glad that, during my 20s and 30s, I read several good books on real estate investing. If I were a recent college graduate now, I would very strongly consider buying a triplex or quadraplex on a 15-year mortgage, managing it, and living in it until it became financially feasible to buy an additional single-family residence. So, by some time in my middle or late thirties, the mortgage would be paid off, and I would have a substantial addition to my monthly income, making a side gig unnecessary. Another good strategy is to have a rental apartment in your house, which may pay half of your mortgage.

If this is interesting to you, you can consider many types of real estate investing, including (1) buying, renovating, and selling fixer-uppers; (2) buying, owning, and renting houses and apartments in houses for income; and (3) buying, owning, renting by the week or month, and occasionally using a resort condo or house. Of course, there are other options. I recommend that you search on the Internet for a book that tells about various real estate investing options. Obviously, getting important details about various types of real estate investing may help you to make a good decision for yourself and your family.

If you are worried about adequacy of income for retirement, you can buy a retirement home 15 years before retirement on a 15-year mortgage. You can rent it until your retirement, when it will be paid off, and use funds from your primary house to help with retirement expenses. For all practical purposes, I succeeded in doing this.

HARP mortgage modification program. You might qualify for this program, which is easily found on the Internet, and reduce your mortgage payment by as much as slightly more than $350 per month.

A warning. In buying real estate, it is obviously important to be well informed and prudent. In the U.S. in the years shortly before the 2007–8 Great Recession, many young real estate investors undoubtedly bought overpriced houses to renovate and flip or rent. Unfortunately, real estate prices dropped so much in the Great Recession that many of these families and individuals lost tens of thousands of dollars. As discussed in chapter 36, some types of investing involve high-risk decision making.

<u>Service in a military service reserve or national guard</u>. Serving in a military service reserve or national guard can have significant financial payoffs. Here is some information most young people probably don't have. If you serve for 20 years in a reserve or national guard and don't have a significant amount of active-duty time, your pension at age 60 will not be very substantial. I had five years of Army active duty and retired at the rank of lieutenant colonel, which made my Army Reserve pension significantly higher than would be the case for a non-commissioned officer (NCO) with nearly no active duty time.

An active-duty Army lieutenant recently told me that, when he leaves active duty, he probably will not try to stay in the Army Reserve. He thinks that many potential employers would not want to hire someone who is in an active reserve or national guard, because of potential conflicts with requirements of civilian employment.

<u>Utilizing your education, talents, and connections</u>. Please forgive me for (again) writing something obvious. Instead of taking the first side gig that is available, maybe you can get a better situation by trying to utilize your strengths and assets, including your education, talents, and connections. Suppose your parents have a friend who owns an expensive restaurant. What would be wrong with using that connection to get a job waiting tables that will pay $30 per hour?

<u>Tradeoffs relating to side gigs</u>. A person who has two side gigs has three jobs. This is generally viewed as a very bad situation to get into.

Having a side gig can interfere with your main job, with your relationship with your spouse, with parenting, and with getting recreation. I was fortunate that my two additional sources of income did not significantly interfere with other aspects of my life.

It seems to me that most people would benefit from finding some income alternative other than having a time- and energy-consuming second job. Recently, Mark Cuban said on *Shark Tank* to three young female entrepreneurs, "Don't get a second job. Live like a college student and sleep on the floor. Make sure you don't accumulate any debt."

One alternative to taking a second job is to move your family to a less expensive city or town, where you can get a job that will more adequately pay family expenses. Another option is reducing family expenses, as discussed in chapter 20 on frugal living.

SECTION 8
Politics and Government

CHAPTER 23
Emergence and Evolution of Political Values

Importance of this subject. Currently, political polarization in the U.S. is, I believe, making traditional democratic compromise very much less likely than as recently as the President Clinton-Speaker Gingrich years (late 1990s). I believe, as discussed in chapter 25, that this is adversely affecting the quality of government on at least the national level.

I recently heard a Republican Congressional leader say that dealing with Obama Care through Congressional legislation cannot possibly occur through compromise with Democrats. In chapter 33 on the origins of religion, I mention that hunter-gatherer bands in Africa during the 200,000 bp to 70,000 bp period nearly certainly had egalitarian band decision making. That had to involve compromise. The point is that compromise was crucial in the governance of, by far, the most successful type of human group, which was the hunter-gatherer band. I think that the approach of Republican leaders now will not succeed.

As I discuss in some other chapters, I think the fact that a high percentage of early Americans with European roots shared adherence to Christian morality was very important and positive. In particular, I believe that the fact that many of them may have genuinely "lived" the Golden Rule ("Do unto others as you would have them do unto you.") had mainly positive effects. Now, the extreme political polarization that has developed in the U.S. is making broad "living" of the Golden Rule much less likely and common. Do we seriously believe that conservative Republicans genuinely care about the wellbeing of poor liberal Democrats or vice versa?

Perceptions of Americans regarding the prevalence of incivility in U.S. society. In December of 2016, a research report by Weber Shandwick and Powell Tate, in partnership with KRC Research, "Civility in America: a nationwide survey," was released. A central finding is that 75% of respondents believed that incivility has risen to crisis levels. That same percentage blame politicians for this erosion of civility.

As I discussed in the previous paragraph, if two people genuinely adhere to the Golden Rule, incivility should not occur. This subject is importantly connected to this chapter and the subjects of chapters 26 through 29.

Author's relevant expertise, experiences, and beliefs.

Expertise. My study in law school and my teaching relating to law have given me substantial information about law and how legal principles emerged in the U.S. As a PhD criminologist, I have had a long-standing interest in various types of human beliefs and had a publication with a PhD anthropologist (Houston & Memory, 2001) about aspects of human cultures, such as norms and beliefs.

Author's relevant experience and belief. With an intelligent, liberal, and well-informed mother, I was exposed to information about politics and government very early in my life. From the time I entered the first grade in 1949 through some time shortly after the turn of the new century, I had the impression that many important Republican and Democratic political leaders ascribed to a large extent to a significant number of "core political values."

Law school has subject matter which allows a motivated student to learn a terrific amount about the evolution of legal principles. So, during law school, I learned a lot about conservative and liberal values. Fortunately, I was able to write a lead law review article (Memory, 1967) about the evolution of the right to counsel in the U.S. and be an associate editor of the law review. As a graduate student at Florida State University, I taught "Constitutional Law."

As I have noted several times in this book, I am a life-long Democrat and have never voted for a Republican.

William F. Buckley, Jr.'s excellent TV show, "Firing Line," aired from 1966 to 1999. Though I knew that he was quite conservative, I watched that show as often as I could. I think that, partly as a result of that long exposure, I have fundamental respect for a high percentage of core conservative values.

Over my life since law school, political values and ideology usually have been significant parts of the "thinking aspects" of my life.

Relevance for young adults. Young adults will live in this politically polarized culture and suffer the adverse consequences. We must hope that they will govern better than some of their elders.

Elaboration. It appears that a high percentage of Americans ascribe to and support primarily either conservative or liberal values. I believe that people who ascribe nearly exclusively to conservative or liberal/progressive values and prescriptions tend to be historically uninformed and politically unsophisticated. The subject matter of a course on this subject should convey that many conservative values are legitimate and important and that many liberal values also are legitimate and important. Consistent with this, I believe that parents should be able to describe positive aspects of conservative and liberal/progressive values.

A proposal. I propose that university and college political science departments include in a three-hour course the emergence and evolution of political values in society. I hereby authorize professors to use any part of this chapter without further authorization by me.

Especially because I did not do a literature review prior to writing the papers in this chapter, I do not assert that this chapter makes a significant contribution to literature concerning political theory. I doubt, however, that many political science professors can provide the detailed thinking in this chapter about specific conservative and liberal values.

A paper I wrote on this subject. Several years after retiring in 2004, I wrote a long concept paper, which was probably fairly close to "publication-quality," describing in detail my hypothesis that liberal values have tended to emerge and evolve in response to excesses and oppression in the implementation of conservative values. In developing and writing that paper, I did not do a review of relevant scholarly literature. That concept paper and handouts I wrote for a talk on the subject follow.

"THE EMERGENCE OF POLITICAL VALUES IN HUMAN SOCIETY"

In this paper, I first present my thinking about how conservative values have emerged in human societies. Then, I present detailed thinking about how particular liberal values have arisen in response to excesses, abuse, oppression, corruption, or other undesirable outcomes in the implementation of conservative values.

Now, some disclosure: Though I have come over my life to embrace many conservative values, I've never voted for a Republican for anything. I did offer to work as a volunteer for the Bob Dole Presidential campaign.

Also, I didn't read any "literature" in developing this paper. I think there are times when one should try to produce thinking that is as original as possible. Kuhn (1996) has argued that it is productive for a scholar from one discipline to transport "paradigms" from his discipline into another discipline. Of course, I did not transport paradigms from Criminal Justice. The point is that I am not a political scientist. Instead, I am a lawyer and social scientist with a PhD in criminology who has tried to do a responsible and good job developing possibly novel ideas within the domain of political science.

You may ask, "How did you derive the 'conservative values' you list in your chart?" I tried, based on my many years as a lawyer, criminologist, professor, and politically aware citizen, to list values which to some degree support maintenance of the existing distribution of power and resources. Of course, I realize that my list is not a perfect listing of conservative values.

More than one scholar has stated (correctly, I assume) that my list of "conservative values" does not correspond to any of the generally accepted listings. I am not wedded to the "conservative" label for these values. I believe that those values are the values of a political establishment that are most likely to emerge in a relatively advanced society prior to liberal counteractions.

One irate, strongly ideological conservative said to me, "Your 'conservative values' alone would produce some sort of autocracy." Precisely!

A wise person said, "Contemplating polar opposites at the same time is very difficult intellectually." That is required in this undertaking. Because of "emotional loadings" concerning many things political, it is also difficult emotionally.

Some common characteristics of human cultures. The following is taken from a chapter (Houston & Memory, 2001) in a commercially published book. I co-authored that chapter with a PhD anthropologist.

When one examines human cultures, several things are practically always found. Since I am a criminologist and have a book on police problem solving (Memory & Aragon, 2001), I tend to focus on the things that involve problematic behavior, social control, and problem solving. This list applies to primitive human groups, human cultures through history, and cultural/ethnic groups existing now. This list does not apply well to advanced, complex, and/or pluralist societies.

Norms—behavior standards. The culture in effect teaches you how to behave by teaching norms. The most seriously maintained norms are mores. Less seriously maintained norms are folkways.

Homogeneity—sharing of race, religion, and other aspects of the culture by members of a group.

Taboos—very important norms which prohibit certain behavior. Several taboos (e.g., incest, killing of group members) are found in practically all primitive human groups.

Internalization of norms through socialization as morality and conscience

Commonly held values, such as ideas concerning what is right or important.

Commonly held opinions. An opinion usually expresses your view of the nature of reality.

Commonly held attitudes. An attitude generally expresses how positive your feelings are regarding something.

Roles. Mother, grandmother, hunter, and priest are roles.

Accumulated problem solutions of many types and important information/ knowledge of many types

Means to accumulate aspects of culture and transmit them to succeeding generations

Customs and traditions, which may involve solving problems or meeting needs.

Rituals, such as initiation of young males into manhood.

Shared religion. Often the shared religion is very central to the culture's means of behavior control. In some primitive human groups, there is no distinction between religious and non-religious aspects of life.

Expected altruism—the expectation that a member will act in certain situations in a self-sacrificing manner to the benefit of members of his or her group.

Reciprocity within the cultural group. "You scratch my back, and I'll scratch yours."

Recognition of the family, including the authority of parents over children.

Hierarchy—a chain of command or "pecking order."

Territoriality—recognition of control of certain territory by certain persons and groups. Control over and privacy concerning a family's living space are common.

Xenophobia—fear and hatred of that which is different.

Ethnocentrism—often exaggerated shared belief that your cultural group is superior to others.

Intentional shunning (ostracism) or exclusion in response to misbehavior

Means to detect and punish "cheaters"

Punishments for unacceptable behavior and reward for good behavior

Art and music

Emergence of conservative values. Sociobiology is the study of the biological bases of social behavior of social animals, including man. (Chapter 32 is about sociobiology.) Sociobiology, as a biological theory, explains certain arrangements and behaviors of social animals including man. The common characteristics of human cultures described above might be seen as arising from phenomena and arrangements described by sociobiology. Arrangements and behaviors that sprang from human nature in primitive human groups might historically and through cultural transmission have led to the existence of similar arrangements and behaviors in progressively more advanced human cultures and societies. Of course, human nature can be operating at any time tending to produce arrangements and behaviors consistent with human nature.

I believe that you find far more precursors of conservative values than liberal values in the common characteristics of human cultures. Though I might say here that conservative values are more primary than liberal values, I've realized that the aggressive responses that generate liberal values and arrangements are rooted in human (and social animal) nature. For example, subordinate male chimpanzees sometimes team up against an oppressive alpha-male chimpanzee. So, one might argue that liberal values are, in a way, more primary than conservative values.

You can find bases for some liberal values in human nature. For example, humans can easily detect if they are treated unequally and/or unfairly, and we often feel a desire to object in those situations.

The following paragraphs relate directly to the lengthy chart.

The emergence of liberal values. I want to make sure you understand the chart. Implementing conservative values involves exercise of power. Unfortunately, the exercise of unchecked power can easily lead to corruption, abuse, and excesses. **I believe liberal values have arisen in response to patterns of corruption, abuse, excess, and oppression in the implementation of conservative values.** It would be sensible to see liberal values as expressive of a desire for justice, including fairness and equality of treatment, which is how I "dumb-down" the thinking of John Rawls (2001). Of course, there are excesses and abuses in the implementation of liberal values which have provoked conservative reactions, such as many of the policies of the Reagan administrations.

Glance over the conservative values listed in the left column of the chart. They represent an inevitably imperfect attempt by me to list conservative values in pure form. It would be impossible to have a stable complex society without implementation of nearly all of those values.

Now, glance over the liberal values in the right column in the chart. Rather than weakening society, they provide great strength and viability to our society, economy, and government.

Remarkably, Republicans have convinced many Americans that it is practically un-American to support anything liberal. I think that, actually, it is un-American to fail to support a substantial number of liberal values.

CONTINUATION OF CHAPTER 21

<u>CONSERVATIVE VALUES</u> >>>>>>>	<u>ABUSES, EXCESSES, OUTCOMES</u>>>>>>	<u>LIBERAL VALUES</u>
Preservation of favorable power and ownership arrangements	Corruption, abuses, ineffectiveness of the conservative "establishment"	Democracy in government and corporations, allowing non-violent transfer of power and property
Allowance of cooperation of the powerful and the "power elite"	Governmental corruption (e.g., Abramoff case); monopolistic practices	Government ethics laws; anti-trust laws
Allowance of communication to the public by "the powerful" in government, business, and industry	Misleading of the public; withholding of information	Freedom of speech and press, which allow dissemination of counter information; freedom of information act statutes (FOIA)

Expectations of conformity with norms and behaviors, opinions, and attitudes consistent with conservative values	Oppression of "the different" and unconventional persons	Tolerance and protection of lawful, non-dangerous behavior, opinions, and attitudes; freedom of action
Enforcement of taboos that are consistent with conservative values	(e.g., prohibition of inter-racial dating and marriage)	"Outlawing" of some taboos
Promotion of male dominance, misogyny	Oppression of women; exclusion of women from positions of power	Women's suffrage; prohibition of discrimination on the basis of sex
Preference for racial homogeneity, consistent with xenophobia	Oppression of members of minority races; discrimination based on race	Prohibition of discrimination on the basis of race; affirmative action; searching for strength in diversity
Preference for religious conformity and homogeneity	Favoritism and oppression on the basis of religion	Prohibition of discrimination on the basis of religion

Implementation through law of religious moral principles	Offending of members of some religious groups	Separation of church and state
Favoritism for members of one's group in government and business	Nepotism in government; less than optimal performance of government	Prohibition of nepotism
Social exclusivity in groups of powerful and affluent conservatives	Exclusion of members of some groups	Prohibition of discrimination in some types of social groups
Protection of ownership and use of property	Harms to society and other persons resulting from property uses	Zoning laws; environmental laws
Enforcement of compliance with directions of constituted authority; all expected to "know their places"	Severe treatment for non-compliance	Protection of "whistle-blowers"; limitations on power to fire
Expectation of hard work by and self-reliance of individuals	Some can't support themselves, even if they work hard and dependably.	Provision of a "safety net"; minimum-wage law

Expectation that individuals obtain resources through lawful activity	Individual failures to meet needs lawfully	Provision of a "safety net"
Reward of individuals for conventional success	Failures of individuals in work and finances	Assistance to individuals with insufficient capabilities and resources to succeed, to avoid casualties (A.D.A.)
Expectation that individuals will meet financial, legal, and social obligations; court and non-official enforcement	Failures to meet various types of obligations	Bankruptcy laws; homestead exemption; only reasonable child-support decrees enforced through jailing
Promotion of heterosexual marriage		Acceptance of other living and sexual arrangements and family
Expectation of protection of self and family	Failures to protect	Protection of "the vulnerable" by governmental agencies and courts; protection of the public by police

Opportunity to prosper through entrepreneurship in the "free enterprise system"		Opportunity to prosper through entrepreneurship in the "free enterprise system"
Opportunity of industries and businesses to profit from work of others, sometimes "have-nots"	Exploitation and oppression of labor; dangerous working conditions	Rights of labor to organize; child-labor laws; safe work conditions laws
Ability of the able and industrious to achieve wealth and an extremely high standard of living and quality of life	Unchecked greed; CEO compensation packages as much as hundreds of times as high as lowest wage worker packages	Expectation of social justice, which includes fair and equal treatment; not implemented to date
Allowing those who earn money to retain it	Need for taxation to fund government operations	Progressive taxation rates implemented
Promotion of economic growth, including reduction of taxes on the wealthy	Widening of gap between rich and poor	Expectation of social justice, which includes fair and equal treatment; demand for non-regressive taxation

Promotion of high spending and "keeping up with the Joneses"	Over-spending, debt, and resulting high incidence of financial destitution	Bankruptcy law; debtors' rights
"Buyer beware" implementation	Fraud, resulting injury of consumers	Disclosure-by-seller laws; responsibility of seller for injury from dangerous or defective goods
Promotion of investment in corporations and businesses	Securities fraud; "insider trading"	Criminalization of "insider trading"; laws protecting investors
Protection of ownership of innovations (patent and copyright laws)	Extreme enrichment of innovators	Statutory provision for expiration of patents and copyrights
Expectation that families will support family members	Failures to support	Provision of "safety net"; Medicaid, food stamps, etc.

Expectation that families will carry out and fund education of family members	Failures to educate	Public education; public universities; community colleges; Pell grants
General antipathy for government	Need for government functions	Creation and expansion of government functions
Emphasis on performance of functions by the private sector rather than government	Inability of the private sector to perform some functions; excessive cost of some "out-sourcing"	Performance of certain functions by government
Avoidance of unnecessary and excessive regulation of business and industry	Harms caused by business and industry	Some governmental regulation of business and industry (e.g., E.P.A.)
Support for "strong executives" in government, business, and industry	Autocratic executive functioning; corruption, nepotism	The Rule of Law; "checks and balances" in government; boards of directors in corporations

Expectation that, in a democracy, the "majority will rule"	Oppression of minorities by majorities (e.g., elimination of home property tax)	Protection of minorities from oppression by majorities, partly through constitutional enforcement
Maintaining security of persons and property	Danger of creation of a police state and resulting oppression; NSA wiretapping	Freedom of movement, assembly, and association
Order maintenance, including prevention and control of riots	Danger of creation of a police state and resulting oppression	Freedom of movement, assembly, and association
Extensive powers for police to achieve legitimate purposes	Invasion of privacy; oppressive and unlawful police action; danger of police state	Freedom from unreasonable searches and seizures, from arrests without probable cause, from detentions without reasonable suspicion; right to recover damages for violations of rights

Sufficient police authorization to use force, including deadly force	Excessive use of force by police; "police brutality"	Limitation on use of deadly force; right to recover damages for excessive use of force
Mistakes by police in search or interrogation should not prevent conviction of the guilty.	Unlawful searches and interrogations	Search and interrogation "exclusionary rules"
Effective and cost-efficient prosecution of defendants	Conviction of innocent persons	Requirement of according of "Due Process of Law" and proof beyond a reasonable doubt in trials
Preference for harsh treatment of inmates	Brutal conditions leading to violence and disorder	Requirement of humane and decent treatment of inmates; right to recover damages by inmates for violations of rights

Implications. "Crossfire" was by far the worst TV show ever. It contributed to an atmosphere of extreme partisanship in the U.S. No adherent to conservatism or liberalism could safely admit to the error of his side or the validity in a perspective of the other side. Also, there are "unmentionables truths" relating to society that conservatives will not acknowledge. The same applies to liberalism and liberals. As a Criminal Justice professor, I have listed and discussed "unmentionable truths" of conservatives and liberals relating to crime and justice. This situation makes intelligent, influential conversation about these issues virtually impossible.

So, the only hope may be that the Presidency and the Congress will be controlled by different parties. An example: Clinton stole conservative initiatives and made them his own. Welfare reform and a balanced budget were passed and were excellent legislative policy for the U.S.

Marxist theorists believe that society is split into competing factions and strata which constantly disagree and conflict because of many deep and serious conflicts regarding crucially important matters. I think the Marxists (Conflict social theorists) greatly overstate their case. I believe that a significant percentage of Americans would support a very high percentage of the values of the right and the left that I list in the handout, if they were presented without a conservative or liberal label.

Importantly, polls near the end of the GWB Presidency (2000–2008) showed that a very high percentage of the public in the U.S. rejected conservative solutions to problems. Excesses, corruption, and oppression by conservatives, especially those in the Bush administration and the DeLay Congress, had made this rejection of some conservative solutions possible.

During the first two years of the Trump Presidency, EPA administrator Scott Pruitt has been abolishing vast numbers of environment-protection measures which had arisen over decades in response to a wide variety of types of "environmental wrongs" by, primarily, U.S. industries. If a Democrat is elected President in 2020 and Democrats have control at least of the House of Representatives, it is predictable that measures to reverse many of the Pruitt actions will be undertaken by the new EPA administrator.

Summary. I have offered some thinking regarding how conservative values have emerged in human cultures and societies and some very specific thinking about how liberal values have arisen in response to abuse, oppression, corruption, and other undesirable outcomes which have occurred in and because of implementation of conservative values. Finally, I discussed several conclusions I have reached related to this subject and line of reasoning.

REFERENCES

Houston, M., & Memory, J. M. (2001). Problem solutions in culture and society. In J. M. Memory & Aragon, R. (Eds.), *Patrol officer problem solving and solutions*. Durham, NC: Carolina Academic Press.

Kuhn, Thomas S. (3rd ed., 1996). *The structure of scientific revolutions*. Chicago, IL: University of Chicago Press.

Rawls, John (2001). *Justice as fairness: a restatement*. Boston, MA: Belknap Press.

— CHAPTER 24 —
The Importance of Moral Courage in Work and Government

Elaboration. The Wikipedia definition of moral courage is, "[T]he courage to take action for moral reasons despite the risk of adverse consequences." So, if you have moral courage, you have courage of your convictions.

While much of this chapter concerns whistle-blowing and "leaking", that is only a small part of this broad subject. I believe that nearly every person who has a job or has a role in government has encountered or will encounter one or more situations in which "doing the right thing" required or requires exhibition of moral courage.

Of course, there can be a need for moral courage in life situations beyond work and government. For example, if a college fraternity engages in severe hazing of its pledges, there will be a need for one or more of the fraternity members to take a moral stand against the hazing.

The book I read as a teenager that influenced me the most was *Profiles in Courage* (1956) by John F. Kennedy. I believe that many Americans have learned a great deal about the importance of moral courage by reading this book.

James Comey's recent book (2018), *A Higher Loyalty: Truth, Lies, and Leadership*, includes detailed description of successful resistance by acting Attorney General Comey and FBI director Robert Mueller to George W. Bush administration continuation of warrantless domestic wiretapping under the Terrorist Surveillance Program. That is an especially vivid example of the moral courage of federal justice officials who were determined to prevent unlawful action by the federal government. I know from my own experience that a government or military lawyer can pay a price for exhibiting moral courage.

A current example of failure to exhibit moral courage concerned the sexual abuse of literally hundreds of female gymnasts by Dr. Lawrence Nassar, a physician affiliated with USA Gymnastics and Michigan State University. Many people affiliated with USA Gymnastics or Michigan State University had strong incriminating information about activities of Dr. Nassar for many years before sufficient public communication of that information occurred.

One can easily develop hypothetical situations that would require moral courage by a teacher or professor, researcher (especially if funded by a corporation), minister, journalist, government official or employee, law enforcement officer, lawyer representing an individual, and persons in a wide variety of other roles. An important book (Null et al, 2011) by a highly qualified team of health professionals reports that annually one million Americans die as a result of some type of error or deficiency of treatment by health professionals. I believe that this definitively establishes that there is very often unmet need for exhibition of moral courage by persons working in the health field.

Importance of this subject. It is difficult to overestimate the importance of this subject. I believe that, for any nation or human group to function constructively, a high percentage of people must be willing to do the right things, especially concerning the treatment of individuals and groups, in spite of possible adverse consequences for themselves. We know of many nations that have overwhelmed any resistance by moral persons and have engaged in horribly immoral action.

The Uniform Code of Military Justice requires that members of military services refuse to carry out unlawful orders. Obviously, this requires moral courage.

Relevance for young adults. As discussed in an essay prior to chapter19 on parenting, it is important for children to develop strong morality that results in moral behavior. A high percentage of young adults have obtained or are seeking employment that they hope will continue and be rewarding in many ways. Obtaining information in a course on this subject might help students to make good decisions about job opportunities and about how to act during employment.

Whistle-blowing and "leaking." Whistle-blowing and "leaking" can involve doing the right thing in spite of possible adverse consequences for yourself. A definition of a "whistleblower" is given in "Whistleblower," which is the title of a Wikipedia article that is worth reading.

"A whistleblower is a person who exposes any kind of information or activity that is deemed illegal, unethical, or not correct within an organization that is either private or public."

On the whistleblower.org website, you can find an article, "A timeline of U.S. whistleblowers." There are other websites that provide extensive information about the history of whistleblowing, starting many centuries ago.

Importance of willingness to be a whistle-blower or "leaker." It is important for a society that information about unlawful and/or destructive functioning of businesses, government agencies, or some other type of organizations can possibly "come to light." If this information about unlawful and/or destructive functioning becomes known by many people or the right people, it may be possible for the unlawful and/or destructive functioning to be ended or greatly reduced. It is important, also, for people to be sophisticated about the possibility of seriously improper functioning within a company, government agency, or other organization. This awareness can help individuals to avoid becoming involved in that type of organization and, if already involved, to avoid a personally traumatic outcome, such as loss of a job and work opportunities as a result of participating in whistle-blowing or "leaking."

Especially in very recent years, the related phenomenon of "leaking" of sensitive information has become common and quite important. There is a Wikipedia article about this with the title "News leak." My recollection is that there was not a significant amount of "leaking" by people in the Obama White House. As we all know, leaking was very significant during the 2016 Presidential campaign and during the first year of the Trump administration. It is possible that some of the leakers were paid to "leak." During recent months, materials have been leaked from investigative agencies. The significance of leaks in recent years is shown by the notoriety or prominence of WikiLeaks, especially regarding the release of Hillary Clinton's emails.

The leaking of the Pentagon papers during the Vietnam War provided information to Americans about the conduct of that war. In my opinion, it was a good thing for the U.S. that a majority of Americans learned about and turned against the Vietnam War.

During June of 2018, the FBI arrested a retired Senate staff person and charged him with criminal leaking of classified material. Leaking of many types of Congressional committee non-classified information would not be criminal.

Some whistle-blowers act altruistically. Many types of human groups can benefit from one or more members exhibiting altruism, which is acting unselfishly motivated by concern for the welfare of others. Sometimes, altruism involves sacrificing your own welfare or survival to protect other members of your group. My impression is that Americans have in recent decades become less likely to act altruistically and that there are progressively fewer people who could be described in a new version of *Profiles in Courage*.

Chapter 26 concerns genocides and "ethnic cleansing." It is unspeakably tragic and horrific that 200,000 Europeans participated in the Nazi "final solution." Obviously, any attempts of these people to be whistle-blowers in that situation were of no consequence.

Whistle-blower protection. To learn about federal statutes that provide protection for whistle-blowers in employment, search on the Internet for "The whistle blower protection programs." Some states, including California, have passed statutes providing employment protections for whistle-blowers.

Author's relevant experience. I provide here possibly more information than you want to have about my personal experiences relating to this subject. I believe I have at least a fairly good understanding of this subject because, during college and my military and civilian careers, I was willing to do the right thing on six different occasions, even if an adverse consequence was possible or even likely for me.

(1) During college at Wake Forest College, I learned that a star

halfback on the football team and one of his fraternity brothers were break-ing into professors' offices, stealing tests, and selling copies of the tests. I had personal morality that was formed in a small-town Baptist church and in Boy Scouting and had read and admired JFK's *Profiles in Courage*. So, I reported them to the WFC Honor Council. They were expelled but returned a year later. I think that the consequences for me were at least as bad. Even way back in 1963, being a "snitch" on an ordinary college campus (not a military service academy) was not accepted by the student culture. There were times when I felt that having reported those two students caused me to be treated as a pariah. Later in life, the star halfback often told people that being kicked out of school was the best thing that ever happened to him.

(2) When I was an active-duty Army defense lawyer, I wrote and sent to the top Army lawyer (the Judge Advocate General) a concept paper arguing that defense lawyers should not have to work for and be rated by their large unit's top lawyer (the Staff Judge Advocate). When my SJA at the time learned of this paper, I was relieved from my position and transferred to another JAG assignment on post. (Fairly soon thereafter the Judge Advocate General changed the assignment structure for defense counsel in the Army in ways that were fully consistent with my recommendations.)

(3) During university teaching prior to being awarded a PhD, I im-prudently gave negative performance ratings to my department chairperson. My guess is that this action very adversely affected my teaching career.

(4) While working in the South Carolina governor's office in the middle 1980s, I became aware that there was a major increase in the prison population occurring, resulting in prison overcrowding. So, I wrote the "S.C. Prison Overcrowding Powers Act," which provided that, if the prisons ex-ceeded their design capacities, there would be a release of inmates until the population was down to design capacity. Excellent Democratic Governor Richard Riley had my bill passed. It was not well received by the law-and-order types. My contract was not renewed. Obviously, I failed to grasp, much less understand, emerging political opinions relating to criminal justice.

(5) When I was later working as a Criminal Justice professor, I

became aware that the police department in the nearby city had entirely stopped reporting aggravated assaults, apparently to qualify to be designated as an All-American City. I reported this by some means and did not have my professor contract renewed, even though my scholarship qualifications were extremely strong (better than those of 10 professors in the Criminal Justice department combined).

(6) In the early 1990s, I was a JAG LTC assigned as the deputy Staff Judge Advocate of the largest Army Reserve unit in the Carolinas. I reviewed a report of an accident, with serious injury, of a military truck that was being driven 20+ miles an hour faster than authorized. I recommended that the driver be court-martialed. Apparently the commanding general and my boss, the Staff Judge Advocate colonel, did not like my recommendation. That may have adversely affected my officer efficiency report (OER).

During my active-duty and reserve military career, I developed a somewhat related impression that an Army officer can survive "taking a stand on principle" one time. I think that doing that more than once tends to result in his or her being branded as a troublemaker, with adverse consequences for the officer's military career.

So, I believe I have several times exhibited moral courage and in every case experienced some type of adverse consequence. Fortunately, in spite of these experiences, I have somehow managed to complete my working career successfully enough to retire comfortably. Many whistle-blowers and others who exhibit moral courage suffer career-ending or other very severe consequences of their only instance of whistle-blowing or exhibition of moral courage.

Speculation about a "whistle-blower personality." I want to clarify that I don't have information about the personalities of particular whistle-blowers. Also, I'm not suggesting that nearly all whistle-blowers suffer from a type of neurosis. My speculation is based on what I know about my own personality and how it led me to do several things that were similar to whistle-blowing.

I think that during my childhood and even late teens, there was significant emphasis on "doing the right and moral thing" in church, Sunday school,

Boy Scouts, and even my college fraternity, Sigma Chi. I don't have the faintest recollection of discussing or hearing a talk or sermon about being careful to avoid doing things that would be likely to result in adverse consequences for yourself.

I have searched on the Internet for good information about an "oppressive superego" or "overactive superego" but haven't found any. Without that information, I will say that, regarding the six incidents I described above, I strongly wanted to do the right thing and wanted to avoid being a coward. My guess is that, until sometime in my 30s, I had a very active conscience (overactive or oppressive superego) that was not sufficiently checked by my ego (rational capacity). Eventually, my ego kicked in and said, "If you shoot yourself in the foot enough times, eventually you will lose the ability to walk."

You may assume that I wish I had not acted as I did in those situations. While I wish I had proceeded more cautiously in some of the situations, I am glad that I took meaningful action in all of those situations.

Some advice relating to potential "moral courage" situations. I don't encourage anyone in the work world to voluntarily confront these types of risks as often as I did. (I'm sure that some people have confronted them much more often than I did.) Instead, I encourage you to find work situations in which you believe you will be unlikely to think you should exhibit moral courage. If that type of situation should arise, I encourage you to work very hard and creatively to come up with a way to act morally and responsibly without jeopardizing your job or your career. It might help to discuss the situation with a person you can trust.

Proposal of an undergraduate course about the importance of exhibiting moral courage in work and government. In my opinion, this subject is important and substantive enough to support a three-hour undergraduate course. I believe that courses on this subject are seldom offered and that the absence of such courses probably occurs for two main reasons: (1) The subject is so broad that it is extremely unlikely that a professor in a discipline and academic department would offer a course with such broad subject matter. (2) This course would involve teaching morality and the importance of exhibiting moral courage in a very wide variety of situations in work and government. My impression is that colleges and universities do not want to focus on teaching morality. University academic tenure was established to protect professors from retribution provoked by their public actions and statements. I think, possibly incorrectly, that display of moral courage by a professor is not a common occurrence in the U.S.

Probable effect on whistle-blowing in the U.S. if the U.S. moves toward tyranny and fascism. As discussed in chapter 25, distinguished scholar and professor Dr. Timothy Snyder fears that the U.S. is moving in the direction of having tyrannical government. Should that occur, obviously the danger of being a whistle-blower or otherwise exhibiting moral courage in government will increase greatly. We know that tyrannical government can be fascist, which involves private ownership of industry. Presumably, whistle-blowing in a company in that situation would be very hazardous. On the *New York Times* website there is an article, "When the boss wants you to do something unethical," by Daniel Victor, dated July 6, 2017.

Feasibility of a nonprofit organization with the goal of assisting potential whistle-blowers and leakers. Such an organization might be worthwhile. It would be difficult to obtain monetary contributions from corporations.

A postscript concerning James Comey. Though I earlier mentioned favorably James Comey's recent book (2018), I do not believe that he has always exhibited exemplary judgment. Near the end of the 2016 Presidential election campaign, he violated very clear and long-standing Department of Justice and FBI policy by issuing a public statement regarding continuing investigation of Hillary Clinton by the FBI. I believe that his flagrant violation of that policy probably resulted in Clinton losing in the election. As discussed extensively in chapter 36, it is extremely important for people to exhibit excellent judgment in making decisions relating to high-risk situations. I believe this was a major misstep by Comey in a long career. Similarly, I believe that, though George W. Bush was a very poor President in many ways, his successful efforts to have the U.S. invade Iraq in 2003 was fully sufficient to establish that he was an extremely bad and deficient President.

REFERENCES

Comey, James (2018). *A higher loyalty: truth, lies, and leadership*. NY, NY: Flatiron Books.

Kennedy, John F. (1956). *Profiles in courage*. NY, NY: Harper & Brothers.

Null, Gary et al (2011). *Death by medicine*. Mt. Jackson, VA: Praktikos Books.

Snyder, Timothy (2017). *On tyranny: twenty lessons from the twentieth century*. NY, NY: Tim Duggan Books.

— CHAPTER 25 —
The Erosion of Numerous Positive Aspects of Government and Life in the U.S.

Elaboration. The central conclusion and prediction of this chapter is that, if important trends in the U.S. since 2000 and since the election of Donald Trump continue, the quality of many important aspects of government and life in the U.S. will decline substantially.

Very recent books and other significant writing related to the subject of this chapter. An important book by Steven Brill (2018) is one of several recent books which argue that many things Americans "hold dear" are gravely jeopardized now. A book about "the plot to destroy democracy" by Malcolm Nance (2018) was published in the summer of 2018.

Of course, many thousands of editorials, opeds, and articles on this subject have been published since early 2017. I will note an article on the Internet in *Slate* by Lili Loofbourow, "The America we thought we knew is gone."

World-wide favorable trends. Credible journalist Nicholas Kristof stated on *Fareed Zakaria GPS* in January of 2018 that 2017 was, worldwide, the best year ever. For example, so much progress has been made against poverty that, worldwide, fewer than 10% of people live in poverty. In attempting to make sense of any subject, you must consider evidence that supports and evidence that doesn't support your pre-conceptions.

Author's relevant experience. My education and career have given me information and ideas relating to this subject. I have always been intensely interested in politics. While I often share with friends something I've written relating to this, I'll mention five of the many people who can talk about this much more intelligently than I can: Fareed Zakaria, Rachel Maddow, Pete Peterson, Nicholas Burns, and Thomas Friedman.

<u>Evidence that erosion of many important aspects of government and life in the U.S. is occurring.</u>

In 2000, U.S. government was excellent. There was a budget surplus, and the national debt was being paid off. Important legislation was being passed through compromise of the political parties. The U.S. was not in a military conflict. U.S. influence was increasing around the globe, and democracy and human rights were increasing in many countries.

Developments concerning the U.S. Supreme Court. The U.S. Supreme Court handling of the <u>Bush v. Gore</u> election case in 2000 suggested to me that significant politicization of the U.S. Supreme Court had occurred. If another conservative Supreme Court justice is soon confirmed by the Senate, many important liberal legal precedents will be jeopardized.

Occurrences during the George W. Bush two-term Presidential administration. I believe that in 2000 many Americans and members of the GWB administration were complacent about the difficulties and hazards involved in conduct of the executive branch of U.S. government. The 9/11 attacks were not prevented. President Bush had Congress pass a major unfunded tax cut. Increase of the national debt resumed. Though it might have been prevented, the Great Recession of 2007-8 was not prevented. At a time when it was important to maintain U.S. attention to the Afghanistan War, Bush commenced the second Iraq War, which was not in any way required or prudent. It is my strong opinion, as a retired Army Reserve LTC, that, for some period of time after the start of the second Iraq War, the U.S. was extremely vulnerable militarily. The Afghanistan and Iraq wars have been and continue to be financially disastrous for the U.S. and have had adverse health consequences for many Americans and for residents of those countries. These two continuing military commitments will nearly certainly have very undesirable consequences for the U.S. for decades to come.

Lack of success in winning significant wars since WWII. As a retired Army Reserve lieutenant colonel, I have felt very hesitant to list this area of difficulty. I believe, however, that, in the greater scheme of things, this is quite significant.

As I discussed above, while the U.S. was engaged in the post-9/11 war in Afghanistan, President George W. Bush managed to commit the U.S. to invading Iraq. Hans Blix, chief U.N. weapons inspector, had stated in public prior to that invasion that in two years the U.S. could complete entirely satisfactory weapons inspections in Iraq. Therefore, there clearly was no military necessity or justification for that war. An expert on national security has told me that alienation of Muslims that was caused by that war has been a central cause of many of the military and national security difficulties the U.S. has encountered in the middle east. To use a golf phrase, the Iraq War caused the U.S. to "take its eye off the ball" in Afghanistan. The result is that it does not appear to be possible, 16 years after the war began, that the U.S. will be able to bring that war to a satisfactory end. This sequence of events showed that there is a serious flaw in the structure of national security decision making in the U.S. Because of the costs of the Iraq War for the U.S., the security situation there now, the extension of Iranian influence there, and other considerations, I believe that the Iraq War certainly cannot be viewed as a "won war" by the U.S.

Developments during the Obama two-term Presidential administration. Republican Congressional leaders announced that their main goal was to prevent Obama's reelection and prevent his Presidency from being successful. Their nearly entirely obstructionist functioning prevented passage of important legislation. I believe that President Obama did not lead constructively concerning to race relations. The national debt increased. For whatever reason, our government did not prevent or terminate the devastating Russian attack on the process of the 2016 election.

Trump administration. Trump is by executive order eliminating many aspects of needed government functioning. He is crippling federal agencies in several ways, such as refusal to appoint many important agency officials and have them approved by Congress. Trump at least acquiesced in Secretary Tillerson's devastation of the structure and function of the State Department. Though the Republicans control the Presidency, Senate, and House, they have been unable to pass any significant legislation, except for the 2017 Republican tax cut. Though the scientific evidence regarding global warming is overwhelming, Trump has withdrawn the U.S. from the Paris agreement relating to climate. He has too little public support to exercise the powers of the Presidency in constructive ways.

Nearly all of Trump's major actions have been by fiat, which is how autocrats govern. **Trump notably fails to exhibit many important types of leadership, including inspirational leadership, moral leadership, leadership in developing national consensus on important subjects, leadership in achieving bi-partisan compromises, and leadership of effective, needed action in federal agencies.**

In October of 2017, a book (Lee et al, 2017) was published which includes discussion by 27 psychiatrists and mental health experts regarding the "dangerous case of Donald Trump." Since early in 2017, many other psychiatrists and psychologists have made detailed public statements to the effect that President Trump is a seriously ill person psychologically and that his service as President poses a very great threat to our government and society.

On December 14, 2017, a major newspaper article told about Trump's adverse reactions during intelligence briefings when there is any mention of troublesome activities of the Russian government. This confirms that Trump is entirely refusing to accept the reality that the Russians have engaged in many types of interference with the 2016 election. It is possible that the truth is that the Russians have information about Trump that gives them a stranglehold on Trump. Either situation–delusional failure of a President to acknowledge very important reality or a President who is to a very large extent controlled by a foreign, very adverse government–will contribute to deterioration of the quality of government in the U.S.

During my career, I worked as an environmental lawyer for 2.5 years. That experience makes me aware that nearly every time Scott Pruitt has eliminated an EPA regulation forces have been put into action that will cause significant, possibly severe, adverse environmental impacts for some number of people living in the U.S.

The danger of development of tyrannical government in the U.S.
A very successful scholar and author, Professor Timothy Snyder, argues in an important new book (Snyder, 2017) that there is a danger that the U.S. is moving toward having tyrannical government. If the U.S. develops tyranny, it will be a failed liberal democratic-republican state.

As recently as the Obama administration, the U.S. was a liberal democratic republic. I believe that, as president, Trump has moved several aspects of government toward authoritarianism and fascism.

(1) The 2017 Republican tax cut is entirely consistent with a tax cut you would expect for a government characterized by authoritarianism and fascism. That tax cut is discussed extensively in chapter 29.

(2) As discussed above, Trump's decision making as president has been nearly entirely by fiat. That is how autocrats rule. As an exception to government by fiat, Trump worked to have passed the 2017 Republican tax cut.

(3) As previously discussed in this book, there are many types of important presidential leadership that Trump is apparently unable to perform. For example, his divisive political strategy and performance as president make leadership in developing national consensus on important subjects impossible.

(4) Trump's intentional alienation from liberal democratic ally nations and his consistent action to curry favor with Putin tend to move the U.S. government toward authoritarian fascism.

(5) The immigrant family separation policy was so intentionally cruel that it was suggestive of action by an authoritarian, fascist government.

(6) As discussed previously, Trump has made nearly all decisions as president in favor of business and against the interests of workers, consumers, and ordinary citizens. That has been especially notable regarding changes in the EPA. It is well known that fascist government is characterized by close cooperation of the authoritarian leader and privately owned industry.

(7) As discussed previously, to preserve liberal democratic republican government, the primary leader and millions of lower leaders and workers must be deeply committed to the democracy, rule of law, due process of law, equal protection of the laws, civil liberties, and civil rights. Trump's behavior as a candidate and president has not suggested that he is in the slightest committed to effectuation and preservation of these aspects of law and values.

Developments concerning functioning of Congress. Political polarization is so great that real political compromise cannot occur. If a member of Congress cooperates with the other party, extremists in his or her party will probably have that person defeated in the next Congressional primary elections. Members of Congress are mainly concerned to be reelected. For decades, there have been no new political "profiles in courage." Influence of lobbyists is very great, and they care only about achieving benefit for their clients. Gerrymandering has been used to decrease political influence mainly of Democrats.

Increase in the national debt. During summer of 2018, I heard a report on NPR that the Republican 2017 tax cut is causing much faster growth of the national debt than had been predicted.

Continued increase of ethnocentrism and xenophobia of ethnic and possibly religious groups in the U.S. Chapter 28 is about the dangers of rampant ethnocentrism and xenophobia of ethnic groups. Just as I think activities of Black Lives Matter partially prompted the emergence of the alt right, I believe the outrageous 2017 Republican tax cut will tend to prompt increase in ethnocentrism and xenophobia of African-Americans.

In human history, the countries that have succeeded and prospered for many years have tended to be ones with a very large, ethnically homogeneous majority group. As discussed in chapter 28, I believe that ethnocentrism and xenophobia of African-Americans have increased substantially in recent years. The emergence of the alt-right appears to indicate that ethnocentrism and xenophobia among White Americans is increasing. Demographers have announced when they believe White persons will become a minority group in the U.S. The U.S. is moving into uncharted, possibly dangerous waters. I believe there is a significant possibility that this will decrease the viability of government in the U.S. I greatly fear that Whites and Blacks in the U.S. are losing their ability to coexist enjoyably and peacefully and cooperate in meeting these challenges.

Changes concerning the U.S. electorate. Democratic government is premised on there being an intelligent, informed electorate with decency and fundamentally positive values. In 2016, the majority of White women voted for Trump, even though he had admitted that he readily sexually assaulted defenseless women. Chapter 34 of this book discusses in detail the many ways in which it has become very difficult for ordinary Americans to obtain correct information and be well informed.

Decrease in percentage of U.S. population who report Christian affiliation. I, an agnostic, believe that the fact that the vast majority of early Americans were Christian and, presumably, behaved primarily according to Christian morality from 1600 ad to some time in the 20th century was a very important factor that led to the success so far of the "American experiment." The Old Testament principle, "Love your neighbor as yourself," merely directs people to love and accept members of their own group. Jesus had the wisdom to articulate the Golden Rule, "Do unto others as you would have them do unto you." That rule directs followers to accept and treat decently even members of other ethnic, religious, and political groups.

It is reported on the Pew Research Center (2015) that from 2007 to 2014 the Christian share of the U.S. population fell from 78.4% to 70.6%. That constitutes a 10% decrease in seven years in U.S. of residents reporting Christian affiliation. McCullough & Willoughby (2009) have reported, based on their review of previous research, that religious parents tend to produce children with self-control. I strongly believe that deterioration of morality of Americans bodes ill for attempts to maintain and improve the quality of government and life in the U.S..

Leaders of Black Lives Matter refuse to acknowledge that all lives matter. This very deeply violates the principle underlying the Golden Rule. A person who genuinely ascribes to the Golden Rule will take action that endangers himself to save the life of a member of another racial, ethnic, or religious group.

I believe that many U.S. Presidents, including most recently President Jimmy Carter, have ascribed to the Golden Rule. I ask you to quickly decide how many of the following characteristics and behaviors are exhibited by President Trump: Catholic 7 virtues (prudence, justice, temperance, courage, faith, hope, and charity) and Catholic 7 deadly sins (pride, lust, envy, gluttony, wrath, and sloth). Of course, doing this doesn't produce a definitive study of Trump's morality. It provides a strong suggestion regarding the extent to which he exhibits morality that was viewed as ideal by the Catholic Church many centuries ago.

Kevin O'Leary, star of CNBC's "Shark Tank," often says, "It's all about the money. Money is the only thing I care about." This is a powerful and potentially significant rejection of human motivation rooted in the Golden Rule and other moral principles.

I want to clarify that I am not confident that, in the U.S. of 2018, Christians exhibit better morality, including ascription to the Golden Rule, than atheists, agnostics, and members of other religious groups. While I am "pro-Christian," it is saddening to me that Evangelical Christians strongly supported Trump during the Presidential primaries and election.

Developments regarding many important functions that are or can be influenced by the federal government. Major problems have developed concerning poor quality of public education, unfunded entitlements, high cost and poor quality of medical care, extreme disparities in income and wealth, and high cost of higher education. The infrastructure in the U.S. is in disastrously poor shape. It appears to me that the Interstate highway system is in many stretches inadequate and in bad condition. Race relations are rapidly getting worse. Interracial violence is increasing. The ravages caused by global warming will dramatically increase funding needed for federal government and state and local governments. If default on national debt occurs, U.S. ability to borrow will end or become much more expensive.

Rapid decrease in ability of Americans reaching retirement age to be able to afford to retire. For several decades, progressively fewer workers in the U.S. have been accruing retirement benefits. As a result, progressively fewer Americans will be able to afford to retire.

Problems regarding the quality of medical care in the U.S. Gary Null, PhD and a team of mainly M.D.'s have a book (Null et al, 2011) in which they claim that annually about one million Americans die as a result of some type of medical mistake or treatment. The point is that there are giant adverse human consequences of failures of traditional medicine in the U.S. Terry A. Rondberg reports in a book (1998) that 60% of surgeries in the U.S. are unnecessary.

Problems regarding availability of medical care. Americans are generally aware that many persons living in the U.S. do not have paid or affordable medical care. Unfortunately, insurance premiums are continuing to increase. A good source on this subject is an article dated September 19, 2017, "Key facts about the uninsured population," on the KFF.org (Henry S. Kaiser Family Foundation) website.

Increase in the cost of government and loss of company profitability as a result of global warming and severe weather events. These two things will increase government expenditures and decrease potential tax revenues.

Decrease in social and economic justice in the U.S. As I discuss in chapter 29, I believe that the 2017 Republican tax cut is extremely socially and economically unjust. This will increase the disparities in wealth and income problems in the U.S. As I discussed in a published oped included in that chapter, major disparities in economic circumstances between the very rich and the very poor tend to exacerbate a variety of social problems. For people in a country to have hope for the future, they need to think that their treatment by the government is just.

Decrease in general quality of life, increase in social problems, and increase in unlawful and otherwise problematic behavior. These things will result from a variety of adverse changes, some of which are described above.

Chapter 29 includes discussion of several worsening problems in the U.S.

Importance of this subject. Many of the developments described in the sections above are very important and either are influenced by or tend to cause deficient functioning of federal government. Recent research indicated that only 25% of Americans believe that the U.S. is "headed in the right direction."

Relevance for young adults. The adverse developments described above influence nearly every aspect of life in the U.S. Nearly all young adults will live in a world influenced by these trends for many decades.

An important relevant book. Peter G. Peterson has a recently published book, *Steering clear: how to avoid a debt crisis and secure our economic future* (2015). Though he is a Republican, I think that for many years he has worked and written intelligently and constructively relating to these types of issues and problems.

The case that America has greatness of many types that will not be lost easily. I always write a handout for discussions with a topic I have suggested. I wrote this for a Unitarian-Universalist church discussion group. U.S. history indicates or suggests that many types of greatness have been, are, or can be exhibited in the U.S.

How Can We Make America Great?

We have many physical characteristics and structures, values, institutions, and aspects of law that are strongly associated with greatness.

Our legal and institutional structures for having constitutional government, with peaceful transfer of governmental power, are strong and unequaled on the planet.

Our federal and state governments have legislative, judicial, and executive branches and meaningful checks and balances.

We have a federal system of government which is characterized by a rational allocation of functions to municipal, county, and state governments and to the federal government.

We have a strong tradition of rule of law and robust capabilities to enforce it.

We have established in law a remarkable array of civil liberties and robust capabilities to enforce them.

We have established in law a strong tradition of due process of law (fundamental fairness) and robust mainly judicial capabilities to achieve it.

We have established in law strong protection of equal protection of the laws and robust capabilities to achieve it.

We have unequaled higher education physical settings and faculty. This includes undergraduate institutions, graduate institutions, and community college institutions, which have the potential to be progressively more valuable.

We have unequaled capabilities relating to advanced medical diagnosis and treatment.

Medicare and Medicaid are viable and affordable and provide high quality medical care to many millions of people.

Social Security is viable and affordable and provides quality of life protection for many millions of senior citizens.

There remains in the U.S. population meaningful adherence to positive morality and common decency.

We have many aspects of governmental regulation, especially at the federal level, that are gravely threatened.

We have very extensive, valuable, remarkable, and, often, spectacular federal and state park systems.

Extensive zoning and city planning have allowed the planning and construction of many thousands of municipalities that offer high quality of life.

While we have extensive and valuable infrastructure (e.g., highways, bridges, tunnels, railroad-related assets, airports, etc.), they need to be very extensively repaired and improved. "Smart" maintenance utilizing the best available methods is needed.

We have very extensive and robust media, human, and technological capabilities and assets.

We have a well-educated population.

We have unequaled military physical and human assets and capabilities.

We have remarkably extensive power generation and distribution structures and capabilities.

We have very extensive computer science and technology structures and capabilities.

We have extensive and capable law enforcement and correctional structures and personnel.

We have extensive and capable legal and judicial institutions and personnel.

We have superb personnel and locales for science, engineering, and technology.

We have promotion and protection of innovation.

We have a President now who arguably has the potential to and appears to be likely to adversely affect many of these capabilities, functions, and assets.

Preliminary thinking about strategies to prevent deterioration of the quality of government and life in the U.S.

The Presidency. It appears likely that Trump will, by some means and fairly soon, be replaced as president. In 2016, the U.S. electorate elected a Republican as president. It will be important for the president for the remainder of the present four-year term to be a Republican. I have always been impressed by the capabilities of John Kasich. Mike Pence, not so much. I believe it is possible that the election of Donald Trump will become the worst occurrence in the U.S. during U.S. history, except for major wars.

It is possible that grassroots outrage about these problems and developments will develop in the U.S. If so, this might result in the election in 2020 of a President who is an ally of Senator Bernie Sanders. How about Elizabeth Warren?

Congress. Just as compromise of the political parties helped to advance responsible government during the second Bill Clinton term, I think it will be crucial for cooperation and compromise to return to Congress.

Federal budget and national debt. As the emergence of this national disaster has been occurring, the financial gap between the very rich and the poor has steadily increased. I believe that there should be a national consensus for dealing with this financial emergency largely by drawing on the exorbitant wealth of the economic elite. How else can Americans deal with this set of giant problems?

Solutions in the health/medical sector. During September of 2017, Democratic senators who will probably be Presidential candidates in 2020 were signing on as co-sponsors of "Medicare for all," which would be single-payer health insurance. As you would guess, I favor that idea.

I would favor rewarding excellent lifestyle and punishing poor lifestyle and unreasonable risk taking in health coverage. I think that implementing this radical idea would be difficult. (If 40% of Americans adopted the approaches recommended in the early chapters of this book, there would be devastating loss of income in the medical sector and disastrous increase in Social Security expenditures for decades.)

REFERENCES

Brill, Steven (2018). *Tail spin: the people and forces behind America's fifty-year fall–and those fighting to reverse it.* NY, NY: Alfred A. Knopf.

McCullough, Michael & Willoughby, Brian (2009). Religion, self-regulation, and self-control: associations, explanations, and implications. *Psychological Bulletin*, Vol. 135, No. 1, pp. 69–93.

Null, Gary et al (2011). *Death by medicine.* Mt. Jackson, VA: Praktikos Books.

Lee, Bandy X. et al (2017). *The dangerous case of Donald Trump: 27 psychiatrists and mental health experts assess a President.* NY, NY: Thomas Dunne Books.

Nancy, Malcolm (2018). *The plot to destroy democracy: how Putin and his spies are undermining America and dismantling the west.* NY, NY: Hachette Book Group, Inc.

Peck, M. Scott (1983). *People of the lie: the hope for healing human evil.* NY, NY: Touchstone.

Peterson, Peter, G. (2015). *Steering clear: how to avoid a debt crisis and secure our economic future.* Portfolio Publishing.

Pew Research Center (2015). America's changing religious landscape. Pew Research Center Religion and Public Life website (May 12, 2015).

Rondberg (1998). *Under the influence of modern medicine.* Published by Chiropractic Journal.

Time staff (2016) "10 Donald Trump business failures." On *Time* website.

Snyder, Timothy (2017). *On tyranny: twenty lessons from the twentieth century.* NY, NY: Tim Duggan Books.

Wolff, Michael (2018). *Fire and fury.* NY, NY: Holt, Henry & Company, Inc.

ADDENDUM ONE
Trump Implementation and Enforcement of an Immigrant Family Separation Policy

In the <u>American Heritage Dictionary</u> (3rd Ed., 1996), the word "punish" is defined as "to subject to a penalty for an offense." Several members of the Trump administration have clearly stated that the immigrant family separation policy is intended to carry out punishment that will deter adults from illegally entering the U.S. or coming to the U.S. border seeking entry and asylum. The purpose of this short paper is to intellectually explore the possibility that that policy violated the Eighth Amendment prohibition of cruel and unusual punishment.

It is assumed in this area of law that punishment is imposed on a person the punishing authority wishes to deter from repeating the punished behavior. In this case, the parents are sought to be deterred, not the children, who are most adversely affected by the punishment. It is important to emphasize that this separation can cause very serious trauma for some children, especially young children. It is predictable that many of the children will later have post-traumatic stress disorder (PTSD) and other more serious adverse consequences.

This analysis allows us to conclude that this punishment of children, who did not commit the offense and are not sought to be deterred, is unlawful in three important ways. First, the punishment is not authorized by law. Very severe punishment cannot be imposed when the underlying authority is a presidential policy. Second, it is not administered in a procedure that accords due process of law protections that apply to the punishment process. Third, in this situation, this punishment of children is cruel by intentionally creating grave risk of severe trauma to some children. It is cruel in that there is extreme disproportionality of the punishment in relation to the behavior of the children. It is cruel and unusual in that it is imposed on young children, many of whom are too young to be held criminally accountable for behavior. It is unusual in that this is intentional punishment of a non-offender to achieve deterrence of other persons. It is unusual in that, as far as I know, this type of treatment does not occur in other contexts. It follows that this treatment is cruel and unusual punishment in violation of the Eighth Amendment of the U.S. Constitution.

I do not believe it would be valid to treat the adverse treatment of children as damage that is collateral to the punishment of the parents. Achieving adverse treatment of children which is intended to result in deterrence of adults is the primary purpose of the immigrant family separation policy.

ADDENDUM TWO
The Adequacy and Acceptability of Donald Trump as President

I have spent many hours trying to think and write intelligently and systematically about President Trump and have concluded that it would take a long book to describe Trump's psychological, moral, intellectual, personality, and behavioral strengths and weaknesses and to describe their known and probable effects. In this addendum, I provide statements or phrases which I believe accurately describe an aspect of Trump's psychological, moral, intellectual, personality, or behavioral problems and deficiencies. I will leave it to others to document and predict adverse effects of these problems and deficiencies.

Many capable and well informed Americans believe that the Trump presidency is likely to be catastrophic for U.S. government, American society, and Americans. **I have concluded that the information described in many of the sections below should standing alone disqualify a presidential candidate or president.**

Psychological. Though I have a PhD in criminology, I do not have doctoral-level expertise concerning psychological diagnoses, which are in the areas of expertise of PhD psychologists and, of course, psychiatrists (who are physicians).

Possible anti-social (criminal) personality. Psychologists and psychiatrist have professional expertise on this subject. My non-expert, well developed and supported opinion is that he does have an anti-social (criminal) personality.

Facade of perfection. Trump maintains a facade of perfection (*People of the Lie* by M. Scott Peck, physician, 1983) and will not acknowledge error by him or apologize for any action, inaction, or mistake by him.

Grandiosity. I believe that Trump generally believes that he is better than he actually is. This is connected with his narcissism.

Self-centeredness and selfishness. Excellent leaders are vastly more concerned about achieving excellent outcomes for their followers than for themselves.

Intellectual

Less intelligence than he claims. Trump has applied his intelligence in unconventional ways, such as achieving financial gain illegally without suffering adverse consequences. Because of this, I think it is difficult to reach conclusions about his level of intellectual ability. My own belief is that he is significantly less intelligent than he claims to be and that he has vastly less intellectual ability than many, probably all, of our great presidents have or had.

Lack of intellectual and personality requirements to perform many types of important presidential leadership. I have tried to think carefully about examples of presidential leadership in U.S. history and, in that process, identified many types of important presidential leadership, all of which I believe Trump does not perform and probably is not capable of performing. Unfortunately, his leading by example may have horrible consequences for the U.S., American society, and Americans.

Failure of many important Trump undertakings. According to an article by the *Time* staff (2016), during his career in development and business, Trump experienced 10 business failures. Trump had managed to protect himself and his organization from major adverse consequences of these failures. Trump's first two marriages failed, and he was having sexual affairs with other women when his current wife was pregnant soon after their marriage.

Trump was very wrong when he announced that North Korea no longer presents a military threat. The immigrant family separation policy was unacceptable in many ways and was loudly rejected by a high percentage of Americans. The point is that many of Trump's important undertakings have failed. I believe that it is nearly certain that some of his undertakings as president will fail with very adverse consequences for the U.S. and Americans.

Naivete. Naivete can be a combination of intellectual and personality deficiencies. For example, Trump is naively influence by personal flattery by other leaders.

I strongly believe that Trump's statement after the Singapore meeting to the effect that "North Korea no longer presents a military threat" is by a giant margin the most naive, uninformed, and stupid statement I have ever heard a U.S. president make about national security.

Moral. Even if Trump does not conform to the requirements of the anti-social (criminal) personality, it is clear that he fails to meet the requirements of being a "morally good" person in many important says.

Conspiracy of Trump and his staff with Russians in their attack on the 2016 presidential election. I strongly believe the available evidence shows that this did occur. The public does not yet have much of the evidence developed by the Mueller investigation. The Mueller investigation may produce evidence that wrongdoing of Trump and his staff was much more serious than the criminal acts of which ordinary Americans are now aware.

Apparent absence of conscience. Many of the other sections support this point.

Pathological lying. By April 30, 2018, the *Washington Post* had documented 3001 lies by President Trump. I believe that Trump has become incredibly proficient at lying to achieve some type of benefit or advantage for himself. During the presidential campaign, he claimed that he had no financial connections with Russia. While saying that, he was attempting to have a Trump tower approved for construction in Russia. This dishonesty was reprehensibly intended to prevent informed voting by Americans. (I am embarrassed to admit that, prior to the presidential campaign, I did not know that the skills and abilities Trump often displays in creating widespread false perceptions regarding truth were even possible.)

Dishonesty. A person who lies as intentionally and frequently as Trump is profoundly dishonest. It appears that Trump is approaching the presidency as a mechanism for increasing his wealth and the wealth of members of his family. In some cases, this is prohibited by federal law concerning emoluments.

As Americans now know, in return for China lending $500,000 to the Trump organization, he is attempting to assist a Chinese corporation. I believe that a comparable act by any previous president would have resulted in removal of the president. Trump receives extremely great financial benefit from the only major legislation he led in having passed by Congress, the GOP 2017 tax cut. Though this is not illegal, it is very outrageous.

Involvement of his presidency and many federal agencies in governmental corruption. Candidate Trump promised to "drain the swamp." Instead, he has caused and allowed expansion and deepening of "the swamp."

Repeated atrocious sexual abuse of women.

Bullying.

His over-estimation of "achievements" of the Trump presidency. Trump brags endlessly about the strong economy and strong job market he has "created." When inaugurated in 2009, Obama faced a disastrously weak economy and extremely high unemployment, which had to a large extent been caused by actions and inactions of the GWB administration. It is nearly entirely President Obama who deserves credit for strengthening the economy and job market after the "great recession" of 2007-8.

Though economics is far removed from my areas of expertise, I will opine that, given the situation President Obama had "handed" Trump, the actual economic accomplishments of Trump as president are minimal. My main point here is that, when a president makes every decision (including the GOP 2017 tax cut) favoring business and against ordinary Americans, it is not remarkable or highly commendable if fairly small improvements in economy and job market occur.

<u>Personality</u>

Lack of commitment to democracy, the rule of law, due process of law, equal protection of the laws, civil rights, and civil liberties. This can result in deficiencies in his leadership and presidential actions and in many types of adverse effects for government and the U.S. I have been deeply committed to these aspects primarily of constitutional law since law school. Though I could never have qualified to be on a Mueller team, I have very deep understanding of this set of Trump deficiencies, which I believe should be disqualifying for a presidential candidate or president.

Racism. By strongly supporting Steve Bannon and Roy Moore, two extreme racists, Trump proved his own racism.

Ruthlessness. Trump is willing to viciously attack and damage many types of organizations, various other types of entities, and persons to achieve advantage for himself. Possibly most importantly, he ruthlessly attacks Mueller and his investigation, the FBI, and the Department of Justice. He has systematically increased racial polarization and animosity in the U.S. and has effectively demolished the Republican Party of Lincoln, Dirksen, Dole, George H. W. Bush, Colin Powell, and Mitt Romney.

The previous addendum is about the ruthlessness and cruelty of the Trump immigrant family separation policy after the references at the end of this chapter.

Intentional destruction. Nearly all of Trump's significant actions as president have involved destruction of something significant by fiat, including the Pacific trade agreement, DACA, Paris Climate Accord, agreement with Iran, vast numbers of agency regulations, and many executive orders of previous presidents. He acts by fiat when he utilizes a power by doing affirmative action, as by imposing a tariff or sanction against another country or granting a pardon. **Autocrats govern by fiat.**

Affinity for autocracy and autocrats.

<u>Behavioral</u>

Laziness. Apparently because of laziness, Trump does not do "due diligence" concerning many functions of a president. Doing due diligence involves exhibiting basic competence. I, as a lawyer captain in the 82nd Airborne Division in the early 1970s and as a criminal justice expert in the South Carolina governor's office of Richard Riley in the early 1980s, was strongly aware of the excellent examples of due diligence that were exhibited by the top leaders and expected on lower levels. It is reported on the Internet that Trump's office in May of 2018 prepared and mailed a letter signed by Trump which seriously failed to meet the requirements for a letter signed by any high-level leader.

It is unquestionably true that, when Trump became president, he had very little of the knowledge a president needs. His lack of due diligence is resulting in a very slow rate of acquisition of needed knowledge.

Trump gave himself an A+ for his handling of the situation in Puerto Rico during and after hurricane Maria. I believe his handling of that situation has been unbelievably incompetent and deficient.

Affiliation with members of organized crime in the U.S. and with members of organized crime in Russia and other foreign countries.

Lack of self-control.

— SECTION 9 —
Crime and Violence

— CHAPTER 26 —
Genocides and "Ethnic Cleansing" in World History

<u>Elaboration</u>. According to the *American Heritage Dictionary*, a genocide is "The systematic and planned extermination of an entire national, racial, political or ethnic group." Of course, many attempted genocides are not entirely successful.

Wikipedia defines "ethnic cleansing" as "Systematic deliberate removal of ethnic or religious groups from a given territory with the intent of making it ethnically homogeneous."

<u>Website articles about genocides and "ethnic cleansing."</u>

Genocides. There is an article, "Genocides in world history," on the Wikipedia web site.

Ethnic cleansing campaigns. There is an article, "List of ethnic cleansing campaigns," on the Wikipedia web site.

<u>Author's relevant expertise and experience</u>. Since genocides involve criminal violence, I have relevant expertise as a PhD criminologist and as a lawyer. (As a JAG captain in the 82nd Airborne Division in 1971–73, I taught "law of war," which prohibits mass killings of civilians by military units,

to 82nd Airborne Division units that had recently returned from combat in Vietnam. Because of their service in Vietnam War combat, some of them understood aspects of that subject better than I did.)

Importance of this subject. Spanish philosopher, poet, and novelist George Santayana (1863–1952) said, "Those who cannot remember the past are condemned to repeat it." While I don't believe that there will be potential for genocide in the U.S. while a government in accordance with the U.S. Constitution continues, as I report in chapter 27, interracial violence is increasing in the U.S. I report my own calculations of rates of White-on-Black and Black-on-White violent crime in the U.S. Unfortunately, race relations have been deteriorating rapidly in the U.S. for several years.

Genocides and instances of ethnic cleansing tell us what human nature and human culture are capable of. It is important for Americans to understand that horribly violent and atrocious treatment of one probably smaller group by another probably larger and stronger group has occurred very often in world history. I believe U.S. history has shown that there is no potential for genocide of Black Americans by White Americans.

Potential for an undergraduate course on this subject. It is likely that few professors would want to teach a course including extensive information about this subject. Also, I doubt that many students would want to take such a course. Therefore, I think that this subject matter should be included in other courses. I have included this chapter because I think it is important for people to know about this horrible aspect of human behavior. It is not accurate to assume that genocides occur very rarely. Tragically, there were many genocides and "racial cleansings" during the 20th century.

Relevance for young adults. I believe that American society is "playing with fire" regarding race relations and the potential for interracial conflict and violence. We can hope that young adults who become influential will help to guide the U.S. toward peaceful existence together of various groups.

The Holocaust. When I was about 6, my twin brother and I accompanied our mother when she visited an elderly couple living near a small North Carolina town. The couple ushered David and me into a non-formal family room, where we were to occupy and amuse ourselves. I found a book of photographs taken during the liberation of Auschwitz and other death camps at the end of WWII. I looked carefully at every photo in the book. Views of those photos were seared into the memory center of my young brain. That day, I concluded that the Holocaust involved unbelievably horrible, systematic, and widespread mistreatment of one group of humans by another group of humans.

A Wikipedia article, "The holocaust," provides detailed information. The Nazis began construction of concentration camps in 1933. The decision by Hitler to exterminate Jews was known as "the final solution of the Jewish question." The systematic murder began in 1941. About 200,000 Germans and persons of other nationalities were "Holocaust perpetrators." About six million European Jews were murdered, and about two million Europeans members of other groups were exterminated. During December of 2017, I viewed on the National Geographic television channel an excellent documentary about the role of the Nazi SS in the worst atrocities by the Nazis.

I believe that a high percentage of people who were children or older in 1945 have clear awareness of many of the facts of the Holocaust. Just as young people now know little about Groucho Marx and other celebrities of the 1940s and 1950s, I think they probably have little knowledge of the Holocaust and of other genocides that have occurred in world history.

—— CHAPTER 27 ——
Interracial Violence in the U.S.

Elaboration.

Political correctness prohibition of publications about interracial violence. My National Criminal Justice Reference Service search about this did not discover any publication(s) about interracial crime. I have not found even one PhD criminologist who would cooperate with me in doing research about or disseminating information about interracial violence in the U.S.

Information on web sites about interracial violence. At least four years ago, I found Internet web sites that reported several of the most important statistical findings I report in this chapter. While I have appropriate qualifications and credentials (PhD in criminology) to report these findings, I found no evidence that the persons who did those calculations had relevant qualifications or credentials. In most cases, their statistical results were consistent with mine. So, white-supremacist groups "figured out" this subject without help from me.

Preliminary information about interracial violence in the U.S. I want to emphasize at the beginning of this chapter that the rates of interracial homicide in the U.S. declined dramatically from 1980 to 2013. The rate of Black-on-White homicide in 1980 was 2.517 per 100,000 per year. (In most years, that rate is about 15 times as high as the rate of White-on-Black homicide.) In 2013, the Black-on-White homicide rate was 1.058 per 100,000 per year. That constitutes a 58% reduction in that homicide rate from 1980, which was a remarkable achievement. That decline was, to some extent, caused by a major increase in prison and jail incarceration. As I report later in this chapter, intraracial and interracial homicides started declining in the 1992–94 period and declined very significantly for 18 to 20 years. U.S. leaders and citizens should have a goal of avoiding loss of very great progress concerning safety of citizens.

It is important to note also that, in 2013 in a city with 100,000 Black residents, the average number of White victims of homicide by a Black person would have been very slightly more than one White person. So, **I don't want to give the impression that Black-on-White homicides occur very often in American cities**. As reported below, in 2012–2013, the rate of Black-on-White non-lethal violent crime was about 33 times as high as the rate of White-on-Black non-lethal violent crime.

Disappointing statement by Michelle Obama. Late in the second term of the Presidency of Barack Obama, Mrs. Obama said in public something to the following effect: "Early in our marriage, my husband and I were humiliated when, as we were walking on a street, White people changed their walking paths to avoid passing near us." While I very strongly worked for the Obama campaign in 2008 and supported him as President, I believe his wife was blaming White people for something that was caused by Black people. Those White people probably were not trying to avoid walking near the Obamas because they, the White people, were racists. They were probably afraid that they might be criminally victimized by Black persons. In many situations, that type of fear is not racist: tragically, it can be the result of awareness of possible significant danger.

Ominous increases of Black-on-White and White-on-Black homicide in very recent years. That is reported in detail later in this chapter. Unfortunately, problems I have experienced in getting correct information about populations of White and Black persons in the U.S. in 2016 have kept me from being confident in reporting interracial homicide rates for 2016. I will report that, White-on-Black homicides increased from 229 in 2015 to 243 in 2016, which was a 6.1% increase in number of homicides. Black-on-White homicides increased from 500 in 2015 to 533 in 2016, which was a

6.6% increase in number of homicides. Since 2014, I have been predicting increase in interracial homicide, and that has occurred and continued in 2016.

Author's relevant expertise and experiences. I hold a PhD in criminology from Florida State University (1981) and have a fair number of scholarly publications. In September of 2016, I presented a paper (Memory, 2016) reporting my extensive calculations on the subject of this chapter at a conference of Criminal Justice professors.

I am a lifelong Democrat and have worked extremely hard in support of liberal/progressive values.

Importance of this subject. In nearly every type of human group, including a society, it is normally expected that a person or persons who become aware of serious danger will warn other people about that danger. Political correctness in the U.S. is prohibiting and preventing that type of warning regarding interracial violence.

As a PhD criminologist, I have had the occasion to discuss interracial violence with many people. An extremely high percentage have said, in effect, "In the U.S., nearly all violent crime is intraracial, by a person against a person of the same race." While rates of Black-on-Black violent crime are tragically high, that statement is incorrect in important ways. As I report in detail below, Black persons select White victims in a much higher percentage of violent crimes than the percentage of violent crimes by White persons in which the offender select a Black victim.

Explanations of tendency of Black Americans to commit violent crimes against White Americans at a much higher rate than vice versa. Criminological theory attempts to explain why patterns of crime occur. I seriously doubt that more than a very small percentage of Criminal Justice professors attempt to explain in class the higher interracial violence rates of Black persons. Criminological theory has never been a strength area for me. My guess is that the higher rates of Black-on-White violent crime than White-on-Black violent crime result partly from more and stronger hatred of White people by Black people than of Black people by White people.

Relevance for young adults. I believe that it would be desirable for young adults and others in the U.S. to have much more accurate information about risks relating to interracial violence than is currently available.

The main reason I developed and am disseminating this information. As discussed in detail later in this chapter and in chapter 28, Black Lives Matter and several young Black male authors have either stated or strongly suggested that African Americans are being violently oppressed and eliminated by White society in the U.S. Several scholars (Whaley, 2004; Grier & Cobbs, 1968) argue that there is cultural paranoia in Black culture in the U.S. This involves prevalent belief among African Americans that they are being persecuted by White society. I believe that the political correctness prohibition of dissemination of information on this subject has the effect of fostering this cultural paranoia in the Black community. For example, political correctness allows African Americans to believe that they are incarcerated at a very high rate because of persecution by White society. Actually, that higher incarceration rate is caused primarily by the much higher crime commission rate of African Americans and by the fact that their offenses are much more likely to be violent than those of members of other races.

I believe availability of information about interracial violence might help in decreasing this paranoia. It would be a step in the direction of better mental health and realism in the U.S. for information regarding interracial violence to be available in various types of publications and websites.

Selected portions of a paper on this subject I presented at a conference of Criminal Justice professors in September of 2016. I have included all of the actual statistical results and have deleted nearly all of the conclusions and implications.

Long-Term and Short-Term Trends of White-on-Black and Black-on-White Violent Crime

The Problem and Introduction

There is now in the U.S. major public concern regarding violence against African Americans perpetrated by white persons, especially by white law enforcement officers. For example, Beyoncé recently had a performance on TV which featured dancers being killed (symbolically) one by one, which apparently was intended to refer to violence against innocent Blacks by White society, especially police officers.

To produce accurate information about interracial violence, the author has obtained the necessary data and carried out the indicated statistical procedures to produce rates of White and Black interracial and intraracial single-offender, single-victim homicide during the 1980–2014 period. Also, White and Black rates of interracial non-lethal violent crime during 2012–2013 were calculated. There were calculations also concerning several categories of non-lethal interracial violence in 2008.

Literature Review

I know from personal experience since starting this effort early in 2015 that political correctness in the U.S. prohibits public reporting of findings about interracial crime. As a result, there is very little published research about interracial crime.

An article by Humphrey and Palmer (1987) reports calculations regarding crime with race of offenders and victims that are based on data from such a remote time that the information is not helpful for the present effort.

A monograph about interracial crime, *Color of Crime: Crime, Race, and Justice in America* (2016), has been written by Edwin Rubenstein, an analyst and writer who does not hold a PhD. It is available on the Internet. Unfortunately, the organization that sponsored the production of this monograph, the New Century Foundation, appears to be involved in "alt-right" activities.

In recent years, it was possible to obtain on the Internet an article by Michael Keene with the title "Interracial crime," *Society and Culture*, September 21, 2009. For reasons I do not know, that journal can no longer be accessed on the Internet. As a result, that publication cannot be accessed.

Table 5 below comes from a Bureau of Justice Statistics, National Crime Victimization Survey 2012–2013 special tabulation. While it was previously available on the Internet, it apparently cannot now be located through an Internet search.

For some percentage of recent years, the National Criminal Victimization

Survey, Bureau of Justice Statistics had a table 42 with the title "percent distribution of single-offender victimizations, by type of crime, race of victim, and perceived race of offender." The most recent year in which that table appeared, as far as I know, was 2008.

If you do an Internet search for "interracial crime," you will be directed to various websites with verbiage relating to interracial crime. While the information on some of the websites may be correct, the presentations generally lack indication of a sufficiently qualified analyst/author. Also, there is generally insufficient information about sources of data, statistical procedures, and findings.

The Black Lives Matter website very prominently displayed until apparently early fall of 2016 the following statement:

> "Black Lives Matter is an ideological and political intervention in a world where Black lives are systematically and intentionally targeted for demise."

As of early November of 2016, the Black Lives Matter website could not be accessed on the Internet.

An African-American journalist, Ta-Nehisi Coates, had an influential book, *Between the World and Me*, published in 2015. Though he has no relevant professional or scholarly qualifications, he has written extensively about police violence against African Americans. Because he is apparently viewed in the Black community as an important emerging leader, a quote from his book is provided here.

> "All you need to understand is that the officer carries with him the power of the American states and the weight of an American legacy, and they necessitate that of the bodies destroyed every year, some wild and disproportionate number of them will be black. Here is what I would like you to know: In America it is traditional to destroy the black body—*it is heritage.*" (Coates, 2015, p. 102)

Though BLM and Coates do not state specifically that Black people are targeted for elimination by white people, white society, white-dominated police departments, and white law enforcement officers, I believe that is their intended inference. Political correctness has not only prohibited development and dissemination of information about interracial violent crime: It has allowed BLM and Coates to create a fictional and false depiction of history and reality according to which white people, white-dominated police departments, and white police officers have been and are selecting and eliminating innocent Black persons.

Two organizations have reported non-published numbers of Black persons lynched in the U.S. The Tuskegee Institute (Tuskegee Institute Archives) numbers are 3446 Blacks and 1297 Whites lynched between 1882 and 1968. Those numbers have changed some in recent years. The Equal Justice Institute (2015, Equal Justice Institute website) number is 3959 Blacks lynched in 12 Southern states during the 1877–1950 period.

There are many reports of analyses relating to the decrease in crime rate in recent decades in the U.S. (e.g., Roeder et al, 2015; Levitt, 2004). The authors of those two articles disagree regarding causes of the decrease in crime.

An important related matter is total incarceration rate in the U.S., which is based on total incarceration in federal and state prisons and jails. It is reported in a Bureau of Justice Statistics report (Kaeble, D. et al, 2016) that the all-time highest rate of incarceration per 100,000 population in the U.S. was 760 in 2007 and 2008. Yearly declines since 2008 resulted in a rate of 690 in 2014. This constituted a 9.2% decline from 2008 to 2014.

Data

The data are primarily from FBI Uniform Crime Reports (now called, for example, *Crime in the United States—2014*) and are of single-offender, single-victim reported homicides from 1980 to the first half of 2015. For many recent years, those data are in "expanded homicide data table 6." Only data regarding Black and White offenders and victims were obtained. A "Black intraracial" homicide rate is a report concerning Black-on-Black homicide. A "White interracial" homicide rate is a report concerning White-on-Black homicide. To be able to calculate rates per 100,000 population per year, yearly population figures were obtained from U.S. Census Bureau publications. To have basis for comparisons and to be able to reach certain illuminating conclusions, it has been important to calculate and report White and Black interracial and intraracial homicide rates. The data, from the Bureau of Justice Statistics, used in calculations reported herein of rates of non-lethal interracial violent crimes are presented in Table 5 below. For some number of years, the National Crime Victimization Survey report included a table 42 with the title "Percent distribution of single-offender victimizations, by type of crime, race of victim, and perceived race of offender." The data in table 42 in the report for 2008 (BJS, 2011) were used in calculation of rates of interracial violent crime.

Methods

The primary method was calculation of White and Black intraracial and interracial homicide rates per 100,000 population for the years 1980 through 2014, as indicated above only for single-offender, single-victim homicides.

For the benefit of non-statistical readers, here is the formula for calculating this.

<u>number of offenses</u>   <u>X</u>
jurisdiction population   100,000

In solving the equation, you multiply the population by X, which becomes the number on one side of the equation, and you multiply number of offenses by 100,000, which becomes the number on the other side. You divide the X number into the other number, and you have the rate per 100,000 population per year. To obtain a ratio of White interracial rates with Black interracial rates, the White interracial rates (which were always lower) were divided into the Black interracial rates.

Results

Table 1. White and Black interracial and intraracial homicide rates 1980-2014

Year	White Interracial	Black Interracial	Ratios of White and Black Interracial Rates	White Intraracial	Black Intraracial
1980	.134	2.517	1:18.78	2.902	21.961
1981	.140	2.500	1:17.86	2.768	20.309
1982	.134	2.052	1:15.31	2.670	18.486
1983	.123	2.110	1:17.15	2.590	17.510
1984	.115	1.910	1:16.60	2.358	14.400
1985	.130	2.036	1:15.69	2.440	15.000
1986	.128	2.109	1:16.48	2.500	17.440
1987	.139	1.947	1:14.01	2.250	15.038
1988	.114	1.909	1:16.74	2.107	14.920
1989	.142	2.095	1:14.75	2.130	15.398
1990	.146	2.023	1:13.86	2.130	16.180
1991	.165	2.217	1:13.44	2.085	16.156
1992	.137	2.510	1:18.32	2.113	16.323
1993	.142	2.638	1:18.58	2.182	16.759
1994	.156	2.418	1:15.50	2.053	15.628
1995	.129	2.124	1:16.46	1.897	13.435
1996	.113	1.675	1:14.82	1.580	10.690
1997	.094	1.532	1:16.23	1.439	9.980
1998\	.092	1.304	1:14.17	1.437	8.908
1999	.069	1.296	1:18.78	1.237	7.670
2000	.078	1.168	1:14.97	1.254	7.626
2001	.078	1.310	1:16.79	1.328	7.730
2002	.098	1.314	1:13.41	1.289	7.761
2003	.096	1.350	1:14.06	1.288	7.720
2004	.097	1.395	1:14.38	1.323	7.423

2005	.097	1.365	1:14.07	1.328	7.891
2006	.087	1.494	1:17.17	1.262	7.910
2007	.102	1.461	1:14.32	1.211	7.498
2008	.095	1.286	1:13.54	1.251	6.943
2009	.086	1.145	1:13.31	1.213	6.569
2010	.090	1.110	1:12.33	1.148	6.101
2011	.079	1.098	1:13.90	1.080	5.996
2012	.079	1.045	1:13.23	1.069	5.846
2013	.077	.980	1:12.73	1.022	5.382
2014	.076	1.058	1:13.92	1.001	5.23

Results of comparing the interracial homicide rates of Whites and Blacks. This table of findings contains many stories, some of which probably have not been told. It is important to understand that the Black intraracial homicide rate in 1980, 21.961, was 8.73 times as high as the Black-on-White homicide rate in that year. The Black intraracial homicide rate in 2014, 5.23, was 4.94 times as high as the Black interracial rate. The ratio figures above are the results of dividing the White interracial rate, which is always in this paper lower than the Black interracial rate, into the Black interracial rate. So, the White ratio number is always 1. The average ratio for the 1980–2013 period was 15.4.

Since data are generally not available regarding multiple-offender, single-victim and single-offender, multiple offender homicides, I am unable to provide any estimates regarding those rates.

Results regarding White and Black multiple-offender, single-victim interracial homicide rates for 1980 and 1981. In 1980 and 1981 FBI Uniform Crime Reports (FBI, 1981; FBI, 1982) there were data for multiple-offender, single-victim reported homicides. Below are the calculated interracial rates and ratios.

Table 2. Results regarding White and Black multiple-offender, single-victim interracial homicide rates for 1980 and 1981

Year	White interracial	Black interracial	Interracial ratio
1980	.075	2.107	1:28.09
1981	.083	2.094	1:25.23

Reduction in Black intraracial rate from 1980 to 2014. There was a very remarkable 76.2% reduction in this rate. This is partly explained by the fact that, from 1980 to 2013, there was a 393% increase in the total (combination of state and federal prison populations) prison incarceration rate in the U.S. (Glaze & Herberman, 2014).

An estimate regarding number of homicides prevented by the immediately above reduction in Black intraracial homicide rate. First, I will note that we cannot know what the violent crime rates would have been in the U.S., if substantial increase in incarceration had not occurred. By 1980 all of the giant Baby Boomer generation were in their "crime-committing" years, so crime rates would have been expected to be high then. The estimates below may overestimate the prevention of homicides in the 1981–2014 period or might possibly even underestimate it.

For the years 1981 through 2014, the number of Black intraracial homicides in each year was subtracted from the number of Black single-offender, single-victim homicides in 1980. Then, those numbers were added, producing a total of 73,236. This provides a very rough estimate of Black single-offender, single-victim intraracial homicides which were prevented by increase in prison incarceration (and other corrections measures) after 1980.

It is reported in a Bureau of Justice Statistics report (Harrell, 2007) that in 2005 there were 7439 Black victims of homicide by a Black offender. It is reported in *Crime in the United States 2005* that there were 2984 Black victims of single-offender, single-victim homicide by Black offenders. To obtain an estimate of the total number of Black intraracial homicides prevented in the 1981–2014 period, I created and solved the following equation:

$$\frac{\text{\#SO, SV bl. intra. hom. 2005}}{\text{\#bl. intra. hom. 2005}} = \frac{\text{\#SO, SV bl. intra. hom. prev. 1981–2014}}{X}$$

$$\frac{2984}{7439} = \frac{73,236}{X}$$

$$2984X = 544802604$$

$$X = 182574$$

This figure, 182,574, is a very rough estimate of the total number of Black intraracial homicides prevented during the 1981–2014 period. (I used two additional mathematical approaches and obtained nearly exactly the same result.)

It is, therefore, estimated that **about 183,000 Black-on-Black homicides were prevented in the U.S. during the 1981–2014 period partly as a result of implemented police, criminal justice, and correctional measures**. Of course, other types of cultural and behavioral factors were operating and probably influenced the amount of homicide during that period to some extent.

While Harrell (2007) reported that in 2005 there were 7439 Black victims of homicide by a Black offender, *Crime in the United States—2005* reports that there were 7125 Black victims of homicide in 2005 and a total of 14,860 homicides. In this situation of contradictory published reports, I believe it is best to emphasize that this entire section is highly speculative. The 183,000 estimate is of intraracial homicides by Black offenders. It is reasonable to assume that there were also a large number of homicides by non-Black persons prevented during that period.

Estimates of numbers of non-lethal Black intraracial crimes prevented during the 1981–2014 period. In 2002 the number and rate per 100,000 population of particular reported offenses were as indicated below (FBI, 2003).

Table 3. Data from 2002 required to estimate number of non-lethal violent Black intraracial crimes prevented during the 1981–2014 period

Crime	# of reported offenses	Rate per 100,000	Ratio with homicide rate
Homicide	16,204	5.61	n/a
Rape	95,136	33	1:5.9
Robbery	420,637	145.9	1:26
Aggravated assault	894,348	310.1	1:55.3

To obtain a very rough estimate of the numbers of these crimes that were prevented during the 1981–2014 period, the relevant ratios would be multiplied by some number that is substantially higher than the estimate of Black intraracial homicides prevented, which was 183,000. Multiplying by the 183,000 number produced the very rough, partial estimates below.

Table 4. Partial estimates of non-lethal Black intraracial violentcrimes prevented during the 1981–2014 period

Crime	Rough partial estimates of non-lethal Black intraracial violent crimes prevented 1981-2000
Rape	1,079,700
Robbery	4,758,000
Aggravated assault	10,119,900

The point of this highly conjectural exercise is that it is not unreasonable to believe that the substantially increased incarceration after 1980, along with possibly other law enforcement, criminal justice, correctional measures, and other factors, resulted in prevention of a large number of homicides and very much larger numbers of rapes, robberies, and aggravated assaults.

Reduction in Black-on-White homicide rate from 1980 to 2014. There was a 58% reduction in the Black-on-White single-offender, single-victim homicide during that period. From 1980 to the previous year, 2013, the reduction was 61.1%. While the other three homicide rates declined slightly from

2013 to 2014, the Black-on-White single-offender, single-victim homicide rate increased by 7.4% from 2013 to 2014. From 2013 to 2014 there was a nine percent increase in the **number** of White people killed in that type of homicide by Black people. This may be the most important finding in this study.

Visual examination of the full-page report of homicide rates above shows that the Black interracial single-offender, single-victim homicide rate went down every year during the Bill Clinton Presidency. Also, the lowest Black-on-White rates of that type of homicide were during the 2009 through 2013 period, which were the first five years of the Obama Presidency.

Reduction in White intraracial rate from 1980 to 2014. There was a 65.5% reduction in this rate. Of course, this also occurred partly because of the increase in prison incarceration rate.

Reduction in White interracial rate from 1980 to 2014. There was a 43.3% reduction in this rate.

Estimating the ratio of rates of White-on-Black non-lethal violent crime with rates of Black-on-White non-lethal violent crime in 2012–2013. I discovered this table in the Rubenstein monograph (2016, p. 13).

Table 5. Violent Victimizations, 2012–2013

Race of victim	Annual average number of victimizations	Race of offender, %				
		White	Black	Hispanic	Other	Unknown
White	4,091,971	56.0	13.7	11.9	10.6	7.8
Black	955,800	10.4	62.2	4.7	15	7.7
Hispanic	995,996	21.7	21.1	38.6	11.6	6.9
Other	440,741	40.3	19.3	10.6	20.3	9.5
Total	6,484,507	42.9	22.4	14.8	12.1	7.8

Data source: BJS, National Crime Victimization Survey, 2012-2013, Special Tabulation

I used the data in table 5 data in calculating the interracial violent non-lethal offense rate for Whites (39 per 100,000 population per year) and the interracial violent non-lethal offense rate for Blacks (1282.2 per 100,000 population per year). Division of the White rate into the Black rate produces the conclusion that during the 2012–2013 period, the rate at which Black people committed non-lethal violent offenses against White people was about 32.9 times as high as the rate at which White people committed non-lethal violent offenses against Black people during that period.

To understand these findings better, I calculated the rate per 100,000 of non-lethal violent offenses for White people (1132.7) and for Black people (3482.4). Dividing the White rate into the Black rate produces a multiple of 3.074. This obviously does not parallel the rates and ratios regarding homicide. Here, the interracial rate multiple (32.9) was very much higher than the overall rate multiple (3.074).

To have basis for comparison, the 2012 rate per 100,000 population of White non-lethal violent victimization of Hispanics was calculated (88.2), and the rate per 100,000 population of Hispanic non-lethal violent victimization of Whites was calculated (918.3) . So, the White rate (88.2) was divided into the Hispanic rate (918.3), resulting in 10.4. So, for 2012, the rate of Hispanic non-lethal violent victimization of Whites was about 10.4 times as high as the rate of White non-lethal victimization of Hispanics.

Estimating the ratio of rates of White-on-Black non-lethal violent crimes with rates of Black-on-White non-lethal violent crimes in 2008. The estimated White-on-Black rate of "completed violence" was 12.6 per 100,000 populations per year, and the Black-on-White rate was 349.6 per 100,000 populations per year. The Black-on-White rate was 27.7 times as high as the White-on-Black rate. It was noted that the White offense total was "based on 10 or fewer sample cases." Since these are NCVS data, the totals are based results of a very elaborate random sample.

The estimated White-on-Black rate of aggravated assault, with the White number of offenses "based on 10 or fewer sample cases," was 6.23 per 100,000 population per year. The estimated Black-on-White rate of aggravated assault was 196 per 100,000 population per year. The Black-on-White rate was 31.5 times as high as the White-on-Black rate.

The estimated White-on-Black rate of robbery, "based on 10 or fewer sample cases," was 2.9 per 100,000 populations per year. The estimated Black-on-White robbery rate was 180 per 100,000 population per year. The Black-on-White rate was 62.1 times higher than the White-on-Black rate.

The estimated Black-on-White rate of rape and rape-related offenses was 49.2 per 100,000 population per year. The indicated number of White-on-Black rape and rape-related offenses was 0.0, apparently because there were either zero or extremely few such offenses reported in the survey.

Increases in other violent crimes from 2013 to 2014. Reported rapes in the U.S. increased from 79,770 in 2013 (FBI, 2014) to 84,041 in 2014 (FBI, 2015), which was a 4,271 increase in reported rapes. Reported aggravated assaults increased from 724,149 in 2013 (FBI, 2014) to 741,291 in 2014 (FBI, 2015), which was a 17,142 increase in aggravated assaults. These increases were counter to a general trend of reduction in reported crimes. (Information on the race of persons reported to have committed rape, robbery, burglary, or aggravated assault is generally not available in the FBI *Crime in the United States* publications.)

Change in rates from first half of 2014 through the first half of 2015. Compared to the first half of 2014, murder increased by 6.2% and rape increased by 9.6% during the first six months of 2015 (FBI, 2016).

Change in interracial homicide rates from 2014 to 2015. From 2014 to 2015, the number of Black-on-White homicides increased by 12.1%, and the Black-on-Black homicides increased by 7.94%. From 2014 to 2015, the number of White-on-Black homicides increased by 22.46%, and the number of White-on-White homicides increased by 3.45% (FBI, 2015).

DISCUSSION AND IMPLICATIONS

Discussion regarding main interracial homicide findings. It is important for me to clarify that 99% of this paper was written before the FBI 2015 crime figures were released. The startling findings obtained through analyses of those data are reported above. So far, I have not developed my other discussion to take those findings into account. I will note that I had predicted in several unpublished papers that, if Black-on-White homicides continued to increase, eventually White-on-Black violence would increase.

My very capable son alerted me to a potential problem in the comparison of calculated interracial crime rates relating to size of potential victim groups. So, I created a hypothetical U.S. in which there were 210,000,000 Whites and 35,000,000 Blacks, which was very close to the actual ratio in the middle 1990s. I assumed that the overall homicide rate was 10 per 100,000 population and assumed that all of the people lived in communities with the 6 White to 1 Black ratio and that White people committed six homicides with White victims for one homicide with a Black victim and that Black people committed six homicides with a White victim for one homicide with a Black victim. The resulting Black-on-White interracial homicide rate was nearly exactly six times higher than the White-on-Black homicide rate. This is not the result of a mathematical distortion. It is the result of the Black people in this model committing a large number of interracial homicides, along with having a small population, and the White offenders in the model committing a relatively small number of interracial homicides, along with having a much larger population. These factors probably contribute some to the high Black interracial violent crime rates in the U.S.

Different from the hypothetical U.S. I created, the overall homicide rate of Black people has for many years been substantially higher than the overall homicide rate of White people. In 2014 the rates were White 1.77 per 100,000 and Black 12.27 per 100,000. Also, whereas the hypothetical situation included an assumption that all Whites and Blacks lived in neighborhoods with the overall White 6, Black 1 population ratio, in reality many poor Black people live in virtually all-Black neighborhoods with very low proximity to potential White victims, and many affluent Whites live in virtually all-White, relatively secure neighborhoods.

I divided the 2014 White overall homicide rate into the Black overall homicide rate for that year, producing a multiple of 6.932. In 2014 there were 187 White-on-Black homicides and 2488 White-on-White homicides. So, the White interracial number was 7.52% of the White intraracial number. There were 446 Black-on-White homicides and 2205 Black-on-Black homicides. The Black interracial number is 20.22% of the Black intraracial number. You divide the White percentage, 7.52%, into the Black percentage, 20.22%, and you get a multiple of 2.69. This is another indicator that the rate of selection of White victims by Black offenders generally exceeds the rate of selection of Black victims by White offenders. The ratio of White-on-Black rate and Black-on-White rate of non-lethal violent crime in the 2012–2013 period was 32.9. This supports an expectation that the interracial homicide ratio would be higher than the ratio of the White and Black overall homicide rates. I believe that these findings provide important information to consider in interpreting the main interracial homicide findings.

So, I have concluded that the main interracial homicide findings are mathematically sound, though they may be significantly influenced by the relatively large number of available White victims and relatively small size of the Black population.

Historic reduction in violent crime in the U.S. The homicide rate findings in Table 1 are generally consistent with reports of historic decline in violent crime in recent decades (e.g., Roeder et al, 2015; *The Economist*, 2013; Levitt, S., 2004). The 76.2% reduction in rate of Black intraracial single-offender, single-victim homicide during the 1980–2014 period is the most dramatic finding derived from Table 1 findings. The finding that from 1980 to 2013 there was a 61% decrease of the rate of Black-on-White single-offender, single-victim homicide is encouraging and should not be ignored. Some of that substantial improvement was lost from 2013 to 2014.

Recent decline in total incarceration rate in the U.S. As noted earlier, the total U.S. incarceration rate per 100,000 population has decreased 9.2% from 760 in 2007 and 2008 to 690 in 2014 (Kaeble, D. et al, 2016). Given that this was a substantial reduction in total incarceration in the U.S., I think that it is remarkable that there was not an increase in single-offender, single-victim homicide rate until the comparison of the first six months of 2014 with the first six months of 2015 (FBI, 2016).

Predictions. I predict that, when the *Crime in the United States—2015* report is released sometime late in 2016, there will be report of a substantial increase in homicides and rapes from 2014 to 2015. Also, I predict that analysis of the homicide data in "expanded homicide data table 6" will show that there has been a substantial increase in Black-on-White homicide and no increase in White-on-Black homicide.

Addendum about causes of crime. You will find a short paper I have written about causes of violence after the immediately following references section.

REFERENCES

Bresnahan, M. et al (2007). Race and risk of schizophrenia in a U.S. birth cohort: another example of health disparity? *International Journal of Epidemiology*, Vol. 36, No. 4, pp. 751–758.

Bureau of Justice Statistics (2011). National Crime Victimization Survey—2008. Washington, DC: U.S. Government Printing Office.

Coates, Ta-Nehisi (2015). *Between the world and me.* NY, NY: Spiegel & Grau/ Penguin Random House.

Federal Bureau of Investigation (1981). *Uniform Crime Reports—1980.* Washington, DC: U.S. Government Printing Office.

Federal Bureau of Investigation (1982). *Uniform Crime Reports—1981.* Washington, DC: U.S. Government Printing Office.

Federal Bureau of Investigation (2003). *Crime in the United States—2002.* Washington, DC: U.S. Government Printing Office.

Federal Bureau of Investigation (2006). *Crime in the United States—2005.* Washington, DC: U.S. Government Printing Office.

Federal Bureau of Investigation (2013). *Crime in the United States—2012.* Washington, DC: U.S. Government Printing Office.

Federal Bureau of Investigation (2014). *Crime in the United States—2013.* Washington, DC: U.S. Government Printing Office.

Federal Bureau of Investigation (2015). *Crime in the United States—2014.* Washington, DC: U.S. Government Printing Office.

Federal Bureau of Investigation (2016). *Crime in the United States—2015,* preliminary semiannual uniform crime report. Washington, DC: U.S. Government Printing Office.

Federal Bureau of Investigation (2016). *Crime in the United States—2015.* Washington, DC: U.S. Government Printing Office.

Glaze, L.E. & Herberman, R. (2014). Correctional populations in the U.S. 2013. Washington, DC: Bureau of Justice Statistics.

Grier, W.H., & Cobbs, P.M. (1968). *Black rage.* NY, NY: Basic Books.

Hacker, D. (2011). A census-based count of the Civil War dead. *Civil War History,* Vol. 57, No. 4, pp. 306–347.

Harrell, E. (2007). Black victims of violent crime. Washington, DC: Bureau of Justice Statistics.

Humphrey, J.A., & S. Palmer (1987). Race, sex, and criminal homicide offender-victim relationships. *Journal of Black Studies,* Vol. 18, No. 1, pp. 45–57.

Jabbar, K.A. & Obstfeld, R. (2016). *Writings on the wall: searching for a new equality beyond black and white.* NY, NY: Liberty Street.

Kaeble, D. et al (2016). Correctional populations in the U.S., 2014. Washington, DC: Bureau of Justice Statistics.

Kennedy, H.G. et al (1992). Fear and anger in delusional (paranoid) disorder: the association with violence. *British Journal of Psychiatry,* Vol. 160, No. 4, pp. 488–492.

Levitt, S. D. (2004). Understanding why crime fell in the 1990s: four factors that explain the decline and six that do not. *Journal of Economic Perspectives,* Vol. 18, No. 1, pp. 163–190.

Lindsay, M. & Lester, D. (2004). *Suicide by cop: committing suicide by provoking police to shoot you.* Amityville, NY: Baywood Publishing Co.

Lowery, W. (2016). *They can't kill us all.* NY, NY: Spiegel & Grau.

Memory, J. M. (1967). N.C.G.S. 15-4.1: "due process of law" under *Gideon v. Wainwright? Wake Forest Law Review,* 3, 1–32.

Memory, J. M. (1999). Some impressions from a qualitative study of implementation of community policing in North Carolina. In M. L. Dantzker (Ed.), *Readings for research methods in criminology and criminal justice.* Woburn, MA: Butterworth.

Memory, J. M., & Aragon, R. (Eds.). (2001). *Patrol officer problem solving and solutions.* Durham, NC: Carolina Academic Press.

Memory, J. M., Guo,G. Parker, K. & Sutton, T. (1999). Comparing disciplinary infraction rates of North Carolina Fair Sentencing and Structured Sentencing inmates. *The Prison Journal,* Vol. 79, pp. 45–71.

Memory, J. M. (2016). Long-term and short-term trends of White-on-Black and Black-on-White violent crime. Presented at the annual meeting of the Southern Criminal Justice Association, Savannah, GA on September 7, 2016.

Null, G. et al (2006). Death by medicine. Monograph available on the Internet. For some number of years after 2006 it was on the website of the Life Extension Foundation.

Rawls, J. (2001). *Justice as fairness: a restatement.* Boston: Belknap Press.

Roeder, O. et al (2015). What caused the crime decline? Brennan Center for Justice. February 12, 2015.

Rubenstein, E.S. (2016). *The color of crime: race crime, and justice in America.* New Century Foundation (available as PDF on Internet).

The Economist (2013). The curious case of the fall in crime. July 20, 2013.

Watson, B. (2015). *Under Our Skin*. Carol Stream, IL: Tyndale House Publishers, Inc.

Whaley, A.L. (2004). Paranoia in African-American men receiving inpatient treatment. *Journal of the American Academy of Psychiatry and the Law*, Vol. 32, pp. 282–290.

Wilkinson, R. & Pickett, K. (2009). *The spirit level: why more equal societies almost always do better*. London: Allen Lane.

—— ADDENDUM ——
Causes of Violence

Many types of causes of violence can operate on virtually all levels of organization and process, which include individual genetics, individual's psycho-biological makeup, the individual person, family, community, city, region, and larger society. Psychologists study causes involving individual psychology and behavior. Criminologists study causes on higher levels of organization and process.

The more of the following things that are found together in an individual, the greater will be the likelihood of commission of violent act(s):

Anti-social (criminal) personality (This involves insufficient superego/conscience.)

Insufficiency of conscience/superego short of anti-social personality

Absence or weakness of impulse control

Deficiency of self-control

Strong unresolved anger and bitterness. Deficiency of impulse control and strong continuing anger can together produce a person with "a bad temper." Arguments lead to many violent crimes.

Lack of hope for the future (An individual's lack of hope for the future increases the likelihood of commission of several types of crime. A person who doesn't have hope for the future is probably depressed.)

Lack of lawful access to sufficient money and other prerequisites for enjoyable living.

Belief that, compared to many others, you are being denied sufficient money or material prerequisites for at least minimally sufficient quality of life.

Paranoid tendencies. Believing that people are "out to get you" can contribute to commission of violent acts.

Addiction to or substantial use of certain illicit drugs and/or alcohol. Of course, being intoxicated on alcohol increases the likelihood of acting violently.

Individual inadequacy of significant types (Genuinely adequate people nearly never commit violent acts.)

Sadistic tendencies (including enjoyment of hurting people)

It is assumed that being violently victimized especially during early childhood increases the likelihood that a person will violently victimize others later in life.

It is possible for a parent or older sibling to teach a child to be violent.

Influence of an impressionable teenager by one or more violent peers

A tendency to be a bully (enjoyment of dominating others)

Strong sex drive can contribute to causation of sexual violence.

Strong xenophobia, probably accompanied by strong ethnocentrism of your group

Membership in a criminal subculture, including Mafia, criminal organizations, gangs (including street, prison, Mexican, immigrant, and motorcycle gangs)

Genetic and developmental tendencies to exhibit some number of these factors may result in a person being a "violent person."

The school shootings present very complex causation issues. I believe that the main prerequisites are lack of hope for the future, which can contribute to some suicidal tendency, and a significant degree of exhibition of an anti-social (criminal) personality or deficient conscience. In the absence of either of these, an individual is extremely unlikely to carry out a school shooting or similar violence. Of course, the shooter probably has anger/resentment for the school and/or students. I believe that, tragically, many hundreds of thousands of males in the 17 to 20 age range exhibit these characteristics. This makes prevention extremely difficult.

Some violent acts are instrumental (to accomplish a probably criminal purpose). Several of the factors listed above ordinarily apply when instrumental violence occurs. A rape is instrumental violence. A robbery is instrumental violence.

Some violent acts are expressive (of anger, rage, resentment, feeling of rejection, etc.). Several of the factors listed above ordinarily apply when expressive violence occurs.

Violent acts can become more likely when there are deficient police actions and response which would have potential to prevent violence. This may contribute to the extremely high violent crime rates in southside Chicago. Deficiencies in pretrial and post-trial incarceration space can increase potential for violence to occur. In the U.S., very dramatic increase in prison and jail incarceration rates started in about1970. According to research I have done, at least by 1980, very substantial decreases in murder rates had begun in the U.S. and continued through 2014, even though some reduction in incarceration rates had begun several years before 2014.

If there are many defenseless, vulnerable potential victims of violence, the likelihood of violence goes up. That is the case in New Orleans, where there are very high violent crime rates.

Research has shown that disparities in income and wealth of the poor compared to the very wealthy tend to be positively associated with higher rates of crime and certain social problems.

Fifty years ago, violent crime rates in African countries tended to be low. So, I believe it is questionable to assume that being of African-American descent without more raises risk of commission of violent crimes. In the U.S., African-American males are much more likely to commit violent crimes in concert with same-race males than is the case with males of other racial/ethnic groups. As reported earlier in this chapter, since 1980, the Black intraracial murder rate in the U.S. has been between five and seven times as high as the White intraracial murder rate.

AN ARTICLE DRAFT ABOUT RECOMMENDATION OF USE OF BULLET-PROOF SHIELDS AGAINST SHOOTERS

The main purpose of this article is to introduce into the dialogue about preventing or stopping shooting incidents, especially those in grade school or higher education institutions, the idea of having volunteers use bullet-proof shields in responding quickly to a shooter, with the goal of overwhelming and disarming the shooter.

I have had several types of relevant experience or expertise: (1) firing expert with a 45-caliber pistol as an MP lieutenant in 1969 and being tasked with giving pistol firing instruction in my company; (2) holding a PhD in criminology and having as my primary career activity serving as a Criminal Justice professor; (3) having policing as my main specialty area, including developing, editing, and being a major contributor to a commercially published book (Memory & Aragon, 1999) about line police officer problem solving; (4) having studied in graduate school sociobiology, which addresses altruistic behavior by members of social animal groups to defend/protect other members of the group; and (5) having responded successfully in all of the life-threatening incidents I have encountered in my private life (deflecting attacking pack of wild dogs, helping drowning boy scout, Heimlich maneuver (twice), and resuscitation of dead bridge player). I am not claiming I ever would have been an excellent firefighter or law enforcement officer. I, however, do have a strong impulse to act constructively in life-threatening situations.

Relevant scientific information. Prodigiously published Harvard University Professor Dr. Edward O. Wilson has for about a half-century known more than any other scientist about how altruism (self-sacrifice) has influenced the evolution of homo sapiens and other social animal species. This scientific knowledge can help a person to predict or explain the outcomes of attacks by lone gunmen on groups of people.

Discussion relating to shootings not in a school or higher education institution. If the members of the attacked group are largely strangers to each other, it is likely that nearly everyone will be concerned with his or her own survival and/or the survival of a loved one. Since there is not a strong sense of community, love, and mutual protection in the group generally, it is not likely that persons will altruistically rush the gunman. As a result, the gunman may be able to walk about unimpeded and shoot people. That was the situation during an attack in a cafeteria in Texas decades ago. No one acted altruistically in defense of the group, and virtually everyone in the dining room was shot to death. It appears that was also the case in an extremely deadly shooting in a movie theater in Colorado several years ago.

You can expect that the outcome will be different if the group members share a strong bond of love and community. That was the case several years ago when a lone gunman entered a church service in Knoxville and started shooting people. A big man rushed directly at the gunman, which helped other men to be able to subdue the gunman. The big, brave and loving man was killed. As a result, there were astonishingly few deaths and injuries. There is no doubt that the people in that sanctuary shared a strong sense of religious and spiritual community.

I believe that you can expect an outcome similar to the one in Knoxville if a lone gunman attacks a hunter-gatherer band (Some exist even now.), a family group in a developed society, a group of police officers or soldiers who have a strong mutual bond, or, I think, members of an athletic team with a strong team spirit. I don't think that most altruistic defenders of groups reach a fairly quick **intellectual** conclusion, "If no one attacks the attacker, many more people will die." (That is what the courageous people on Flight 93 realistically concluded.) Rather, I think (not contrary to the ideas of Dr. Wilson) that these defenders generally act driven by a strong, nearly instinctual impulse. (About 45 years ago, a group of apparently wild dogs started very aggressively charging a small family group I was in near an old house in the country in North Carolina. Without the slightest conscious decision to do so, I started running toward the dogs with my arms outstretched, yelling at them. They stopped and ran away.)

When a shooting is occurring, in which there is no strong mutual bond of the group members, physically capable people need to realize that group defenders are not going to instinctively come forward. Then, when there is an opportunity, such as a misfire or reloading, one of the group members can shout loudly, "Misfire!" or "He's reloading! Let's get him!" Of course, that shout should occur as the shouting person is rushing at the gunman. In the Texas cafeteria, some men and women, strengthened by a burst of adrenaline, could have picked up a chair and rushed the gunman. With angry people wielding chairs rushing quickly toward him, the gunman probably would have been overwhelmed and disarmed.

I am delighted to add that, during the April 22, 2018 shooting in a Waffle House in Nashville, TN, James Shaw, Jr., a 29-year-old African-American man, heroically did exactly what is urged in the previous paragraph, preventing many additional deaths. When the shooter was reloading, Shaw grabbed the rifle and took it away from the shooter.

<u>Discussion relating to shooter incidents in a school, college, or university</u>.

Measures that may work. I think measures to prevent entry by shooters and to allow students to hide safely should be improved and expanded.

Measures that I think are unlikely to work. Tragically, it appears very unlikely that law enforcement "first responders" or "school resource officers" will prevent or quickly stop deadly attacks that cause many deaths very quickly.

I strongly believe, based on experiences with pistol firing and my long experience as a Criminal Justice professor, that it cannot be sensibly assumed that one or even two or three school teachers, each armed with a pistol, would be able to stop a shooter armed with an AR-15. In 2016, an Army veteran ambushed armed police officers in Dallas, Texas. He killed five officers and injured nine other officers. All or nearly all of the officers were armed with a pistol. Officers eventually used a robot to kill the attacker.

Discussion concerning use of bullet-proof shields during school/ college/university shooting incidents. I need to explain that I would not expect that use of these shields would entirely prevent deaths and injuries. The primary goal would be substantial reduction of deaths and injuries.

I believe that I would probably be much more effective and safe against a shooter when I had a bullet-proof shield than when I had a pistol, especially when there were several other shield wielders.

You can find on the Internet tall (and not-so-tall) bullet-proof shields manufactured and marketed by several American and Chinese companies. Fortunately, the shields have a bullet-proof glass vision slot high on the shields. There are sturdy handles on the user side.

I would favor having a communication device wirelessly connected to the school intercom system mounted on the user side of each shield. This would allow effective communication by, to, and among the shield-wielders. (They will be referred to as "S-W's" subsequently in this article.)

It would be possible to recruit for a school maybe between 10 and 20 school employees or possibly even students who would be willing to be shield wield-ers. Money to buy the shields could come from the school budget, teachers, parents, and monetary contributions. I think it would be important for selected S-W volunteers to have fairly great body power and foot speed. There should be training and drills regarding use of the shields. During a shooting incident, the special communication devices could be used to inform S-W's and school administration and coordinate S-W activities. Of course, the shield wielders could wait until the attacker is reloading, unless deadly shooting is continuing. Obviously, the goal would be for several shield wielders to charge the shooter at the same time and physically overwhelm him. If the shooter is overwhelmed by S-W's, the S-W's should, if needed, kick him to disarm and disable him.

School districts would need to get expert advice about how effective particular shields can be in stopping various types of bullets.

I am not asserting that bullet-proof shields can be a panacea regarding school shootings. I do strongly believe that school districts and law enforce-ment agencies need to carefully consider them, along with other products and strategies.

Potential for use of bullet-proof shields in incidents other than shooter incidents. I believe that, if schools were to purchase and prepare to use shields in school shooter incidents, they would discover that the shields could be used in dealing with much more common and less dangerous situations, such as a student wielding a knife and refusing to drop it. In such a situation, it would be much better for a school resource officer and teacher, both with a shield, to rush the student and overwhelm him, as opposed to the school resource officer shooting the student. You may not know that law enforcement agencies generally do not have policies that require officers to "shoot to wound."

REFERENCES

Memory, J. M. & Aragon, R. (Eds.). (2001). *Patrol officer problem solving and solutions*. Durham, NC: Carolina Academic Press.

SECTION 10
Race and Justice in the U.S.

CHAPTER 28
Dangers Posed by Rampant Ethnocentrism and Xenophobia

Elaboration. Ethnocentrism is an exaggerated belief in the superiority of your group, which can be a racial, ethnic, religious, or other type of clearly defined group. Xenophobia is the fear and hatred of that which is unknown or different.

I believe that virtually all ethnic and religious groups tend to exhibit ethnocentrism and xenophobia to some degree. So, it is logical to conclude that the tendency to exhibit ethnocentrism and xenophobia had survival value for early human hunter-gatherer bands for hundreds of thousands of years prior to the exit of humans from Africa starting in about 70,000 bp (before present).

Here's my main point in this chapter: I believe that Black Lives Matter, the four young Black male authors (Coates, Watson, Butler, and Lowery) I mention several times, Rev. Sharpton, the lynching memorial, Black athletes "taking a knee," and a recent one-hour MSNBC program, *Everyday Racism,* are teaching Black Americans, including children, to hate, distrust, and fear White people and white society. This will tend to accelerate our currently occurring disastrous deterioration of race relations and increase Black-on-White violence. As discussed in chapter 27, a recent increase in Black-on-White homicide apparently triggered a pronounced increase in White-on-Black homicide. Since I have information about this that few people have, **I**

am trying to sound an alarm. I believe that persons of all races and religious in the U.S. need to consciously work on living peacefully and enjoyably with persons of other races, religious, and political groups. I try to do that every day.

Likely adverse effects of ethnocentrism and xenophobia. Being personally in the grips of ethnocentrism and xenophobia can cause a person to not have empathy and compassion for members of other groups. This tends to cause substantial reduction of likelihood that the individual will treat members of other groups with courtesy. Just that seemingly inconsequential tendency can cause the person to move down a slippery slope from discourtesy to rudeness, to inconsiderateness, to incivility, to indecency, and, possibly, to intentionally harmful behavior.

Extremely racist remark made by Steve Bannon. On March 10, 2018, I heard on public radio a report that Steven Bannon said the following in a speech in Europe: "Wear racism as a badge of honor." I have confirmed that he actually uttered that imperative sentence. It is entirely consistent with sentiments of far-right white nationalist parties Bannon favors in Europe and did favor before expulsion from Breitbart. I think it is outrageous that Fareed Zakaria featured Bannon on a recent Zakaria *GPS* television show.

Though the early drafts of this chapter emphasized the dangers of the Black Lives Matter brand of Black racism, I want to express my strong belief that the Bannon/Breitbart brand of White racism is even more objectionable and dangerous than the BLM version. It is more dangerous because it has during the last two years strongly influenced the policies and actions of Donald Trump.

I very strongly believe that racism, ethnocentrism, and xenophobia of all groups in the U.S. will tend to make it more difficult for our country to achieve a more peaceful and enjoyable quality of life for its citizens and residents or even retain the now rapidly deteriorating relations of persons of various races in the U.S.

Racism involves making important decisions because of the race of a person or persons. As an Army company commander and lawyer, civilian prosecutor, Governor's office employee, and professor, I have been strongly opposed to that product of racism. I have never known a decent Army NCO or officer, government employee, or professor who disagrees with me about this.

Though the potentials for ethnocentrism and xenophobia among Black and White Americans have existed during my lifetime (1943–present), Americans are being exposed to those phenomena more now, with the emergence of Black Lives Matter, antifa, and the alt-right. It appears to me that one consequence of this shift is a continuing increase in the sale of firearms, including assault rifles, such as the AR-15.

You can learn some about the alt right by reading an article, "Alt right," on the Wikipedia website and learn some about the antifa by reading an article on the *Washington Post* web site, "Who are the antifa?" (August 16, 2017) by Mark Bray.

A circumstance I did not predict. I believe that, since Black Lives Matter appeared several years ago, its leaders, along with several other Black activists and authors, have exhibited rampant ethnocentrism and xenophobia. About the time of the 2016 Presidential election and for no obvious reasons, Black Lives Matter disappeared. Even though that has occurred, I am leaving in this chapter important content relating to Black Lives Matter.

Trump's intentional causation of animosity between White and Black Americans. I believe that, when candidate and President Trump has made outrageous racist remarks, he has been "playing to his base" of White supporters. This is having the effect of decreasing the potential for "peaceful coexistence of the races" in the U.S. I could write a full page about ways in which his "shithole nations" comments were wrong and harmful.

I will make an obvious distinction we need to remember. Because there is a tendency of cultural groups (racial, ethnic, religious, etc.) to exhibit ethnocentrism and xenophobia, there is a strong tendency for members of cultural groups to develop some prejudice against members of other cultural groups. Just as many White people are prejudiced against Black people, a high percentage of Black people, I am very sure, are prejudiced against White people. Decent and honorable people will not allow that type of prejudice to influence a significant action or decision. A high percentage of police officers in the U.S. are prejudiced against Black Americans. The genuinely fine officers are extremely careful to keep that from influencing their decision making. The same applies to military officers and noncommissioned officers. **The Golden Rule I learned as a child and made a part of my morality strongly urges me to be courteous, kind, fair, and helpful with members of other races, religions, nationalities, and political persuasions.**

Author's relevant expertise and experiences.

Author's relevant expertise and qualifications. Aspects of human cultures, such as norms, beliefs, ethnocentrism, and xenophobia, are part of the subject matter addressed by a PhD criminologist. I have had a publication with a PhD anthropologist (Houston & Memory, 2001) on that subject.

My career primarily involved working as a Criminal Justice university professor during the 1976–2004 period. I occasionally taught "Police-community relations," which involved the subjects of this chapter. Of course, many aspect of criminology and academic criminal justice are significantly concerned with race and race relations.

I, however, am not a social-psychologist and do not have expert-level understanding of African-American culture in the U.S.

Since law school, I have been deeply committed to democracy, the rule of law, due process of law, equal protection of the laws, civil liberties, and civil rights. This is shown in many of my scholarly and non-scholarly publications. Trump is not committed to advancement of any of those things. Unfortunately, it often seems that he is committed to reducing some or all of them.

Author's relevant experiences. I grew up from age five in a rural family-owned community where eight Black families lived in what were or had been tenant-farmer houses. Especially during those years (1949–61), my immediate family and many in my extended family were liberal/progressive and strongly supported improvement of the circumstances of African Americans. My education, working career, and retirement have been nearly entirely in the South, especially North Carolina and South Carolina.

As a result of living now in a substantially integrated suburb of a city of about 100,000, I have developed a strong impression that day-to-day interactions between Black and White people are gradually becoming less friendly, which is also suggested by research about race relations.

During 2015 there was a meeting on the University of South Carolina campus at which only Black Lives Matter leaders were scheduled to speak. I was denied admission to that meeting, apparently at the request of BLM people.

Using skills I discuss in a published scholarly article (Memory, 1999) about qualitative (non-statistical) research, I have tentatively concluded that race relations are significantly worse in Greenville, SC than in Columbia, SC. A high percentage of African-Americans I encounter in substantially integrated northeast Columbia, SC are courteous with me. It's not very unusual for one of us to share a brief humorous or friendly comment. I have found African-Americans in Greenville, SC to be distinctly "cold" in brief encounters with me.

Author's impressions concerning Trump, Bannon, and Roy Moore. By saying that America was most recently great before slavery was abolished, Roy Moore demonstrated that he is not fit to serve in any governmental role or be accepted in "decent society." Doug Jones' win over Roy Moore was one of my five all-time favorite election results. By selecting Moore to back, Bannon acted in accordance with the remark on March 10, 2018, that was discussed earlier. Trump's support for Moore was just one of many demonstrations that he is not fit to serve as President. Rampant ethnocentrism and xenophobia of the right is just as dangerous as rampant ethnocentrism and xenophobia of Black activists (especially BLM), writers, and leaders. Fortunately, recent events are tending to marginalize the Bannon variety of white supremacists. I believe that, if BLM had intruded itself into the Alabama Senatorial election in a major way, Moore might have won.

Importance of this subject. As I was writing this on August 12, 2017, with my television on, I learned about the violent conflict in Charlottesville, VA, between white supremacists and others, including people affiliated with Black Lives Matter and the antifa. As you know, white supremacists were protesting the decision to remove a statue of Robert E. Lee. Events on that day very vividly demonstrated that strong ethnocentrism and xenophobia were found among the white nationalists and their opponents, most notably Black Lives Matter and antifa.

Ongoing deterioration of race relations in the U.S. Recent research has indicated that there is currently occurring in the U.S. a precipitous decline of race relations. A *New York Times*/CBS News poll ("What do Americans feel about race relations?) released on the internet on July 23, 2015, found that 68% of black people said that race relations are bad, while 56% of white respondents said they are bad. On the Gallup website, there is a report ("Gallup poll on race relations") of several years of polling results regarding race relations. One question was, "Would you say relations between (whites and blacks) are very good, somewhat good, somewhat bad, or very bad?" In 2013, 72% of white respondents answered "very good" or "somewhat good." In 2015, 45% of white respondents answered "very good" or "somewhat good." The Gallup poll results show that between 2013 and 2015 there was a 27% drop in White Americans rating race relations between white and black Americans as "very good" or "somewhat good." On April 11, 2016, there was on the Gallup website an article with the title "U.S. worries about race relations reach a new high." The percentage of Americans who worry "a great deal" about the problem of race relations increased from 17% in 2014 to 28% in 2015 to 35% in 2016.

Since the death of Trayvon Martin in 2012, I have occasionally initiated conversation with an older Black person about race relations. The great majority of these people have said something to the effect that the situation regarding race relations among younger Blacks is extremely bad.

Relevance for young adults. Information provided above indicates that the potential for cross-ethnic antagonism and violence is becoming greater in the U.S. Young adults will be aware of this potential in the U.S. for the rest of their lives.

Public opinion regarding Black Lives Matter. On June 27, 2016, the Pew Research Center made available on its website an important article about race relations, "On views of race and inequality, Blacks and Whites are worlds apart." It was reported that 65% of Black Americans support Black Lives Matter, including 41% who strongly support Black Lives Matter. Of Black Americans, 12% oppose Black Lives Matter. Among White Americans, 40% support Black Lives Matter, and 28% oppose BLM.

Chapter 34 of this book concerns problems in the U.S. regarding being able to stay well informed. In recent years, a progressively smaller percentage of people have been agreeing to respond to a public opinion survey. Consequently, we cannot be sure that the results of recent Gallup and Pew Research Center research accurately reflect the opinions of members of various groups in the U.S.

Political incorrectness of some of my views on this subject. Undoubtedly, virtually all professors view it as politically incorrect and forbidden to make public statements (oral or published) about the dangers associated with increases of ethnocentrism and xenophobia among African Americans. I believe that the activities of Black Lives Matter prompted the emergence of the alt-right, and I believe that Hillary Clinton's enthusiastic embracing of Black Lives Matter was one of the significant causes of her loss in the electoral college vote in 2016.

A letter I sent to 22 leading African-American leaders and public figures late in 2016. You will find in this letter some information and ideas I have provided elsewhere in this book. Because I wrote and mailed this letter in late 2016, some of its information could be updated in light of events in 2017. I believe this letter shows that I was trying to influence the related dialogue in the U.S. in constructive ways.

Subject: **Warning regarding potentially disastrous developments regarding race relations and interracial violence in the U.S.**

Dear Ladies and Gentlemen:

This letter has been sent only to important American Black leaders, journalists, and officials because I think only respected Black leaders can exert needed influence relating to the subjects of this letter.

Though I retired from university teaching in Criminal Justice in 2004, I have, since the killing of Trayvon Martin, been paying close attention to race relations in the U.S. Also, I have since early 2015 done very extensive statistical study of interracial violence in the U.S. **This work has convinced me that we are headed for substantial worsening of problems in the U.S. concerning race relations and interracial violence**. I feel duty-bound to attempt to disseminate this information.

Additional information about my qualifications. I was an associate editor of the *Wake Forest Law Review,* wrote a lead law review article about right of counsel in criminal cases, had a commercially published book about police problem solving, and had several articles published in refereed journals. You can find one of my refereed journal articles by doing an Internet search for "Juvenile suicides in secure detention facilities: correction of published rates," which was published in *Death Studies.* I was a consulting editor of a refereed journal. In September of 2016, I presented a scholarly paper mainly about interracial violence. A retired PhD economist favorably reviewed my statistical work reported in that paper. Much of the crucial information in that paper is also in this letter. If you want to receive that paper (which will be updated, with all appropriate references), you can email me at the address above. I am authorizing distribution of this letter only to well-qualified and responsible persons. I am not authorizing any distribution of my conference paper.

Information about my politics and ideology. I, a nearly 73-year-old Southern white male, have never voted for a Republican and in 2015 and 2016 tried to assist the Hillary campaign as much as I could. The belief that the only moral and feasible way forward for the U.S. is as a pluralistic nation with the rule of law protecting members of all racial, ethnic, and religious groups is a central part of my ideology. That belief is the most important motivator for my work. Also, I am motivated by concerns regarding public safety and quality of life for Americans.

I believe that various Black groups and individuals and other persons and organizations on the radical right are especially responsible for causing or allowing this situation to develop. I very strongly condemn actions by Donald Trump which have caused further dissemination and acceptability of white supremacist materials and ideas.

A reader of this letter may think, "This information will help the white supremacists." Black Lives Matter and its colleagues have provided important causation of the present potentially disastrous situation in the U.S. I am hoping that my interjection of sound information can help Americans and our leaders to find the right path to "a better place" for Americans to enjoy living and working together.

I will now provide brief presentations of important information and ideas.

(1) **Rapid deterioration of race relations in the U.S.** In very recent years a rapid deterioration of race relations in the U.S. has occurred, and it is continuing. (A brief Internet search will show this. If you receive my conference paper, see page 14.) I have been extremely worried by this development partly because I know that there will be emotional and behavioral consequences. As examples of consequences, I will note that from 2014 to 2015 there was a 10.8% increase in murder in the U.S., which is a very significant departure from the decades-long major decrease in violent crime in the U.S. From 2014 to 2015 rape increased by 6.3%.

I believe that race was the most influential variable in the recent Presidential election. Trump was embracing Bannon and Breitbart, and Clinton was embracing Black Lives Matter. I believe that the rapid deterioration of race relations influenced the outcome.

(2) **Interracial homicide in the U.S.** Because it is important to understanding of the subjects addressed in this letter, I will report findings of my own calculations which indicated that between 1980 and 2013 the rate of Black-on-White homicide in the U.S. averaged 15.4 times as high as the rate of White-on-Black homicide. It is important to know that increase in Black-on-White homicide is nearly certainly accompanied by very much greater increases in other violent Black-on-White crimes. Findings in section (4) below for 2008 suggest that increase in White-on-Black homicide probably will not be accompanied by major increases in White-on-Black rape, aggravated assault, and robbery.

Now, I will provide the most startling and possibly the most important information in this letter.

From 2013 to 2014, the number of Black-on-White homicides increased by 9%, and the increase from 2014 to 2015 was 12%. From 2014 to 2015, the number of White-on-Black homicides increased 22%. In several unpublished papers I have predicted that eventually White-on-Black homicides would increase.

I believe that the combination of rapid deterioration of race relations

and rapid increase in interracial homicide indicates that a national disaster is in the process of developing. I will predict here that, unless there are significant counter-measures, race relations and interracial violence will continue to worsen in the U.S.

(3) **Potential for rioting**. During the summer of 2016, a Black police officer in Milwaukee repeatedly ordered a Black man armed with a very dangerous pistol to drop the pistol. When the subject failed to drop the pistol, the Black officer shot and killed the armed subject. Very serious and violent rioting followed in Milwaukee. During September of 2016, a Black police officer and other officers in Charlotte, NC, repeatedly ordered a Black man armed with a pistol to drop the pistol. When the subject failed to drop the pistol, the Black officer shot and killed the armed subject. Very serious rioting followed in Charlotte.

The fact that serious and violent rioting occurred in Milwaukee and Charlotte, even though in both cases an armed Black man who refused to drop a pistol was shot by a Black police officer, suggests that there is now great potential for Black-resident violence and disorder in some percentage of U.S. cities.

(4) **Felonious killing of law enforcement officers**. An FBI report indicates that during the 2005 and 2014 period 563 law enforcement officers in the U.S. were feloniously killed. The number killed by Black subjects was 224, which was 40% of the total number killed. It is, therefore, clear that Black persons are heavily over-represented among felonious killers of law enforcement officers. The number of officers feloniously killed in 2013 was 27. The number feloniously killed in 2014, 51, was up nearly 100% from the previous year.

(5) **Strongly inflammatory action of Black Lives Matter and others**. The sentences that are most strongly associated with Black Lives Matter, with Black journalist and author Ta-Nehisi Coates, and with Black journalist and author Wesley Lowery all can reasonably be interpreted as saying that White people in the U.S. now are killing Black people at a fast rate. It is important to note that all three of these sentences fail to specify who is committing the violent acts. None of the sentences is limited in applicability

to police officers. I believe the obvious intent in every case was that Black persons would assume that the killers of Black people are American White people, not just White police officers.

The Black Lives Matter website, which was no longer accessible on the Internet at least by early November of 2016, very prominently displayed the following statement:

> **"Black Lives Matter is an ideological and political inter-vention in a world where Black lives are systematically and intentionally targeted for demise."**

An African-American journalist, Ta-Nehisi Coates, had an influential book, *Between the World and Me*, published in 2015. Having carefully read and reread the book, I will confidently state that the following quote is the emotional center of the content of the book.

> **"Here is what I would like you to know: In America it is traditional to destroy the black body—*it is heritage."***
> (Coates, 2015, p. 102)

During November of 2016 a book by Wesley Lowery, *They Can't Kill Us All*, was published. Lowery is a reporter for the *Washington Post*. The cover of the Lowery book shows a young Black male who is confronting two White police officers who are in riot gear. Everyone with whom I have discussed the Lowery book agrees with me that the title is extremely inflammatory and irre-sponsible. Millions of Black Americans will hear or read the title, *They Can't Kill Us All*. I believe that a high percentage of them will infer from the title that White people, especially White police officers, have recently been wrongfully killing a large number of Black persons and would like to kill many more.

The three leaders of Black Lives Matter and Ta-Nehisi Coates have often been referred to as important new leaders of Black Americans. The Lowery book has been widely publicized. In his book, Lowery tells in very great detail about the efforts of Black activists during and since Ferguson to create a new Black civil rights movement. Obviously, they have been attempting to make violence by White persons against Black persons the subject of this new civil rights movement.

I very strongly believe that Black Lives Matter activities, supported by Reverend Al Sharpton and, since 2015, by the Ta-Nehisi Coates book, *Between the World and Me*, are achieving nearly nothing positive and are causing a wide variety of significant problems in the U.S., including worsening of race relations. Worsening of race relations is apparently contributing to an increase in interracial violence.

(6) **Crucial falsehood of the Black Lives Matter and Coates message. Black Lives Matter and author Coates are totally wrong in asserting that there is violent oppression and/or elimination of Black people by White people in the U.S.** The opposite is very much closer to being true. I obtained the necessary data and, using my statistical skills as a PhD criminologist, calculated offense rates for several categories of White-on-Black and Black-on-White violent crime. (I don't know of any other qualified scholar who has done these analyses with the very limited available data. I will be glad to mail a copy of my data as requested.)

Here are brief presentations of my statistical findings regarding interracial violence in the U.S.

1980–2013. The Black-on-White single-offender, single-victim homicide rate averaged 15.4 times as high as the White-on-Black rate. The data were from FBI uniform crime reports.

2012–2013. The Black-on-White rate of non-lethal violent crime was 32.9 times as high as the White-on-Black rate. The data were from the National Crime Victimization Survey.

2008. The Black-on-White rate of completed violence offenses was 27.7 times as high as the White-on-Black rate. The data for all of the 2008 findings were from the National Crime Victimization Survey.

> The Black-on-White rate of aggravated assaults was 31.5 times as high as the White-on-Black rate.

> The Black-on-White rate of robbery was 62.1 times as high as the White-on-Black rate.

The Black-on-White rate of rape and rape-related offenses was 49.2 per 100,000 population per year. The rate reported for White-on-Black rape and rape-related offenses was 0.0, apparently because there were no such offenses reported in their survey.

These findings together overwhelmingly prove that there is no violent oppression or elimination of Black people by White people in the U.S. Tragically, these findings indicate that Black people in the U.S. select White people to be violently victimized at an astonishingly high rate, which is vastly higher than the corresponding rate of White-on-Black violent crime.

(7) **Research about killing of Black subjects by law enforcement officers**. In an October 16, 2015, article ("Police killings of blacks: here is what the data say") in the *New York Times*, Harvard PhD economist Sendhil Mullainathan concluded that there is no evidence that police in the U.S. are using deadly force against Black subjects at a higher rate than against White subjects. Similar conclusions were reached by Harvard economist Roland Fryer, who is Black, in an article in the *New York Times* on July 11, 2016. Information about killings of persons by police in the U.S. during 2015 collected by *Washington Post* employees appears to be consistent with the Mullainathan and Fryer conclusions. An important point made is that, generally, there is, because of high Black offense rates (especially high violent crime rates), an over-representation of Black persons among offenders and suspects that police encounter, detain or arrest. The percentage of subjects killed by police who are Black is generally close to the percentage of Blacks persons among persons encountered, detained and arrested by police.

Having for many years in the past been an expert on patrol policing in the U.S., I will share my belief that there is no evidence that White law enforcement officers tend to act influenced by racial hatred or bias in use of deadly force against Black subjects. I do believe, however, that in a very small percentage of cases, a law enforcement officer, not at all because of racial hatred or bias, fails to exercise sufficient restraint in the use of deadly force. I believe that there should be improvement in training and officer control relating to use of deadly force.

Also, I strongly favor prosecution of persons, including law enforcement officers, who commit chargeable homicide. Of course, recovery in a civil law suit may be possible in cases of police use of deadly force.

(8) **A suggestion from me about disarming armed and dangerous subjects**. I believe that it would be helpful for police to have available a device which could be used in reliably disarming armed and menacing subjects. Such a device might be similar to a long rifle or gun and might fire a very hard ball that would quickly inflate after being fired. When the ball hits the subject's hand and firearm, the impact would be sufficient to fully disarm and disable the subject. Effects could include breaking of hand, wrist, and/or arm bones. This would obviously be less severe than killing the subject.

(9) **Complaints by NFL players**. Some of the currently protesting/demonstrating football players are complaining about denial of social justice. A long list of laws, measures, and programs have been established in the U.S. to overcome problems and help Americans to attain a high quality of life. This process tends to increase social justice in the U.S. Especially progressive/liberal Presidents Lincoln, Teddy Roosevelt, FDR, and LBJ worked terrifically hard and effectively with strong voter support and support in Congress in making these types of improvements. I think it is not justified for these football players to make a broad complaint about denial of social justice in the U.S., especially given the pattern of interracial violence I have reported.

In several of the numbered sections below I try to show that deterioration of race relations and worsening of interracial violence in the U.S. will be likely to be especially harmful for Black persons in the U.S.

(10) **Hesitancy of police officers regarding approaching of potentially dangerous Black subjects**. Regular CNN contributor Van Jones refers to a "Black Lives Matter revolt." I call it a Black Lives Matter furor and frenzy. That furor and frenzy is apparently causing police officers in some cities to be more hesitant regarding intervention in situations involving possibly dangerous Black subjects. Apparently the current catastrophically high homicide rate in Chicago is partly the result of this phenomenon. The Black community obviously needs effective police service more than any other demographic group in the U.S. I have in my conference paper estimated that

the increase in incarceration after 1980 may have resulted in the prevention of 183,000 Black-on-Black homicides.

(11) **Worsening of mental health problems of Black persons in the U.S.** In the U.S., the Black schizophrenia rate is three times higher than the White schizophrenia rate. The totally false and widely disseminated assertion that White people violently oppress and eliminate Black people in the U.S. has very great potential to cause increase in paranoia in the Black community. There is a positive association of paranoid schizophrenia with the commission of violent crime. The title of the Lowery book, *They Can't Kill Us All*, will feed into and worsen Black cultural and individual paranoia in the U.S. Lowery mentions several times in his book that **a high percentage of shootings by police in the U.S. involve mentally ill and/or suicidal subjects**. There is here a "perfect storm" of existence of vast numbers of especially Black males who are mentally ill and/or suicidal who hate police and may be drawn to committing "suicide by police."

(12) **Likely effects on Black children**. I believe that the effects of the BLM furor and frenzy on Black children can be extremely devastating. We can predict that, as a result of the BLM furor and frenzy, including the demonstrations of football players at NFL games, Black children will like White people less and fear them more. I believe that this can very adversely affect the ability of Black children to learn from White teachers, coaches, and police officers.

(13) **Possible effects regarding Black employment in the service sector**. For many decades a high percentage of African Americans have worked successfully in the service sector, which generally requires friendliness and courtesy. Recently I talked with an owner of a business near my home who knew of two young Black persons, each of whom had recently lost a job in the service sector because of rudeness with customers. This may be an indicator of a major national trend, which would obviously be disastrous.

For many decades, large numbers of African Americans have worked very well and successfully in policing and other aspects of the criminal justice system. Increased hatred by Black persons of police can result in a great reduction in this successful working. Our country needs many excellent

Black police officers, prison and jail guards, probation and parole officers, and prosecutors.

(14) **Likely adverse effects regarding interactions between Black and White persons**. I grew up in the 1950s in a rural community in North Carolina where eight Black sharecropper families lived. During every era of my life, I have enjoyed interacting with Black people. Of course, we have used the skills and practices that have allowed White and Black persons to coexist enjoyably and peacefully with each other. Coates ridicules those skills and practices in his book. I greatly fear that especially Black persons are setting aside those skills and practices, which will end the learning of those skills and practices by young persons. This can eliminate an important "social lubricant" in encounters of Blacks and Whites. In a highly pluralistic nation, such as the U.S., people of many different races, ethnicities, and religions need to be able to enjoy working, learning, playing, and living in close proximity with members of other groups. I fear that BLM and Coates, who promote intense Black ethnocentrism and xenophobia, are in the process of making this enjoyable and peaceful living more unlikely.

(15) **Unintended support of BLM for the arguments of white supremacists**. As previously noted, white supremacist ideas and proposals have recently been disseminated in the U.S. more than at any time for many decades. The BLM-driven furor and frenzy, involving inflaming of Black hatred of White people and rapid deterioration of race relations in the U.S., can only support the arguments and goals of white supremacists. As Black people hate White people more and communicate this through their actions, such as unfriendliness, hostility, and violence, White people can be expected to like Black people less and fear them more. This may drive many White people into the arms of white supremacists.

Since I strongly support having a pluralistic society with legal protections for members of all racial, ethnic, and religious groups, I view growth of support for white supremacists as an extremely undesirable development.

(16) **Possibility of Black support for Islamic extremism**. Should alienation of Black and White Americans continue to worsen, there will be increased potential for Black Americans to develop identification with and

support for Islamic extremism and terrorism. I cannot think of any way that this would be helpful for Black Americans.

(17) Absence of need for the Black Lives Matter furor and frenzy. This point is hard to express adequately. Slavery was a horrific institution that could not exist in a decent society. Prior to the start of the Civil War, corrective action regarding slavery was necessary. The Great Depression of the 1930s created vast financial hardship, and many types of remedial action were necessary. The 9/11 attacks necessitated meaningful action by the U.S. government and military against terrorism directed against the U.S. and Americans. The purely fictional assertion of White violent oppression and elimination of Black persons entirely fails to exhibit any of the aspects of this type of situation. For example, my impression is that, in the average year, possibly between 25 and 50 subjects are wrongfully killed by police in the U.S. (This is a very rough estimate. I'm sure that current experts can provide better estimates than I.) In 2015, there were 2380 reported Black-on-Black single-offender, single-victim homicides. There is a very credible, professionally prepared report on the Internet that annually about one million Americans die as a result of medical or pharmacological error or neglect. We can roughly estimate that, annually, 120,000 of these people are Black.

Based on my study and observation, Black people in the U.S. have recently come to like White people much less and hate them more, to a significant extent because of the BLM/Coates fictional and false depiction of history and reality according to which Whites in the U.S., especially White police officers, are violently oppressing and eliminating Black persons. Of course, there probably have been some other contributing causes. For example, there may have been things relating to the Obama Presidency which have contributed to this causation. Also, I am sure that White people have generally come to like Black people less.

Support for the statement that hatred of White people by Black people has recently increased significantly is found in a statement by Oprah Winfrey during the Presidential campaign. She noted that a lot of Black people don't like Hillary Clinton and said, "You don't have to like Hillary: She's not coming to your house." I will very seriously ask, "If American Black people don't like Hillary Clinton, what White person will they like?"

Since this furor and frenzy is not the result of a real and seriously undesirable pattern of human behavior, I greatly hope that the furor and frenzy and its horrible consequences can be ended. Otherwise stated, I don't think there's anything "White society" can do to obtain discontinuation of the furor and frenzy. After creating the vast array of government programs and entitlements listed earlier, "White society" then established affirmative action in favor of Black people in education and employment. Then, a Black President was elected. I seriously ask, "What further can 'White society' do?"

(18) **Where can these developments and forces take the U.S. and Americans?** The American people, our leaders, and our government are attempting several things that I believe have never been achieved for a long period of time in a large society: (1) Achieving peaceful and fulfilling living of members of many racial, ethnic, and religious groups together in the same country, states, cities, and neighborhoods. (2) Guaranteeing of civil rights, civil liberties, equal protection of the laws, and due process of law to people in the country regardless of racial, ethnic, and/or religious group membership. It is entirely possible that the trends I have reported and noted will result in substantial reduction of success in achieving these important goals.

BLM and Coates have strongly encouraged Black ethnocentrism (belief in the superiority of your group) and xenophobia (fear and hatred of that which is different). Of course, white supremacists strongly encourage ethnocentrism and xenophobia of White persons in the U.S. I will repeat that I greatly fear that these things have created a situation in which disastrous worsening of relationships and interactions of members of various racial, ethnic, and religious groups is occurring. I have observed and believe that there is occurring some withdrawal of common courtesy in interactions between White and Black people. As a criminologist, I am particularly concerned regarding continued worsening of interracial violent crime in the U.S.

How can responsible and caring Americans of good will deal with this worsening situation? While I have many ideas about this, I believe that the addressees can develop many more and better ideas on this subject than I can. I hope that many of the recipients of this letter will take action or speak in public in ways that may help in ameliorating these severe difficulties.

In my own life, I try to go the extra mile in courtesy in interactions with Black persons, which occur frequently for me. For example, while I was waiting to talk to a manager at a Home Depot store recently, I said to the nearest customer-service person, "Why don't you assist this gentleman (who was Black) while I'm waiting?" She did.

Here's the most important rule: "Do unto others as you would have them do unto you." Historically, in the U.S. it has been a big plus for race relations that a high percentage of Blacks and Whites have been Christians. This has reduced the potential for Black v. White ethnocentrism and xenophobia.

I will end with two unfortunate conclusions I have reached. First, I think Black people hate White people very much more than White people hate Black people. How else can the differences in violent crime rates be explained? Second, I strongly believe that Black persons, especially the BLM leaders, Sharpton, and Coates, have created a vast and destructive furor through their nearly entirely fictional story, with concern only for their own gains thereby and without concern regarding adverse effects for America and Americans.

Sincerely yours,

John M. Memory, PhD, JD
(LTC, JAGC, USAR (ret.))

Motivations and effects of activities of Black Lives Matter, other Black activists, and Black authors. Ida B. Wells (1862–1931) was a very influential Black journalist, newspaper editor, and suffragette and was one of the founders of the National Association for the Advancement of Colored People. She said, "Somebody must show that the Afro-American race is more sinned against than sinning." I believe that, among other things, BLM, Black activists, and some Black authors are answering her call to action. I believe that the National Memorial to Peace and Justice established in Montgomery, AL in 2018 will tend to increase Black hatred and distrust of White people, tend to worsen race relations, and tend to increase interracial violence. These trends involve increase of ethnocentrism and xenophobia in the African-American community.

I strongly believe that the activities since about 2015 of BLM, some other Black activists, and some Black authors have constituted an action, and the growths of support for the alt right and for other white supremacist groups have constituted an opposite reaction. My own impression is that, even since the recent emergence of the alt right, White people in the U.S. do not support white supremacist perspectives nearly as strongly as Black people support the ethnocentric and xenophobic perspectives of Black Lives Matter.

I have been a southern white male all of my life and have never known anyone who displayed a Confederate flag. I've never heard a pro-white supremacy remark by a person in my presence. Those people intuitively sense that I'm not in their camp.

Speculation about a possible reason for behaviors and emotions of some African Americans. Some scholars (Whaley, 2004; Grier & Cobbs, 1968) believe that African Americans exhibit what they call "cultural paranoia," which is a greater sense of members of a racial and/or ethnic group of being persecuted than actually is the case. I strongly believe that the BLM movement, the Coates book (2015), the Lowery book (2016), the Butler book (2017), and the Watson book (2015) are contributing, along with repeated television stories about black men being killed by a police officer, to increase of cultural paranoia in the African-American community.

It seems to me that many African Americans have psychological needs to blame, complain about, and hate White Americans and not experience and/or communicate appreciation for positive treatment by "White society." It is possible that these beliefs and behaviors serve to some extent as a cultural and individual "defense mechanism." "Our problems aren't our fault: They're caused by White people." Blaming other people, especially incorrect blaming, nearly always fails to contribute to solution of an individual's or group's problems.

Result of the 2016 Presidential election. Hillary Rodham Clinton has had a new book (2017) published, *What happened*. You will notice that there is no question mark at the end of the title. Incidentally, I wrote many documents, including a published op-ed, in support of Secretary Clinton during the campaign.

I believe that candidate Clinton enthusiastically embraced Black Lives Matter during the Presidential primaries and general election campaign. BLM has refused to acknowledge that all lives matter. So, their effective message is, "Only black lives matter." I believe that many White Americans viscerally sensed that the BLM message is very un-American and even dangerous. I think that message precludes genuine ascription to the Golden Rule. So, I think that many White Americans sensed that Clinton was taking the U.S. down a dangerous path regarding race relations, and I believe that Secretary Clinton's embrace of BLM contributed substantially to her loss in the election.

I believe that prominence of BLM and Maxine Watters in election campaigns in 2018 and 2020 will increase the likelihood that Democrats will suffer major defeats. Unfortunately, I believe that, if White people in the U.S. view the Democratic Party as primarily the party for Black people, the likelihood of major political victories for the Democratic Party will be greatly reduced.

Putting Black rage and furor regarding some killings of African Americans by police into perspective. My rough estimate is that in recent years many Blacks have become enraged by between 10 and 20 killings of Black men annually by police officers. In virtually all of those cases, the man who was killed had resisted police, had committed a dangerous act, or was committing "suicide by cop," which means that the person wanted to cause himself to be killed by a police officer. The Black Georgia Tech student who was killed by a campus police office during September of 2017 left suicide notes and was recorded saying to police officers, "Shoot me."

Here is my point: Many Black people have become enraged, some violently enraged, regarding between 10 and 20 killings of Black men by police officers annually, often under the indicated types of circumstances, while, as reported in chapter 27 of this book, the rate at which Black-on-White homicide occurred from 1980 through 2013 in the U.S. was 15.4 times as high as the rate of White-on-Black homicide. During 2012–13, the rate of Black-on-White non-lethal violent crime was about 32.9 times as high as the rate of White-on-Black non-lethal violent crime. African Americans obviously are much more concerned about those 20 "questionable" deaths per year than they are about the very high Black-on-Black violent crime rate. It seems that they don't care at all about the high rate of Black-on-White non-lethal violent crime.

Counter-productive effects of the "furor and frenzy" created by Black activists, especially BLM, and Black authors, since 2015. The deafening furor, accompanied by some rioting by mainly Black persons in some cities, is not producing positive outcomes for the African-American population of the U.S. Instead, it is producing negative outcomes.

Emergence of the alt right. I strongly believe that this "furor and frenzy" was a major cause of the recent increase in prominence of the white-supremacist movement.

Election of Donald Trump. As I have mentioned several times, I believe that Hillary Clinton's embracing of Black Lives Matters and related developments resulted in the election of Donald Trump, whose goals and policies are, to a very large extent, contrary to the interests of Black Americans. The 2017 Republican tax cut demonstrates not a hint of concern for African Americans and their problems and does demonstrate concern nearly exclusively for corporations and the wealthy.

Withdrawal of police from potentially dangerous encounters in predominantly Black communities. The complaints about police killings of Black males since the death of Trayvon Martin are resulting in some hesitancy of police to engage in encounters with potentially dangerous Black males. Because of the extremely high Black-on-Black violent victimization rate reported in chapter 27, Black Americans need the protection of police more than any other group.

Substantial increase in Black-on-Black violent crime. As I report in chapter 27, **the substantial increase in prison and jail incarceration rates in the U.S. that started in about 1980 resulted in preventing many millions of Black-on-Black violent crimes, including the prevention of possibly as many as 183,000 murders**. Complaints by Black activists about the high incarceration rate of Black males is contributing to some reduction of the incarceration rate. The homicide rate in the U.S. increased by 10% from 2015 to 2016. If these trends continue, a high percentage of the increase in violent crime will victimize Black persons. As reported in chapter 27,

Black-on-White homicide has increased for several years. White-on-Black homicide increased by 22% from 2014 to 2015.

Rapid deterioration of race relations in the U.S. As discussed in this chapter, I believe that this deterioration is producing many types of adverse effects, a high percentage of which will negatively affect Black persons. I believe that many African Americans are enjoying this increase in Black ethnocentrism and xenophobia. Still, this will not produce positive effects that are nearly as strong as the negative effects.

Here are some things that White people with the relevant knowledge might feel angry about. In some cases, only I and extremely few other people have "the relevant information."

(1) Since the Civil War, many wonderful White people in every part of the U.S., including the South, have worked as hard as they could to improve the circumstances of African Americans. Though a White person could detect gratitude of African Americans during previous decades, I doubt that White persons more than very infrequently detect any gratitude in the Black community concerning this favorable treatment. Instead, there is a continued impulse to complain about treatment by White people, maybe because, for a long time, complaining has gotten positive results.

(2) Especially the Black-on-White rate of non-lethal violent crime, which, as indicated above, in 2012–13 was about 33 times as high as the rate of White-on-Black non-lethal violent crime.

(3) In recent years, African Americans have complained vehemently about the small number of African Americans nominated for Oscars. They believe that is an important problem that should be solved. They do not appear to be concerned about the high rate of Black-on-Black violent crime or the high rate of Black-on-White non-lethal violent crime, mentioned above.

(4) A reasonable person could conclude that BLM, some other Black activists, and some Black authors are very strongly motivated by desire to stoke Black rage to increase their own ability to achieve major financial

rewards. I believe this effort has constituted brainwashing. Lowery (2016) discusses that phenomenon in his recent book.

Now, speaking for myself, I will say that I seriously doubt that these African-American activists and authors care about Black Americans as much as I do. For example, I have for years hoped that my study and writing about heart and brain health can be used to benefit African Americans, which is the group of Americans who have the highest rates of heart and brain disease. As discussed in my letter in this chapter, I want African Americans individually and collectively to prioritize well and spend time, energy, and money solving major problems, such as health problems (It is quoted in chapter 3 that 48% of African-American adults are obese.), problems in achieving optimal education, the availability of affordable housing, problems regarding the availability of jobs (including the effects of mechanization, automation, robotics, computerization, and artificial intelligence), and the outrageous disparities in wealth and income of the richest and poorest Americans. Instead of working terrifically hard trying to reduce these incredibly serious problems, some Black leaders, as previously mentioned, have complained most about lack of Black nominees for an Oscar or Emmy.

REFERENCES

Bresnahan, M. et al (2007). Race and risk of schizophrenia in a U.S. birth cohort: another example of health disparity? *International Journal of Epidemiology*, Vol. 36, No. 4, pp. 751–758.

Butler, P. (2017). *Chokehold*. NY, NY: The New Press.

Coates, Ta-Nehisi. (2015). *Between the World and Me*. NY, NY: Spiegel & Grau.

Grier, W.H., & Cobbs, P.M. (1968). *Black rage*. NY, NY: Basic Books.

Humphrey, J.A., & Palmer, S. (1987). Race, sex, and criminal homicide offender-victim relationships. *Journal of Black Studies*, Vol. 18, No. 1, pp. 45–57.

Kennedy, H.G. et al (1992). Fear and anger in delusional (paranoid) disorder: the association with violence. *British Journal of Psychiatry*, Vol. 160, No. 4, pp. 488–492.

Lowery, W. (2016). *They can't kill us all.* NY, NY: Little, Brown and Company.

Memory, J.M. (1999). Some impressions from a qualitative study of implementation of community policing in North Carolina. In M. L. Dantzker (Ed.) (1999). *Readings for research methods in criminology and criminal justice.* Woburn, MA: Butterworth.

Watson, B. with Petersen, K. (2015). *Under our skin: getting real about race.* Carol Stream, IL: Tyndale Momentum.

Whaley, A.L. (2004). Paranoia in African-American men receiving inpatient treatment. *Journal of the American Academy of Psychiatry and the Law*, Vol. 32, pp. 282–290.

—— CHAPTER 29 ——
Social, Economic, and Criminal
Justice in the U.S. since 1900

Elaboration.

Content of this chapter. This chapter is concerned with the extent to which different levels of government accord justice to citizens and persons in the U.S. For example, in my opinion, gerrymandering and attempts to disenfranchise voters are outrageous denials of political justice. It would be desirable for a wide variety of types of denial of justice to be addressed in an undergraduate course on this subject.

Social contract theory. In discussing the extent to which justice is achieved in the U.S. in the 20th and 21st centuries, one needs to start with discussion of the "social contract theory."

Though Greek philosophers discussed related concerns and issues, English philosopher Thomas Hobbes (1588–1679) first clearly articulated the social contract theory in his important book, *Leviathan* (1651). During the Enlightenment of the 1700s, English philosopher John Locke and French philosopher Jean-Jacques Rousseau further developed thinking concerning social contract theory. According to that theory, people in a society enter into an agreement that a government will be formed and that, in return for acceptable and adequate functioning of the government, the people will obey the laws and mandates of the government.

Twentieth century scholarship relating to justice. By far the most important modern American scholar concerning justice was John Rawls. To read an outline relating to Rawls' thinking about justice, you can do an Internet search for "A theory of justice by John Rawls." The outline is by Professor Dick Piccard. Rawls developed a "Kantian version of social contract theory." Shortly before his death in 2001, Rawls had a book (2001) published that elaborated on some of his earlier published work.

Some scholars in the field consider Rawls' writing somewhat "dense." I think it would be helpful for a scholar in the field to provide a brief and "dumbed down" version of Rawls' thinking about justice. I "dumbed down" justice in my teaching in Criminal Justice by defining justice as "fairness and equality of treatment."

Explanation. I am proposing a course concerned with the period since 1900 because I don't think there is any doubt about the brutality of slavery and the treatment of former slaves, especially in the South during Reconstruction under Jim Crow laws.

By including this chapter, I am to some extent taking "author's license." I believe that economic and criminal justice, and to a lesser extent social justice, are covered some in undergraduate courses. I want to include in this chapter several points of view that I believe are nearly never communicated in university and college undergraduate courses.

You may be surprised that I include in this chapter my strident criticism of the recent Republican tax cut and of actions of Black Lives Matter and other Black activists and authors. In this book, I am not trying to defend or promote any group. Instead, I am trying to provide correct information and valid perspectives.

Author's relevant expertise, experience, and belief. As a lawyer and fairly well-published PhD criminologist with strong expertise in criminal justice, I have had extensive information on this subject. I taught Constitutional Law at Florida State University when I was a graduate student in criminology there.

I will remind the reader that I am a lifelong Democrat and have never voted for a Republican. I worked very hard assisting the Obama campaign in the NC mountains in 2008 and attempted to assist the Clinton campaign in

2016. In my civilian professional life, my military life, and my private life, I have worked very hard to advance achievement of social and criminal justice. As mentioned in the previous chapter, I have since law school been deeply committed to democracy, the rule of law, due process of law, equal protection of the laws, civil liberties, and civil rights.

During my 50 years since completing law school, I have developed a strong belief that people in the U.S., including lawyers, have very little notion concerning how important good laws, good courts, and good lawyering have been and are now in getting and keeping a very high percentage of important things in the U.S. I could easily give an extemporaneous hour-long talk about this.

"Sliding scale of due process of law." It's important to know that the extent of due process procedural protections (e.g., right to counsel in criminal cases, right to jury trial, right to confront witnesses) depends on the possible severity of adverse governmental action. The fullest form of due process protections is available in death-penalty murder trials. A vastly less extensive set of protections apply when only a small civil monetary penalty is possible.

In recent years I wrote a proposal for a 14-chapter book I would write with the following title: *The sliding scale of due process of law: flexibility in government social control*. Fortunately, just the information I have provided above can introduce a person to the "sliding scale of due process" concept.

Importance of this subject. There is an extensive body of important scholarly literature about social, economic, and criminal justice. It is possible for me to cover only a small amount of that subject matter in this chapter.

I believe that, for people in a country to have hope for the future, they must believe that they are being treated justly by the government.

Relevance for young adults. It is important for young adults to understand what justice is and to have correct information about whether justice has been and is being dispensed in their country.

During 2003, I wrote a handout about social justice for a Criminal Justice class at a North Carolina university. The class was made up exclusively of Criminal Justice majors, nearly half of whom were African-American. To my amazement, the students seemed distinctly uninterested in that subject. While I have not supported the NFL players' refusal to stand for the "National Anthem," I very strongly believe that young adults, especially African Americans, should be intensely interested in achievement of social justice in our society.

Social justice and, most importantly, the gross social injustice of the Republican tax cut. On the Internet, "social justice" is defined as "Justice in terms of the distribution of wealth, opportunities, and privileges within a society." It is important to fully address the social injustice of the 2017 Republican tax cut. To do so, the first step will be the provision of an op-ed I wrote on social justice that was published in 2012. Then, I provide detailed discussion relating to the Republican tax cut.

I believe that severe denial of social justice in a country can constitute violation of the underlying "social contract." This can lead to a revolution. At the end of 2017 and beginning of 2018, Iranian citizens have been demonstrating expressing serious dissatisfaction concerning aspects of conditions in Iran.

A published newspaper op-ed by me about social and economic justice. This op-ed was published in the *Asheville Citizen-Times* in 2012.

Effects of Economic Inequality

"One of the important issues that were discussed in the Presidential campaign was: **Should the very wealthy in the U.S. be required to pay a significantly higher share of federal taxes?** In order to discuss this sensibly, one needs to have information about disparities in income and wealth in the U.S. and effects of several types of socioeconomic disparity.

"That subject has been addressed in very helpful ways by several superb scholars and writers, including Nobel Prize winning economist Paul Krugman, Pulitzer Prize winner and author Nicholas Kristof, University of California-Berkeley professor Emmanuel Saez, and economist Timothy Smeeding. It is generally agreed that income and wealth disparity/economic inequality in the U.S. has risen dramatically since 1980. Richard Wilkinson and Kate Pickett are the authors of an important book on the subject, *The Spirit Level: Why More Equal Societies Almost Always Do Better* (2009). They conclude that a wide variety of negative social phenomena, such as shorter life expectancy, higher disease rates, homicide, infant mortality, obesity, teenage pregnancies, emotional depression, and prison population, correlate positively with extent of socioeconomic inequality. ((As inequality increases, these problems (and possibly others) tend to increase.))

"As a PhD criminologist, I have expertise concerning social and behavior control in societies. The problems listed above involve human behavior. I have studied extensively human (homo sapiens) hunter-gatherer existence in Africa between 200,000 and 50,000 years ago. During that period and probably during hundreds of thousands of earlier years, our ancestors generally lived in bands that probably were between 20 and 80 in number and nearly certainly were **remarkably egalitarian** (fn 1). Adults in those bands very likely ordinarily were fairly equal in power, living conditions, and availability of food. I believe that hoarders of food and other valuables usually were sternly dealt with, possibly with shunning. I think that the egalitarian nature of these bands was very important in allowing enough of the bands and their members to survive.

"So, the later part of evolution of "human nature," during some number of hundreds of thousands of years, occurred in social conditions of equality. Because of this, **equality is the situation in which humans will be most likely to flourish.** The corollary of that statement is that humans will tend to encounter problems functioning in social conditions of severe social and economic inequality, such as inequality in living conditions.

"Such problems in functioning are exactly what we have observed in the U.S. as the extent of income and wealth disparities between the "haves" and "have-nots" have increased since about 1980. **Incarceration has increased by more than 400% since 1970.** Simple calculations I have done suggest that there may be many times as many genuinely dangerous (but not necessarily violent) people in the U.S. now, compared with 1970. Addictions have increased. Self-destructive behavior is rampant. An entrenched underclass has developed. It exhibits many social and behavior problems, including high unemployment.

"My idea that humans are not evolved to exist in conditions of extreme social and economic inequality is supported by information concerning crime of black persons in the U.S. and in Africa. While Black males in the U.S. currently have very high rates of violent crime and incarceration, in less advanced countries in Africa several decades ago, they had notably low rates of violence and other problematic behavior.

"Like many of the writers mentioned above, I strongly believe that **these serious social and behavior problems are, to a very significant extent, the results of incredibly great disparity in living and economic circumstances.** The causal processes involved probably are very complex.

"**I believe that there is a danger that, if such extreme disparities and the GWB-era reductions in tax rates of the very wealthy continue, eventually many people in lower socioeconomic classes will develop very strong resentment toward the very wealthy and for politicians who protect their interests.**

"Research on happiness has shown that, above the $75,000-income level, increased income has little ability to produce greater happiness. Therefore, should the very wealthy in U.S. society be required to pay taxes at a higher rate, there is little reason to think that they will experience much reduction in happiness, except as this might result from resentment concerning paying higher taxes.

"**Our society is playing with a powerful corrosive, divisive, poisonous, and potentially explosive force by allowing severe socioeconomic inequality to develop and increase.** Some will say that this sounds like a threat of class warfare. The truth is that, especially since 2000, many of the very affluent and powerful in the U.S. have been engaging in intense class warfare. The published proposals of the Romney campaign and of Congressman Ryan would, if they were ever implemented, dramatically advance this class warfare with, I predict, disastrous consequences.

"Instead of straight-forward wealth redistribution, we need cost-efficient policies and programs that will help as many people as possible to be successful, responsible workers, entrepreneurs, taxpayers, spouses, parents, and community members."

Footnote 1. An excellent, easily accessed introduction to the egalitarian ways of life of hunter-gatherers is a 2011 article in his "Freedom to Learn" blog by Peter Gray, PhD, entitled "How hunter-gatherers maintained their egalitarian ways: three complementary theories." The article is on the *Psychology Today* web site.

Author's impressions concerning the December 2017 Republican tax cut. The closest thing I know of to this tax cut is a financial grab by a group who want to establish a fascist oligarchy that is dominated by an autocrat. Two important recent books argue that Trump is intentionally moving the U.S. in that direction. One is by Snyder (2017). The other is by Madeleine Albright (2018).

It is very difficult to obtain accurate information about the Republican tax cut, partly because it is impossible to predict some of the effects. I am inclined to believe *New York Times* op-ed writer, David Leonhardt, who is strongly critical. Leonhardt reports that now the top 1% have 40% of the wealth in the U.S., and the bottom 90% have 27% of the wealth. The Tax Policy Center predicts that 80% of the benefits of the Republican tax cut will go to the top 1% in the U.S.

On November 13, 2017, Christopher Tidmore wrote in the *Louisiana Weekly* that a family of four in Louisiana with an income of $59,000 will receive a tax benefit of $1182 per year. The Tax Policy Center projects that families of four with income more than $1 million will average a benefit of $70,000. If you divide the Louisiana family of four $1182 benefit into the $70,000 benefit of the $1 million income people, you get about 59, which tells us the $1 million and higher income people will get nearly 60 times as good a benefit as the $59,000 income folks.

The night before the final vote in Congress, Trump said on TV, **"I will be hurt very badly by this tax cut. I have many rich friends who are very mad with me."** Though he is, by far, the biggest liar in American political history, this is his biggest and possibly most consequential lie. In genuinely democratic, representative government, the leader does not lie to the people about important matters. **It is reported that on Christmas day of 2017 he said to friends at his Mar-a-Lago Resort, "You all just got a lot richer."** Since Trump's income is vastly more than the $1 million income level, we can assume that his tax cut annual benefit will be many times as high as the $70,000 for the higher than $1 million income group. I am astonished that lower income Americans have not strongly expressed outrage concerning the amount of his projected benefit and about his repulsive, outrageous lying about it.

Though I am not an economist, I will list two major reasons why it is unlikely that the tax cut will provide benefits for Americans generally. (1) The tax cut is another example of "trickle down" economics, which never work. (2) On television, credible economists argue that it is extremely unlikely that the tax cut will "pay for itself."

I will compare this tax cut monetary grab to somewhat similar actions in the contexts of several types of human groups. In hunter-gatherer bands millennia ago, hoarding probably was prohibited. If an individual or family took much more (for example, three times as much) than their share of valuable things, it is likely they would have been expelled from the band, which probably would have resulted in their deaths. In the tribe context, a chief has traditionally gotten more than his share of good things, but not vastly more. I am confident that tribal chiefs who attempted a major grab of valuable things would, in many cases, have been killed. In the context of a ship in olden times, if the captain made a major grab of valuable things, there might have been a mutiny, resulting in the death of the captain. Even in the animal kingdom, if an alpha male chimpanzee attempts to take much more than his share, he probably will be dislodged as alpha male by several cooperating males.

Great American presidents have had deep concern for the welfare of the poor. Teddy Roosevelt developed liberal/progressive concepts. FDR championed the New Deal. LBJ obtained passage of important liberal/progressive measures. This Republican tax cut money grab, which is expected to result in the reduction of Social Security, Medicare, and Medicaid, is entirely contrary to the democratic and egalitarian concept of American government.

Problems in the U.S. that should be addressed through concerted action. I want to make the point that, by enacting the tax cut, the Republicans are intentionally ignoring very significant and pressing national problems. The Buzzle.com website on August 14, 2016 listed "Major social issues prevalent in the U.S." They were the following:

Unequal distribution of wealth. During the Great Recession of 2007–2009, the Dow Jones index went down to slightly more than 6000. Many less affluent persons had their houses foreclosed during the Great Recession, and banks received very great financial assistance from the federal government. Now, the index is around 25,000, which represents more than a 300% gain. An extremely high percentage of that gain enriched the top 1%, exacerbating the wealth and income disparities problem.

As I expressed in my 2012 op-ed, I believe that these disparities are extremely unjust socially and economically and cause very great behavioral and social problems. As an experienced attorney, I would support and believe it would be constitutional for there to be a Democratic tax bill that significantly alleviates some aspects of these disparities.

Poverty. It is reported that between 13% and 17% of Americans are below the federal poverty line. I assume (but may be wrong) that tens of millions of Americans who are poor will receive no benefit from the tax cut. Because the cost of living is going up more than wages are going up, the poverty problem is getting worse. Since it is expected that Obama Care will be abolished, Social Security will be reduced, and Medicare and Medicaid will be reduced, the GOP fully intends for these developments to worsen the circumstances of the poor in the U.S.

Unequal educational funding. Affluent jurisdictions spend much more on public schools than poor jurisdictions. Schools in poor jurisdictions have a high rate of school dropout. It is reported on the Brookings.edu website ("Ten economic facts about crime and incarceration in the U.S.") that 70% of African-American men without a high school diploma are incarcerated in prison by their middle 30's. Disparities, which will be worsened by the Republican tax cut, will make this problem worse.

Crime and incarceration. The writers of this Buzzle.com article have a different view from mine. I believe that, if major reduction in prison incarceration in the U.S. continues, there will be a resulting major increase in intraracial (e.g., Black-on-Black) and interracial (e.g., Black-on-White, White-on-Black) crime. The poor of all races will be victimized the most. I report findings relating to this in chapter 27.

Health issues. The Republican tax cut apparently will eventually have the effect of ending Obama Care. As a result, it is predicted that 13 million Americans will lose their health insurance. As a result, health insurance premiums will go up. Hospitals will perform expensive medical care and procedures without compensation. This can result in higher local tax rates or even the closing of some hospitals.

Gary Null, PhD, and a team of mainly MDs have a book (Null et al, 2011) in which they report that annually about one million Americans die as a result of some type of medical mistake or treatment. The point is that there are giant adverse human consequences of failures of traditional medicine in the U.S.

There is no doubt that health care in the U.S. costs much more than health care in other countries and is of lower quality than the health care in a high percentage of industrialized nations. The Republican tax cut will tend to make the terrifically bad situation concerning health and health care in the U.S. significantly worse. Medical bills often cause bankruptcy, which increases the poverty problem.

Additional major problems in the U.S. that Republicans have ignored in favor of giving giant benefits to corporations and the wealthy.

The budget deficit. It is inevitable that the tax cut will increase the annual budget deficit significantly. This will result in a significant increase of the national debt, which will have adverse consequences.

Degraded infrastructure in the U.S. I will predict that the fact that the Republicans have enacted the tax cut, with a major increase of the deficit, will be viewed as making it not feasible to have a major infrastructure bill. Trump will have led in vastly enriching corporations and the already very rich instead of working on solving a giant multi-faceted problem that adversely affects quality of life and the economy in the U.S.

The opioid and total drug overdose problem. Opioid overdoses increased from 2500 in 2013 to 20,146 in 2016. It was reported on TV that the number of opioid deaths in 2016 was 42,000. As an experienced social scientist, I will state that this is the most startling health-related trend I know of. The drug overdose total in 2016 was 64,070. The end of this trend is not in sight. I believe this trend tells us that there are giant underlying human problems in the U.S. Those problems may be related to economic disparities.

Increase in obesity, type 2 diabetes, and hypertension, especially among the young and young adults. In 2002, 65% of Americans were overweight (National Center for Health Statistics, 2003), and, in 2001, 30%

of adults had hypertension (National Center for Health Statistics, 2002). In the 1990s, a major increase in child obesity occurred, which has been associated with major increase in type 2 diabetes, hypertension, and cardiovascular disease among that group when they are young adults (Lee, 2008). Instead of addressing this, the GOP "paid back their donors."

Suicides and suicide attempts in the U.S. In 2013, there were 41,149 suicides in the U.S. The rate was 12.6 per 100,000 population. Males commit suicide at four times as high a rate as females. Among students in grades 9–12, 17% seriously considered committing suicide (22.4%, female; 11.6%, male). *In grades 9–12, 8% of students (10.6%, female; 5.4%, male) attempted suicide one or more times in the previous year.* ("Suicide: facts at a glance in 2013," Centers for Disease Control (CDC))

Mental health. Funding relating to mental health services is grossly deficient. Several of the alarming problems described above are partially caused by mental health problems of Americans.

Deterioration of race relations and increase in interracial violent crime. Chapters 27 and 28 are about these major problematic developments. It is very likely that the Republican tax cut will cause African Americans to hate White people more, increasing the problems concerning race relations and interracial crime. As I report in my 2012 op-ed, increase in economic disparities results in higher crime and other problematic behaviors and conditions. As discussed above, the Republican tax cut will increase those disparities.

The Republicans admit that the tax cut was intended to help friends and hurt enemies, such as liberals in California and New York. Seen this way, the tax cut was a White attempt to hurt Black people. It will have that effect. This can result in more hatred of White people, especially Republicans, by Black people in the U.S., which will further worsen race relations.

Trends affecting availability of jobs and qualification of Americans to take available jobs. Since the Industrial Revolution in the 1800s, the availability of jobs has been decreased by mechanization, automation, computerization, robotics, and artificial intelligence. Not only are jobs continuing to be eliminated as a result of these phenomena, available jobs have come to be more likely to require high tech skills. Of course, readers know that unemployment (including that of African-Americans) has decreased since Trump became president.

In the U.S., there is a major problem of high unemployment of teenagers. In this job market, many people who are not able to develop high tech capabilities are to a large extent excluded from high paying jobs. I very seriously believe that dealing with this phenomenon should be a high federal government priority. I have no notion what the solutions might be.

The economy. Ordinarily, stimulant tax cuts occur when there is a sluggish economy. This one is occurring during a strong economy. It is likely that this will cause problematic inflation. An over-heated economy and stock market may result in a bubble that eventually will burst, causing giant problems for Americans. If so, the banks will be protected, and the middle class probably will be hurt the most.

Global warming and destructive weather events. Trump and the Congressional Republicans are allowing these problems to worsen, which will impose even greater economic and quality-of-life problems on Americans in coming decades.

Reminder concerning the potential for ethnocentrism, xenophobia, and genocide. It is important to mention that ethnocentrism (belief your group is superior) and xenophobia (fear and hatred of that which is different) tend to cause members of one group to treat badly, even violently, members of substantially different groups within the same country. For example, Shiite and Sunni Moslems treat each other very viciously and violently, though they are genetically the same. Starting in 1915, the Ottoman government and Turkey massacred 1.5 million Armenians, many of them Christians, who probably were genetically quite similar to the Turks.

Vast improvement of the feasibility of achievement of justice in the U.S. since the Civil War. We know that slavery in the U.S. was deeply immoral and violated the Golden Rule ("Do unto others as you would have them do unto you."). After the Civil War, Congress passed and enough states adopted the Fourteenth Amendment of the Constitution. Both of the major clauses of the Fourteenth Amendment have been vitally important to achievement of justice in the U.S. I believe that the requirements of those clauses are consistent with the Golden Rule.

Relevant provisions of amendments of the U.S. Constitution. Below is part of the Fifth Amendment and two clauses of the 14th Amendment.

(1) Part of the Fifth amendment. "No person . . . shall be deprived of life, liberty or property, without due process of law."

(2) Due process of law clause of the Fourteenth Amendment. ". . . nor shall any State deprive any person of life, liberty, or property without due process of law."

(3) Equal protection of the laws clause of the Fourteenth Amendment. ". . . nor deny to any person within the jurisdiction the equal protection of the laws."

Due process of law clause of the Fourteenth Amendment. This clause made the Bill of Rights amendments applicable against the states. So, state governments were required to comply with those amendments in their official actions. The due process clause operates significantly to improve fairness of government action. John Rawls in his last book (2001) emphasized that "justice is fairness."

Equal protection of the laws clause of the Fourteenth Amendment. Initially, this clause mainly prohibited state government action that discriminated on the basis of race or religion. Fortunately, it was later held that discrimination on the basis of sex also was prohibited.

Leaders who helped to expand the functions of federal, state, and local government that improve the treatment and quality of life of citizens and other persons in the U.S. This is one of the great and inspiring American stories, which would take a long book to tell.

Lincoln led in eliminating slavery in the U.S. Recently developed "new" estimates of death tolls of the Civil War are 431,250 of the Union and 318,750 of the Confederacy. (These figures are based on information in an article in the *New York Times*, April 12, 2012, "New estimate raises Civil War death toll.")

The progress since the Civil War in dispensing justice in the U.S. was accomplished when there was a very powerful white majority. I believe that the conduct of the Civil War and the establishment of many types of government benefits since the Civil War, especially since 1900, were expressive of broad ascription to the Golden Rule among the White majority in the U.S. I think that they also did not want the "judgment of history" to be that White Americans horribly oppress and abuse Black persons in the U.S.

Congressional leaders knew after the Civil War that meaningful amendment of the Constitution was required. So, they had the Congress in 1868 adopt and enough states ratified the Fourteenth Amendment.

Theodore Roosevelt was a very important developer of progressive/liberal strategies. His cousin FDR oversaw Congressional enactment of many statutes that Teddy foresaw. President John Kennedy died too soon to contribute very importantly to this effort. His successor as President, Lyndon Johnson, risked his own political future and the future of the Democratic Party by pushing many progressive/liberal statutes through Congress. Of course, this telling of the story is far too brief.

So, what programs, guarantees, and entitlements resulted?

<u>Partial list of government statutes, programs, and measures that have made having high quality of life in the U.S. more achievable:</u>

- The Fourteenth Amendment of the U.S. Constitution, which includes a due process of law clause and an equal protection of the laws clause.
- Progressive income tax. Social Security.
- The GI Bill.
- Medicare.
- The Civil Rights Act.
- The Voting Rights Act.
- Medicaid.

- Government assistance regarding housing, such as public housing and government-guaranteed loans.
- Protections against discrimination in hiring (EEOC) and education.
- Affirmative action regarding employment and higher education in favor of African Americans and women.
- Free public education.
- Integration of public education.
- Public colleges and universities, including community colleges.
- Pell grants.
- Food stamps (SNAP).
- Allowance of tax deductions for charitable contributions.

The availability of these measures tends to increase the social justice in our country.

It is very important to understand that citizens or even persons of all races are equally entitled to receive these benefits. I will provide the caveat that eligibility for a type of program or entitlement can sometimes be an important matter. We know, however, that White and Black citizens have equal rights (except in the case of affirmative action, which discriminates in favor of Black persons).

The importance of the civil rights movement. It would not be accurate to suggest that all of these beneficial rights and programs were created without strident complaints by Black persons, especially during the civil rights movement of the 1960s and 1970s.

An attempt to put this in historical perspective. During August of 2017, five months before the outrageous Republican tax cut, I emailed letters to two tenured, very successful history professors and asked them the following question: "During recorded world history, has a large and dominant majority population in a country ever treated a fairly large, culturally and visibly very different minority population nearly as well as white society in the U.S. has since 1900 treated Black Americans?" I have not gotten any response from either of them. Though I majored in history in college, I am not an expert on world history and cannot authoritatively answer that question. Obviously, political correctness would prohibit teaching the negative answer I would give to that question. Also, I would guess that any professor at a "mainstream" university or college who publicly communicated a negative answer to that question would be nearing the end of his or her teaching career. I recently talked about this with a retired U.S. Army colonel who grew up in India. His comments indicated that he substantially agrees with me about the treatment of African Americans by "White society" since 1900.

I regret making here a comment that is quite severe. Black Lives Matter is suggesting what their priorities would be if they could influence U.S. government controlled by an African-American majority. Their most important message is, "Black lives matter." They will not even agree that all lives matter. I believe that many Americans, including many African Americans, feel and think that is a very un-American and divisive stance for Black Lives Matter to take.

Substantial increase in incarceration rates in the U.S. Steep increases in U.S. prison and jail incarceration rates began in about 1980. My calculation is that between 1980 and 2007 the state and federal prison population increased by about 400% (The Sentencing Project, 2016).

Estimates of Black-on-Black violent crimes prevented by the substantial increase in incarceration rate from 1980 through 2014. In chapter 27, I report results of my calculations which indicate that this increase in prison incarceration rate was accompanied by a very substantial decrease in the homicide rate in the U.S. I will not repeat here my elaborate mathematical method for developing very rough estimates of Black-on-Black violent crimes prevented by the increase in incarceration rate and other police and criminal justice policies. The rough estimates of numbers of **prevented** Black-on-Black violent crimes from 1981 through 2014 are as follows:

Estimate of Black-on-Black homicides prevented	**183,000**
Estimate of Black-on-Black rapes prevented	**1,079,700**
Estimate of Black-on-Black robberies prevented	**4,758,000**
Estimate of Black-on-Black aggravated assaults prevented	**10,119,900**

Inevitable increase in Black-on-Black violent crime. From 2015 to 2016, there was a 10% increase in murder rate in the U.S. Of course, many of the increased number of homicide victims must have been Black. Also, because of the strident complaints about police handling of Black male subjects, apparently police in some cities have to some extent withdrawn from potentially difficult encounters with Black males. That, also, will tend to increase the rate of Black-on-Black homicide and other violent crime.

Criminal justice reform. For decades, U.S. liberals and Black activists have been complaining about the high rate of incarceration of African-American males. That strident complaint has not, as far as I know, been accompanied by acknowledgment that a giant amount of serious Black-on-Black violent crime has been prevented.

Republican support for criminal justice reform. Starting in 2010, several Republican Congressional leaders have expressed support for criminal justice reform, which includes some decrease in the prison incarceration rate.

Fortunately, a fairly small decrease in prison incarceration rate since 2007 was not through 2015 associated with increase in violent crime rates in the U.S. This suggests that this effort has been carried out carefully.

I wrote the following paragraph before the release in September of 2017 of *Crime in the United States—2016* (Federal Bureau of Investigation, 2017). It reported approximately a 10% increase in murder rate in the U.S. from 2015 to 2016.

I am not an expert concerning criminal justice reform. I will here express my opinion that, should substantial additional decrease in prison-incarceration rate occur, it is very likely that there will be a resulting substantial increases in rates of violent crime in the U.S.

REFERENCES

Albright, Madeleine (2018). *Fascism: a warning.* NY, NY: HarperColli9ns Publishers.

Federal Bureau of Investigation (2017). *Crime in the United States—2016.* Washington, DC: U.S. Government Printing Office.

Hobbes, Thomas (1651). *Leviathan*. Oxford: Oxford University Press.

Lee, Joyce (2008). Why young adults hold the key to assessing the obesity epidemic of children. *Archives of Pediatric and Adolescent Medicine*, Vol. 162, No. 7, pp. 682–7.

Rawls, John (2001). *Justice as fairness: a restatement*. Belknap Press: Boston, MA.

Snyder, Timothy (2017). *On tyranny: twenty lessons from the twentieth century*. NY, NY: Tim Duggan Books.

The Sentencing Project (2016). Trends in U.S. corrections.

Wilkinson, Richard G. & Pickett, Kate (2009). *The spirit level: why more equal societies almost always do better*. NY, NY: Bloomsbury Press.

— SECTION 11 —
Miscellaneous Science

— CHAPTER 30 —
Geography and History since 200,000 bp (before present)

<u>Elaboration</u>. The starting date indicated in the title of this chapter, 200,000 bp, was selected because it is the date many experts give as an approximation of the date of first evidence that homo sapiens existed as a separate species. The first part of a course on this subject could cover from 200,000 bp to about 4000 BC (before Christ), which is about when writing was invented.

I believe that geography and history tend to be inextricably connected. Knowing the geography of an area can greatly improve your ability to understand historical events that occurred there.

While I doubt this is very often the subject of a university or college course, I have discovered through Internet searches for available high school textbooks that this is sometimes the subject of a high school course. I have bought an excellent high school textbook, *World History & Geography* (Spielvogel, 2013).

<u>Author's relevant experience</u>. I majored in history at Wake Forest College (1961–65) and was invited to take and did take the History Honors courses during my senior year.

How have I acquired some information on this subject? During my adult life, I have watched too much TV. I have, however, generally tried to avoid the situation comedies (American and British) and tried to watch as many documentaries as possible about history, geography, science, technology, and other "serious" subjects. I've estimated that I watched around 3400 of these documentaries. My 1½ years studying the origins of religion made me much more aware of hominid species from which man is descended and of the circumstances of humans in Africa prior to 60,000 bp. Of course, watching those types of documentaries and studying origins of religion don't provide expertise needed to develop and teach a course about geography and history.

Importance of this subject. I don't think it is very often or well communicated that there are extremely important connections between geography and history. A course about this could be a wonderful way of communicating very vividly and understandably a giant amount of important information about the history of man and related geography. The instructor would need to be very careful in selecting maps to use along with lectures. The sequencing would help students to have nearly lifelong knowledge regarding the sequencing of important cultural groups, dynasties, empires, etc. This course could count in a history major and/or geography major.

A criminologist/lawyer's suggestion about history education. In chapter 35 about thinking and writing well in the professions, I mention that sometimes a writer needs to answer the classic questions, "who, what, when, where, why, and how?" The maps and related verbiage in a geography and history course might also do that. Those bits of information might increase a student's ability to learn and remember important historical information. So, I am suggesting important connecting of the spatial, temporal, sequential, behavioral, cultural, political, and military in classroom use of particular maps and related historical information. (Since one of my very distant ancestors was one of William the Conqueror's dukes, I think I should do a better job of this for myself relating to the Norman Conquest.)

Relevance for young adults. This is relevant for young adults who want to have a sound educational grounding in geography and history.

A strong argument for connecting geography and history in public education. To read an excellent discussion of the desirable connections of geography and history in public education, go to the ericdigests.org website and find "Geography in history: a necessary connection in the school curriculum."

I continue to doubt that this type of course is taught very often in universities and colleges. There could be several reasons. It would require broad knowledge of geography and history and would cover content of many other geography and history courses.

<u>Candidates for inclusion of particular maps in this course.</u>

Current map of South America showing rivers. It is fascinating to me that eons ago rivers that rose west of the center of the northern part of South America flowed west to the ocean. When the Andes mountains rose, the direction of flow of many rivers reversed. It is fascinating also that the volume of the Amazon River is so much greater than the volume of any other river. This map would explain much concerning the central and eastern parts of South America.

Map showing location of Carolina bays in the U.S. southeast. These are about 500,000 depressions in the U.S. southeast with consistent elliptical shape and consistent orientation. Some scientists believe they were formed about 75,000 years ago and other scientists think about 13,000 years ago, when an extra-terrestrial body broke up as it entered Earth's atmosphere over what is now Canada moving in a southeastern direction. Other scientists believe that area was hit by a comet. I believe that many millions of Americans live near one or more Carolina bays but have no information about Carolina bays. During the 1800s, my ancestors in Riverton gave names to the four nearby Carolina bays.

Map of north Africa after 70,000 bp when, instead of constituting mainly dessert, there were lakes, rivers, and much lush vegetation. This map might help students to understand timing of human migration from Africa.

Map showing the locations of Mayan cities at the height of Mayan culture. Information about that culture is, to me, very astonishing.

One or more maps showing the height of influence of the Goths and Visigoths.

Map at height of Genghis Khan (1162–1227) empire after his death.

World map at the height of the British Empire. This might be the most amazing map of all. It would juxtapose the minute size of Great Britain and the incredibly great size of the British Empire. The map would beg the question, "How could so few people impose their will on giant numbers of people inhabiting such vast areas?"

The French and Indian War. That war was fought by Britain and France in North America during the 1756–1763 period. It would make sense to include a map at the beginning and another at the end of the war.

Distribution of Indian tribes in U.S. about 1400. There could be a map of North America in 1400 showing the locations and populations of various Indian tribes. Probably the most startling information would be the total number of indigenous humans in North America then.

Distribution of Shiite and Sunni Muslims. There could be a current world map indicating, for countries with a high Muslim population, the percentage that are Shiite and the percentage that are Sunni.

REFERENCES

Spielvogel, Jackson L. (2013). *World History & Geography*. NY, NY: McGraw Hill Education.

—— CHAPTER 31 ——
Multi-Disciplinary Study of Futurology

<u>Elaboration</u>. Information about past trends and predictions for the future are reported and studied in many disciplines, including meteorology, geology, sociology, social-psychology, psychology, criminology, education, public health, medicine, holistic medicine, pharmacology, economics, business administration, marketing, recreation, athletics/sports, military science, religion, political science, city planning, oceanography, agriculture, anthropology, various sciences, computer engineering and various other engineering fields, computer science, other high-tech disciplines and fields, and, no doubt, other fields.

The complexity of future studies results partly from the fact that changes and trends in each of these areas can influence developments in many other areas. One of the virtually infinite number of examples would be that a financial recession in a country will predictably result in many bankruptcies of businesses and individuals.

An example of the vast number of subjects regarding which important predictions have been made is water supply. There are several places on the planet where limited underground aquifers of high quality water are being depleted. When depletion is completed in an area, the area's habitability by humans will be greatly reduced, unless innovations and inventions overcome that problem.

Vast array of research and statistical methods used in these futurology studies. A major subject addressed in a course on futurology could be the extremely great variety of scientific, social scientific, and behavioral science research and statistical methods utilized in the generation of predictions of future developments and occurrences.

A crucial issue relating to this subject. A person who would undertake teaching an undergraduate course on this subject would need to make a well informed judgments concerning how effective the methods of futurology and futuristics have been and possibly can be in predicting important aspects of the future. I do not have sufficient relevant knowledge to answer that question. If future prediction efforts have often been notably unsuccessful, it would seem that there would be limited justification for this course. Obviously, a course could justifiably be limited to especially high quality work.

<u>Author's relevant experience</u>. When I was considering leaving Army active duty in 1974, I read *Future Shock* (Toffler, 1971). That gave me important information that helped me to make reasonably good decisions about additional education and civilian working career.

As a Criminal Justice professor, I often taught research methods. The information I had on that subject would have allowed me to discuss fairly intelligently the various types of research and statistical methods referred to above.

During retirement I, like many other retirees, have tried to pay attention to and, sometimes, obtain information about trends and predictions reported in various disciplines. I will admit that this information is so vast that I do not now have the sets of knowledge needed to teach a course on this subject. This challenge may be a reason why this type of broadly structured course is apparently not offered very often. Professors want to teach courses within their area(s) of expertise.

<u>Importance of this subject</u>. I will describe four pre-historical and historical stages of importance of this subject. (Since I developed this information, I can receive the credit or blame for including it here.)

(1) Archeological evidence indicates that, for about two million years before 60,000 bp (before the present), humans and our ancestor species had an extremely slow rate of introduction of new tools and other inventions. So,

those hominins had little reason to try to predict the future. The future was likely to be very much like the past and the present.

(2) Spanish philosopher, poet, and novelist George Santayana (1863–1952) said, "Those who cannot remember the past are condemned to repeat it." Since long before the appearance of Santayna, intellectuals were aware of the importance of recording and learning history and attempting to predict future events and developments.

(3) *Future Shock* (Toffler, 1971) made readers aware of the rapid pace of change in many aspects of life in the U.S. for several decades prior to the publication of that extremely important book.

(4) I believe that the pace of change now is very much more rapid than during a few decades before *Future Shock* was published. For that reason, **I believe that multi-disciplinary futurology is the most important subject addressed in this book**.

A good course about multi-disciplinary futurology could shed light on the subjects of nearly all of the chapters of this book.

Relevance for young adults. Taking a course about multi-disciplinary futurology should help students to gain information about the likely availability of particular jobs during her or his working career and, possibly, about real estate markets in selected areas. As global warming continues and, possibly, conditions in the U.S. deteriorate, many current young adults may want to migrate to Canada. If so, they will search on the Internet for projections of job and real estate markets in Canada.

Levels of organization and process. In many aspects of human activity and existence, there are what are called levels of organization and process. For example, in biology you find on the lowest level the components of individual cells, then the cells, then organs made up of the cells, and so on. In human society, you have at the lowest level the individual person, then the family, then the neighborhood, and so on. Of course, you have levels of organization and process in many types of hierarchical businesses and aspects of government.

We need to remember that developments and trends on one level of organization and process can be causally connected with developments and trends on higher and lower levels of organization and process. Of course, this adds to the complexity of future studies.

A course and books about futurology. If you do an Internet search concerning things such as "futurology" and "future studies," you will find information about a few university/college courses on that subject. For example, you find "Introduction to Future Studies" by Dr. Linda Groff and Dr. Paul Smoker at California State University, Dominguez Hills; Future Studies at University of Texas, Clear Lake; and the Hawaii Research Center for Future Studies at the University of Hawaii.

There are many recent books about futurology. You can find a list, "Popular futurology books," on the goodreads.com website. Well down in the list you will find a book (about the subject of a chapter of this book) by Aubrey deGrey (2007), *Ending aging: the rejuvenation breakthroughs that could reverse human aging in our life time.* The book that has the highest average rating is *Sapiens: a brief history of humankind* by Yural Noah Harari (2014). You will remember the most important scholar concerning sociobiology, Harvard professor Dr. Edward O. Wilson. On the list is a book (2003) by him, *The future of life.* I believe that every young adult who wants to be genuinely well-informed should read at least one book on that list.

Major organization concerned with futurology. A major organization concerned with future studies is the World Future Society, which has 40,000 members. About 1,200 of the members are "professional members" who work exclusively in that area. It's obvious that there are tens of thousands of researchers and statisticians in the U.S. who spend some of their time working in that area. I have learned that some full-time "professional members" refer to themselves as "empirical futurists."

An article with predictions of the future. On the Guardian website, there is a relevant article, "20 predictions for the next 25 years." Reading that article may help you to decide whether to get one of the books listed above.

Examples of trends and predictions.

Trends regarding mechanization, automation, robotics, computerization, and artificial intelligence as they impact availability of jobs. I recently heard a radio report on NPR in which an expert stated that no one can confidently describe the job market in the U.S. 30 years from now.

The future of golf in the U.S. I have in several chapters promoted golf, specifically walking golf, as high quality recreation that doesn't have to cost very much. Recently, the U.S. has in the average year lost 3 million golfers. Not many years ago, there were 125 golf courses in the greater Myrtle Beach, SC, area. Now, there are 85. If you are young and interested in having golf as an important recreational activity or area of employment for yourself, it would be prudent to think about the future of golf in the U.S. I think that inexpensive public courses have more of a future than private country club courses that require payment of very high dues. I own and live in a house on a golf course that has been in jeopardy of no long operating as a golf course.

The phragmites invasion. There are four varieties of phragmites, which are plants that originated in other countries and are now considered invasive plant species in the U.S. They out-compete native desirable vegetation. This would probably be discussed briefly in a "Multi-disciplinary futurology" course. (I wonder what the future of kudzu is. Why don't some smart people make their fortunes using kudzu?)

Reduced interest in antiques. For many decades, I have often watched "Antiques Road Show" on ETV. After the Great Recession of 2007–8, there was a substantial drop in value of many types of antiques. Beside a road I often take driving home, there is a big antique mall, with probably 25 booths. About half of the time, there is one car there, owned, no doubt, by the business owner or an employee. About half of the time, there is one additional car. I think this is very strong evidence that interest in antiques has plummeted in the U.S., especially since the Great Recession. A Columbia area antique dealer agrees with my thinking about this.

Erosion of positive aspects of government and life in the U.S. This, the subject of chapter 25, could be importantly illuminated by multi-disciplinary futurology.

Extent of rising ocean levels by 2050. A course on multi-disciplinary futurology could include a map of the east coast of the U.S. some number of years in the future, possibly 2050. Obviously, the map would reflect expected effects of rising ocean water levels as a result of global warming.

The future of race relations in the U.S. I believe that intelligent, knowledgeable, and sensible people would have predicted that race relations would improve during the administration of any African-American U.S. president. The unfortunate truth is that race relations worsened substantially during the second Obama administration. What can be predicted now?

REFERENCES

de Grey, Aubrey & Rae, Michael (2007). *Ending aging: the rejuvenation break-throughs that could reverse human aging in our life time*. NY, NY: St. Martin's Press.

Harari, Yural (2014) *Sapiens: a brief history of humankind*. London: Harvill Secker.

Toffler, Alvin (1971). *Future shock*. NY, NY: Bantam Books.

Wilson, Edward O. (2003). *The future of life*. Portland, ME: Abacus.

— CHAPTER 32 —
Sociobiology

Elaboration. Sociobiology is the study of the biological bases of social behavior. The central idea of sociobiology is that the evolution of social animals does not occur only at the level of the individual: It occurs also on the group level. If, for example, a member of a hunter-gatherer band sacrificed himself to protect his band, his own genes would not survive, but the gene for altruism which he shared with other band members would survive. His willingness to act altruistically, resulting in his death, actually would have enhanced the survival prospects of genes for altruism.

The most important developer and scholar of sociobiology has been Harvard biology professor Dr. Edward O. Wilson. Dr. Wilson has had so many books published, including a book on the future of life, that you can search for "books written by Dr. Edward O. Wilson," and Amazon will give you full information.

I have not found on the Internet information about books that obviously were written to serve as texts for a course about sociobiology.

The importance of the hunter-gather band in sociobiologists' theories about the evolution of man. For many hundreds of thousands of years before about 40,000 bp, our human and pre-human ancestors existed nearly exclusively as members of hunter-gatherer bands. It was in that context that some aspects of human nature evolved. In chapter 33, I discuss the importance of sociobiology in the study of the origins of the precursors of religion in the hunter-gatherer context.

It's interesting that scientists, including sociobiologists, are discovering that genetic evolution can occur much more quickly than once thought.

Why is the sociobiology sub-discipline of biology no more influential than it appears to be? I read the course descriptions of all of the graduate biology courses in a semester at a major university in the Southeast. There was one very brief reference to sociobiology. To me, this seems to be a significant scientific and academic oversight.

I believe that professors in the U.S. strongly tend to want to operate in their discipline on their customary "level of organization and process." Thomas S. Kuhn (1996) argues in the *Structure of Scientific Revolutions* that it is good for professors to transport paradigms of their discipline to other disciplines. I think it is remarkable and admirable that Dr. E. O. Wilson is comfortable in addressing phenomena on several levels of organization and process in his work relating to sociobiology.

Importance of this subject. I believe that every person who wants to work as a social or behavioral scientist should study sociobiology. Social sciences include sociology, anthropology, criminology, economics, political science, public health, and demography. As a criminologist, I am a social scientist. I suggest that social scientists concentrate on developing information about their primary subject or phenomenon on many levels of organization and process, rather than learning about other subjects and phenomena on their primary level of organization and process. Consistent with this, I have tried to develop meaningful information about the psychology of crime. Psychology and social-psychology are two of the behavioral sciences. Psycho-biology is importantly connected with the subject matter of sociobiology.

Relevance for young adults. Many of the most important experts regarding difficult subjects started their study of their subjects during their early teen years. It follows that, if a person wants to develop strong expertise concerning sociobiology, the person should study it in courses and/or independently at as early an age as possible.

Author's relevant experience. A very important part of my education was studying sociobiology in a doctoral course in the School of Criminology at

Florida State University in the middle 1970s. I couldn't possibly have done the work needed to write the chapters of this book on origins of religion and on the emergence and evolution of political values if I had not had that an excellent introduction to sociobiology.

An Internet encyclopedia article about sociobiology. The best introductory article I have found on the Internet is "Sociobiology" in the *Encyclopedia of Science and Religion* (2003), the Gale Group.

Concepts and principles of sociobiology from a scholarly paper I presented (Memory, 1979).

Sociobiology is the study of the biological bases of social behavior. It is based on scientific study of primitive human groups and non-human social species. It can contribute to understanding of human nature. Sociobiology has nothing to do with race or racial differences or "social Darwinism." With regard to homo sapiens, the focus is on the evolution of the species, not man in complex, modern society. It is concerned with the behavioral tendencies of normal human beings, not "disturbed" persons. Sociobiology argues that, if heredity tends to produce certain behavior of members of a group and that behavior improves the survival prospects of the group, then the members of the group are more likely to survive and their genes are more likely to get into the next generation. Below are some manifestations of social behavior which are viewed as having had survival value for social animals, including homo sapiens.

Hierarchy—the tendency of social animals to organize into groups with a chain of command or "pecking order."

Competition/competitiveness. This helps to shape the hierarchy. Also, there is some "survival of the fittest" on the individual level.

Submissiveness to hierarchical power. This makes existence of hierarchy possible.

Capacity to cooperate as required by circumstances. Male hunters and female mothers/gatherers needed to be able and willing to cooperate.

Nurturing, especially of infants and other young children by parents and others in the group, such as aunts and grandmothers.

Serial monogamy—the tendency of human males and females to go through a sequence of intimate and parenting relationships.

Altruism—the tendency to be self-sacrificing to the benefit of close relatives and other close members of one's primary group.

Favoritism for blood relatives

Reciprocity within the group—"You scratch my back; I'll scratch yours."

Territoriality—the protection of your home turf and certain other space and territory.

For some species, the capacity to develop, learn, preserve, and transmit problem solutions and other aspects of culture, such as language

Means to detect cheating, which includes failing or refusing to reciprocate, for example, through sharing of food.

Means to punish individuals for cheating and other misbehavior. This can be meted out by the highest-ranking male. Shunning or exclusion are much more likely than highly dangerous physical aggression. (If the highest ranking male fought to the death with another male, the survival prospects for the group would be reduced.)

Sibling rivalry. There is some survival of the fittest on the individual level here also.

Division of labor. Some species have division of labor, which can increase survival prospects.

Behavior control. In primitive human groups and in non-human social species, individual animals are very likely to behave in ways that are acceptable to the high-ranking animals. Those behaviors are likely to advance the prospects for the survival of the group.

Some common characteristics of human cultures. The following information is not taken from writing about sociobiology. It is importantly related information from anthropology.

Since I studied criminology and sociobiology, I have been interested in the **common characteristics of human cultures,** which flow from the part of human nature that sociobiology is concerned with. I co-authored with a PhD anthropologist the published article (Houston & Memory, 2001) from which this is taken. This list applies to primitive human groups, human cultures through history, and some cultural/ethnic groups existing now but does not apply well to advanced, complex, and/or pluralist societies. This is provided because it offers an interesting comparison to the less-complex arrangements of social animals described by sociobiology.

Norms—behavior standards. The culture in effect teaches you how to behave by teaching norms. The most seriously maintained norms are mores. Less seriously maintained norms are folkways.

Homogeneity—sharing of race, religion, and other aspects of the culture by members of a group.

Taboos—very important norms which prohibit certain behavior. Several taboos—e.g., incest, killing group members—are found in practically all primitive human groups.

Internalization of norms through socialization as morality and conscience

Commonly held values, such as ideas concerning what is right or important.

Commonly held opinions. An opinion usually expresses your view of the nature of reality.

Commonly held attitudes. An attitude generally expresses how positive your feelings are regarding something.

Roles. Mother, grandmother, hunter, and priest are roles.

Important information/knowledge of many types, including accumulated problem solutions of many types

Means to collect aspects of culture (e.g., tools, problem solutions, language) and transmit them to the next generation

Customs and traditions, which may involve solving problems or meeting needs.

Rituals, such as initiation of young males into manhood.

Shared religion. Often the shared religion is very central to the culture's means of behavior control. In some primitive human groups, there is no distinction between religious and non-religious aspects of life.

Expected altruism—the expectation that a member will act in certain situations in a self-sacrificing manner to the benefit of members of his group.

Reciprocity within the cultural group. "You scratch my back, and I'll scratch yours."

Recognition of the family, including the authority of parents over children.

Hierarchy—a chain of command or "pecking order."

Territoriality—recognition of control of certain territory by certain persons and groups. Control over and privacy concerning a family's living space is common.

Xenophobia—fear and hatred of that which is different.

Ethnocentrism—shared belief that your cultural group is superior to others.

Intentional shunning (ostracism) or exclusion as a result of misbehavior

Means to detect and punish "cheaters"

Punishments for unacceptable behavior and reward for good behavior

Art and music

REFERENCES

Houston, M., & Memory, J.M. (2001). Problem solutions in culture and society. In J.M. Memory & Aragon, R. (Eds.), *Patrol officer problem solving and solutions*. Durham, NC: Carolina Academic Press.

Kuhn, Thomas S. (1996, 3rd ed.). *The structure of scientific revolutions*. Chicago, IL: University of Chicago Press.

Memory, J.M. (1979). *Sociobiology and the metamorphoses of criminology: 1978–2000*. Presented at the annual meeting of the American Society of Criminology.

━━━ CHAPTER 33 ━━━
Use of Sociobiology and Anthropology in Thinking about Origins of Religion

An admission. As you will observe, this is not a conventional book chapter. Instead, it is a work in progress. I hope later to produce an article on this subject and submit it for publication.

Elaboration. This chapter reports extensive work and thinking I have done on this subject, which included doing a thorough review of literature. Some scholars (e.g., King, 2007) who have studied "origins of religion" have emphasized evolution and behavior of some of man's related species, such as chimpanzees. Instead, I have focused on information about the apparent origins of precursors of activities and aspects of religion among humans in Africa between 200,000 and 60,000 years ago. **I believe that the interaction of the effects of these activities and aspects resulted in the great importance pre-religious and religious activities and beliefs have had for humans since that time**.

You may ask, "How can a competent scholar study behavior that occurred tens of thousands of years ago?" There are methods available in behavioral archeology, which is a sub-discipline of archeology.

Author's relevant expertise, experience, and belief.

Expertise. As a PhD criminologist, I have studied and had a publication with a PhD anthropologist (Houston & Memory, 2001) about aspects of human cultures, such as norms and beliefs. During criminology doctoral studies, I received an excellent introduction to sociobiology, which is the subject of chapter 32. I believe origins of religion provides the best opportunity to use sociobiological theory in relation to homo sapiens.

My study of this subject during 2009–2010. For about 1½ years starting in 2009, I did scholarly work about equal to that needed to earn a master's degree developing information and hypotheses on this subject. I made significant progress in outlining and writing chapters for a reader on the subject. Two PhD scholars with relevant expertise who reviewed the work I had done urged me to develop and be the senior editor of and a major contributor to an international reader on this subject. The fact that I, a long-retired PhD criminologist, was urged by well qualified and knowledgeable scholars to undertake that effort suggested to me that there is a lack of excellent scholarly work on this subject. During my work on this, I had the impression that many of the ideas in nearly all of the books on this subject are seriously flawed.

Because an extremely high percentage of persons "believe in God," religion professors may want to avoid disseminating information that contradicts the ideas of a high percentage of people about existence of God. This may involve adherence to a type of political correctness.

Author's relevant experience and belief. I feel very fortunate that my mother was a Christian and that I, from age 5 through 17, attended church every Sunday morning for Sunday school and the church religious service. On a high percentage of Sunday evenings, my twin brother and I rode with a neighbor family to a Sunday night church activity. I greatly value having learned and internalized Christian morality. During those years, the Southern Baptist Sunday School Board was quite progressive, as opposed to being fundamentalist.

I believe that my father's tragic death when I was five years old made me much less likely to believe that there is a knowing, loving God who is protecting me. Since my late teens, I have been a religious agnostic.

Whether there is or isn't a God is immaterial to my thinking on this subject. I strongly believe that atheists have no better proof that there is no God than believers have that there is a God.

Importance of this subject. I believe that "origins of religion" is an important, interesting, and even uplifting story about which a high percentage of people know nearly nothing.

Before the 20th century, in virtually all known human cultures and societies a very high percentage of people engaged in what we would agree were religious activities. Since religious beliefs and activities have previously been ubiquitous, we have strong reasons to believe that those types of beliefs and activities have had some type of "survival value" at least in the later evolution of man and the development of human cultures.

It appears to me that some of the benefits of religion are being lost in many cultural groups existing now. Though I am an agnostic, I think it is very undesirable for positive characteristics and practices of religion, such as the teaching of morality, to be lost. After chapter 18 there is an essay I have written about teaching moral behavior to children.

Relevance for young adults. Studying this can be beneficial for young adults in several ways. It can help a person to understand human nature, human behavior, and human cultures.

An interesting contrarian view concerning innovation during the Stone Age. While it is often stated by scholars, and has been repeated by me, that there was very little innovation during the Stone Age, you can find on the Internet a very readable article with a different view, "Stone age innovations and inventions," by Barbara Soper. Reading that brief article will help you to "make sense of" materials I have written, which are found below.

Two different ways for you to learn about my study and conclusions. Below, I first provide handouts I wrote for a discussion about origins of religion. Then, I provide a short paper I have written about the subject.

HANDOUTS FOR A DISCUSSION ON THE ORIGINS OF RELIGION

"What were the origins of religion?" is a big, complex, difficult, and, I think, important subject. My work relating to the origins of religion involved trying to figure out to what extent there were precursors of present-day religion's characteristic activities in hunter-gatherer groups in Africa between

200,000 bp (before present) (when scholars think homo sapiens first existed as a separate species) and 70,000 bp. If those precursors probably existed, why did they exist, and how did they influence (maybe strengthening) each other? How did those precursors impart a survival advantage to individual believers or to hunter-gatherer bands consisting nearly entirely of believers?

My list of activities and aspects of contemporary religion and religious groups which are found in many types of religion. (Of course, a book could be written about the extent to which precursors of these activities and aspects existed among hunter-gatherer bands in Africa during the 200,000 bp-70,000 bp period.)

Belief in a god or gods. Worship of the god or gods.

For many believers, membership in a caring and mutually supportive "spiritual community" or cell between 20 and 80 in number.

Strong bonds of members of "spiritual communities" and cells, including mutual compassion and love.

Reciprocal altruism within fairly small groups, including cells, of believers. (In about 2006, an armed man entered a Unitarian-Universalist church in Knoxville, TN, and started shooting at people. A large male member of the church rushed at the shooter, altruistically sacrificing himself. That allowed other men to subdue the shooter, which saved many lives.)

Individual experiencing of "spiritual experiences," which may enhance belief in a god or gods.

Spiritual leaders of groups of believers.

Theology. Shared beliefs about the god or gods and about things such as the creation of the world.

Important shared beliefs about morality. This includes taboos, which strongly prohibit certain behaviors.

Teaching children about moral precepts and aspects of theology.

Attempts to achieve behavior control over members of the religious group.

Religious rituals. These may be attempts to cause shared experiencing of spiritual experiences.

Sharing of music in religious contexts.

Shared ethnocentrism (exaggerated belief in the superiority of your group) of adherents to a particular type of religion.

Some degree of xenophobia (fear and hatred of that which is different) relating to adherents to other types of religion.

SOME ADDITIONAL RELEVANT INFORMATION

The Middle Paleolithic era (and Middle Stone Age) is sometimes dated to fall from 300,000–30,000 bp. Elsewhere, the Middle Paleolithic era is dated between 200,000–45,000 bp.

Homo sapiens emerged as a new species about 200,000 years ago in Africa. (Note by author in 2018. Experts disagree about some things discussed below.)

All humans have a common female ancestor who lived probably about 150,000–140,000 years ago in Africa.

Prior to about 100,000–50,000 bp, humans did not have the ability to speak to communicate. (Alec MacAndrew, "Foxp2 and the evolution of language," evolutionpages.com website) (I'm guessing that, prior to that time, humans and recent ancestor species whistled to communicate.)

There was definitely a major homo sapiens population bottleneck probably between 140,000 and 70,000 bp. We cannot know whether the precursors of religion were commonly exhibited by homo sapiens before the bottleneck. I believe that it is extremely likely that those precursors were common at least after the bottleneck.

For many hundreds of thousands of years prior to about 70,000 to 40,000 bp, there was a relatively low frequency of innovation of tools and other things by our earlier ancestor species and homo sapiens.

About 80,000 years ago, there was a very large population in Africa. Prior to 40,000 years ago, homo sapiens and other hominid species in Africa probably lived in hunter-gatherer bands which usually had between 25 and 80 members.

Prior to about 40,000 bp, human hunter-gatherer bands were not warlike.

Rather than being ruled by one or more powerful males, these bands probably were egalitarian, which involved major influence of females on group decisions. It follows that male-dominated bands tended to be less successful than egalitarian bands in surviving.

Though there probably often was a shaman (witch doctor), he/she probably did not have general leadership power.

Hunter-gatherer bands of homo sapiens started walking out of Africa in a northeastern direction probably about 70,000 bp. Other hominid groups, including Neanderthals, had exited Africa very much earlier.

In some hunter-gatherer bands during recorded history, band members have shared singing, percussion, and dancing for many hours, sometimes all night. At times, these probably somewhat spiritual experiences helped with conflict resolution.

All known hunter-gatherer bands have exhibited many of the precursors of aspects of religion, such as belief in spirits.

Because xenophobia is exhibited by virtually all types of racial, ethnic, and religious groups, xenophobia must have had at least group survival value during the evolution of man.

Because ethnocentrism is exhibited by virtually all types of racial, ethnic, and religious groups, ethnocentrism must have had at least group survival value during the evolution of man.

Identical-twin research has indicated that 50% of variation in strength of religiosity of humans is attributable to genetic variation. Since the "god gene" may determine about 1% of this variation, I will not discuss it.

Scholars believe that the tendency of early hominins and humans to try to determine what entity caused something important, which is referred to as the agency tendency, has been an important cause of belief in spirits by early hominins. (If the cause of something was not apparent, they might have concluded that spirits were the cause.)

Experts argue that the neurological mechanisms that are involved in an orgasm are also involved in spiritual experiences.

SOME HYPOTHESES

(Things that I think at least probably had "individual survival value" are marked ISV. Things that I think at least probably had "group survival value" are marked GSV.)

Belief in spirits. This probably had ISV in that believing in spirits allowed a person to be accepted in a band composed predominantly of believers. Other than this, I doubt that belief in spirits had much ISV. Research now shows that becoming religious does not enhance a person's self-control.

I believe that, connected to tendency to exhibit xenophobia, there is a tendency of humans to want to have significant affiliations with people with whom they share important characteristics (ISV). During recorded history, humans have often thought that the belief in spirits, a god, or gods is an important characteristic. This tendency would have between 200,000 and 70,000 bp brought together in bands humans who shared belief in spirits. Xenophobia would have tended to exclude non-believers (GSV).

Individual experiencing of spiritual experiences probably increased individual belief in spirits (GSV, maybe some ISV). Because the capacity to have spiritual experiences is very often associated with belief in spirits, these bands of believers in spirits must have had individual and shared spiritual experiences (at least GSV). Group sharing of spiritual experiences, as in all-night singing, percussion, and dancing, would have enhanced group sharing of belief in spirits and would have strengthened the bond in the band (GSV). Commitment of individuals to membership in the band would have increased (GSV). All of this would have caused these hunter-gather bands to constitute mutually supportive spiritual communities (ISV, GSV). (I believe that is the most important thing people are seeking in religion now.)

All of this would have "strengthened the bond" in the bands by increasing altruism (GSV), increasing mutual compassion (at least GSV), increasing mutual understanding and trust (ISV, GSV), nearly certainly increasing happiness (ISV, GSV), reducing boredom (probably ISV, GSV), and probably helping band members to sleep better (ISV, GSV). Like many religious people now, these band members in Africa may have been made to feel happier and possibly safer by being given spirit-laced answers to unanswerable questions (e.g., What causes thunder? What happens when a person dies?).

Altruism, promoted by the effects above, could have had a negative survival effect for the altruistic person but GSV for the band.

Increased mutual trust and understanding resulting from strengthening the bond and increased compassion may have had ISV and GSV, in that mutual trust probably helped band members in cooperating in dealing with a wide variety of extremely challenging situations. Mutual trust, knowledge, and understanding is always crucial when two or more persons engage together in high-risk decision making. I strongly believe that our homo sapiens ancestors in Africa had astonishingly great ability to deal effectively and safely with high-risk situations. A minor misjudgment could sometimes have resulted in deaths of band members and failure of the band.

Sharing of belief in spirits probably increased shared support for norms and taboos (GSV). Some bands may have believed that particular spirits would punish violations of certain taboos, which would have had GSV. Strengthening of the bond, as by increasing mutual compassion, probably enhanced behavior control, which would have had ISV and GSV. Recent research indicates that children who have parents who have religious belief tend to develop self-control. Self-control of band members would have had ISV and GSV.

Belief in spirits, by strengthening the bond in bands, probably made it more likely for xenophobia, triggered by non-belief of individuals, to occur. Being excluded from a band because of inadequate belief in spirits probably would have resulted in the failure of the non-believer to survive. Research indicates that among modern humans, women tend to be more religious than men. In the evolution of man, men with inadequate belief in spirits probably had trouble finding a mate, which would have tended to exclude from the gene pool genes that tend to produce non-belief in spirits.

Improved bond in the band, which involved increased mutual compassion, trust, and understanding, would have improved aspects of cooperative child care and socialization (ISV, GSV). This would have allowed children to learn from the examples and teaching of several women and men.

If the capacity and tendency to have spiritual experiences were highly associated with compassion on the individual level, the most important thing regarding individual and group survival might have been the enhanced compassion instead of the enhanced belief in spirits. Capacity to have spiritual experiences would have been a **spandrel**. A spandrel is something that appears to have had survival value but actually did not.

Early hominins and homo sapiens with agency tendency may also have had a strong ability to identify problems and identify their causes, which are important in group problem solving. If so, this enhanced ability to identify and solve problems might have been more important regarding survival than the belief in spirits, which would have been a spandrel, triggered by the agency tendency.

Prior to the population bottleneck, it is possible that bands sharing belief in spirits had superior survival. This might not have been because of this sharing of belief in spirits but because of greater influence of women in band decision making. (Even then, women probably had more pre-religious tendencies than men.)

Faith v. rationality. I think that early humans had a continuing balancing act concerning this. To meet formidable challenges and threats, they had to be capable of impressive rationality. Assuming that belief in spirits and in the abilities of shamans emerged some number of hundreds of thousands of years ago, it seems certain that our ancestors needed to keep faith and belief in spirits from intruding destructively on rationality and the utilization of advanced intelligence.

During the Middle Paleolithic era, humans must have retained, even in their egalitarian social organization without a dominant, guiding, and punishing leader, a social-animal impulse to look in their environment for the powerful being(s) they would need to avoid incurring the wrath of and to whom they could look for protection, guidance, and assistance. This could have led easily to belief in (fabricated) spirits of various types.

Research suggests that people with religious beliefs tend to be healthier and live longer than those who don't. Maybe this is primarily because they probably belong to a close-knit religious group, which provides healthful emotional support and assistance, which could have been the case for humans 200,000–70,000 bp in Africa.

It was noted earlier that experts believe that the same neurological mechanisms and responses involved in human orgasms are involved also in individual spiritual experiences. If, during late human evolution in Africa, there was a very high correlation on the individual level of belief in spirits, ability to have spiritual experiences, and the ability of men and women to have and enjoy orgasms in heterosexual sex, the most important factor in survival of hunter-gather bands might have been ability of members to have and enjoy orgasms. If so, belief in spirits would have been a spandrel. These individuals would have wanted to have maybe serially monogamous relationships with a mate or mates. They would have wanted to do whatever would have been necessary for their band to survive and for their ability to have a continuing ability to enjoy sex. High birth rate and good child care and socialization could have resulted.

A Short Paper on the Precursors of Aspects and Activities of Religion among Hunter-Gatherer Bands of Humans in Africa between 200,000 and 50,000 years Ago

The "precursors of aspects and activities of religion" which I address include, but are not limited to, rituals which were likely to produce spiritual experiences, the spiritual experiences themselves, spiritual communities, behavior control, and compassion.

Many Americans no doubt believe that, if one could be transported back to see our ancestors in Africa between 200,000 and 50,000 years ago, she or he would observe a horribly brutal existence including human sacrifice, cannibalism, killing of step children by their mothers' new mates, severe oppression of women by men, frequent wars with other bands, and a very hierarchical social structure with a powerful, possibly polygamous male at the top. I believe that, partly because of the considerable influence of women and several precursors of aspects and activities of religion, what the time traveler would have observed would have been vastly different from that.

Scholars agree that for hundreds of thousands (possibly millions) of years, including the Middle Paleolithic period between 200,000 and 50,000 years ago, our ancestors lived in Africa in egalitarian hunter-gatherer bands characterized by monogamy, at least serial monogamy. Conformity was not compelled through threats or violence by dominant males. Important band decisions often would have been reached through discussions in which women very likely were able to participate. This process would have been the precursor of democracy.

For women, living in a small egalitarian band involved exercise of greater power, in comparison to the power of men, than in the vast majority of other human social organizations over the eons. The fact that women were closer in size to men than is the case for many other primates influenced this allocation of power. Women also gathered more than half of the food, prepared much of the food for eating, controlled the availability of heterosexual sex to men, did the great majority of child rearing and early teaching of children, and no doubt did other important tasks where the band slept and ate. Some women had giant troves of valuable knowledge. My guess is that this great power of women was crucial, in a wide variety of ways, in allowing our ancestors to survive and advance some in culture during that period. For example, I believe that women probably generally opposed optional wars with other bands, which could easily have resulted in the failure of a band.

Since women today are consistently more religious and spiritual than men, we can justify an assumption that women were somewhat more responsible than men for the gradual emergence of the precursors of aspects and activities of religion. Many scholars believe that a type of spirituality permeated nearly every aspect of life of those ancestors in Africa. This would have been promoted by participation in rituals, including singing, dancing, and percussion, that must have induced some degree of spiritual experience for many of the band members. Also, it must have been spiritually moving for band members when they realized that they had succeeded in overcoming a great threat to survival. Sharing spiritual experiences and joy would have tended to make the bond within the band even closer. A closer bond would have enhanced cooperation, communication, reciprocity, willingness to act altruistically, willingness to forego individual advancement in favor of advancement of the band, group problem solving, and even high-risk decision making. All of this was necessary for bands to overcome great challenges and survive.

The strong bond within the band probably included a strong element of mutual empathy, love and compassion. Actions expressive of empathy, love, and/or compassion could have enhanced the survival prospects for particular individuals, such as injured persons, and even survival prospects for the band. The protection, rearing, and teaching of children, motivated partly by love, would have been to some degree altruistic. (Love and compassion are central in world religions.) The socialization of children and control of behavior of band members had to operate incredibly effectively in order for members to learn the required information and skills and for them to do the required work. (Behavior control is a crucial function of religion.)

I believe that shared spiritual experiences were important enough to the social organization and process of bands for us to view them as mutually caring and supportive spiritual communities. Spiritual communities share with families, soldiers in a small unit, and police officers in the same department a valuable willingness of group members to altruistically sacrifice themselves in defense of the group.

Simple math indicates that bands in the normal size range from 25 to 80 would not have fought optional wars at all frequently. So, sacrifice and cannibalism of captives probably was not common. Because band members were probably valued, I greatly doubt that, in this atmosphere of mutual compassion, there was much sacrifice and cannibalism of band members.

Because of the great power and influence of women, I **doubt** that a woman's new mate would have viewed elimination of stepchildren as a safe activity. Rather, I think that new mates generally saw stepchildren as important helpers or future helpers.

This social organization and process worked so well that some bands at times experienced a type of affluence and leisure. They appreciated and enjoyed the genuinely good, but simple, things they had.

Humans and even churches today can learn a great deal of value from these ancestors and their ways of living. Many of the worst things in human history have been done in the name of male-led religion. They were not done, however, in the name of the precursors of aspects and activities of religion embraced and practiced by our hunter-gather ancestors in Africa in the Middle Paleolithic period.

Postscripts for emphasis. While there are, I think, many important lessons from the study of precursors of aspects of religion among hunter-gatherer bands in Africa between 200,000 bp and 70,000 bp, I want to emphasize two.

The roles, importance, and influence of women. As I hope you read and remember, we have every reason to believe that band governance was quite egalitarian, with women participating on approximately equal terms with men. I believe that Hillary Clinton's loss in the 2016 Presidential election was partly the result of deep misogyny among the American voters. It seems unlikely that misogyny was common in Africa between 200,000 bp and 70,000 bp. It seems extremely likely that, during those years, women did a high percentage of the important work and other behaviors in bands. Speculating about how misogyny of American voters emerged is beyond the scope of this chapter.

Emotional suitability to be in a mutually supportive spiritual community. The hunter-gatherer bands in Africa 100,000 bp functioned as mutually supportive spiritual communities, which many churches in the U.S. now want to offer. The fact that our ancestors for many hundreds of thousands of years functioned well in mutually supportive spiritual communities suggests that suitability for that is probably part of human nature. I enjoyed growing up in that type of Baptist church and in my extended family, which, to a significant degree, functioned that way. When I was a member of the Unitarian-Universalist Fellowship of Columbia (SC) (1981–88), it undoubtedly functioned as a single-cell mutually supportive spiritual community.

As progressively fewer Americans are affiliated with conventional churches, one can wonder how non-affiliated people will meet those needs. Can having a few drinks in your friendly neighborhood bar partially meet those needs? That is not as frivolous a question as you may think. For people with human nature that adapts well to being a member of a mutually supportive spiritual community, living without that can cause one's life to be somewhat emotionally barren. Is it possible that this partially explains the current opioid overdose epidemic in the U.S.? A reality of Christian churches in the U.S. is that it is very difficult to affiliate with a church if you can't make substantial monetary contributions. When I was young, many people tithed, which was contributing one tenth of your family income. I expect that now many opioid addicts couldn't afford to contribute $15 per month to a church.

BIBLIOGRAPHY

Ambrose, S. H. (1998). Late Pleistocene human population bottlenecks, volcanic winter, and differentiation of modern humans. 1998. *Journal of Human Evolution*, Vol. 34, pp. 623–651.
(Extract carefully read and reviewed.)

Boyer, P. (2001). *Religion explained: the evolutionary origins of religious thought.* NY, NY: Basic Books.
(Because the verbiage is very extremely obtuse, I read only especially applicable sections.)

Houston, M., & Memory, J. M. (2001). Problem solutions in culture and society. In J. M. Memory & Aragon, R. (Eds.), *Patrol officer problem solving and solutions*. Durham, NC: Carolina Academic Press.

King, B. J. (2007). *Evolving God: a provocative view of the origins of religion*. New York: Doubleday.
(All relevant chapters carefully read and reviewed.)

Klein, R. G. (2000). Archeology and the evolution of human behavior. *Evolutionary Anthropology*, Vol. 9, Issue 1, pp. 17–36.
(Carefully read and reviewed.)

McClenon, J. (2002). *Wondrous Healing: Shamanism, Human Evolution, and the Origin of Religion*. DeKalb, Illinois: Northern Illinois University Press.
(Nearly all carefully read and reviewed.)

McCullough, M. D., and Willoughby, B.L. (2009). Religion, self-regulation, and self-control: associations, explanations, and implications. *Psychological Bulletin*, Vol. 135, pp. 69–93.
(All carefully read.)

Newberg, A. et al. (2001). *Why God won't go away: brain science and the biology of belief*. NY, NY: Ballantine Books.
(All carefully read.)

Smith, H. (1991). *The world's religions*. NY, NY: Harper One.
(Chapter on primal religions carefully read and reread.)

Wilson, D. S. (2002). *Darwin's cathedral: evolution, religion, and the nature of society*. Chicago, IL: The University of Chicago Press.
(Relevant parts carefully read and reviewed.)

Wright, R. (2009). *The evolution of God*. NY, NY: Little, Brown and Company.
(Relevant parts carefully read and reviewed.)

— SECTION 12 —
On Good Thinking, Communicating, and Deciding

— CHAPTER 34 —
Problems and Assists in Trying to Stay Well Informed

<u>Elaboration</u>. I believe that there are dozens of factors which tend to make it much more difficult than decades ago for an American to be well informed.

<u>Relevant expertise and experience of the author</u>. In my extensive education, in my civilian and military working careers, and in my numerous intellectual projects, I have tried to obtain high quality information. Now, 14 years after retirement, I continue to work very hard to determine what the truth is relating to important subjects and issues.

<u>Importance of this subject</u>. Nearly all types of effective action and problem solving are unlikely to occur without correct information. In a high percentage of work fields, being well informed is needed to be successful. Our democratic government is premised on having intelligent and well informed voters. Tragically, it appears that it is now extremely difficult for an American voter to be well informed. I believe that this is a tremendously serious and complex problem.

All of us have heard this quote from the writings of Thomas Jefferson:

"[W]ere it left to me to decide whether we should have a government without newspapers or newspapers without a government, I should not hesitate a moment to prefer the latter."

Prior to the drafting of the U.S. Constitution and Bill or Rights, Thomas Jefferson and other Founding Fathers discussed in detail the rationales for various constitutional rights. This quote is part of Thomas Jefferson's writings concerning the importance of freedom of press.

Of course, newspapers are just one type of source of information. In our complex, rapidly changing society, there are major problems regarding the quality of information from many types of sources.

Relevance for young adults. I strongly believe that young adults are now confronting much more numerous and more serious problems regarding access to and quality of information than we confronted when I was a young adult in the 1960s. A crucial skill of young professionals is the ability to recognize and collect correct information.

Possible outcomes when a powerful person, company, or organization does not want important truthful information to be disseminated. The first three of these short accounts are from my life.

Hacking of a computer to destroy documents. In 2013, I incorporated a nonprofit concerned with heart and brain health and within a year had written 500 pages of what I believe were high quality documents. Apparently someone connected with the drug industry found out about my work: In late 2014 there was a major hacking of my computer, resulting in the destruction of all of my documents. Who other than someone affiliated with the drug industry would have wanted to go to the expense and trouble of having that done?

Failure or refusal of Google Scholar to report the most important research in searches. In 1989 I had published in a refereed health journal, *Death Studies*, an article (Memory, 1989) correcting statistical findings regarding rate of suicides of juveniles in adult jails. I reported that the actual rate was 165 times as high as the rate reported in the article (Flaherty, 1983) I criticized. In recent years, the article I corrected has usually been the first article given in Google Scholar searches regarding "suicide of juveniles in adult jails." Usually, my article is not on the first page of the search report. I do not know why this occurs.

To me, it is hard to comprehend that the astonishingly inaccurate Flaherty suicide rates were published in 1983, and I apparently was at least the first scholar who corrected those rates in print.

Fraudulent change of article abstract. In 1999, I was the senior author of an important article (Memory et al, 1999) in the *Prison Journal* reporting findings regarding inmate disciplinary infractions. We found, as expected, that, the greater the possibility of severe prison disciplinary punishments, the lower the disciplinary infraction rate of inmates tended to be. Apparently, this finding is somehow politically incorrect. Several times, someone has managed to fraudulently substitute on the Internet an entirely incorrect abstract for the actual article abstract.

The point is that, in our complex international world, some people who do not want the truth to be disseminated will not hesitate to act ruthlessly to keep that from occurring.

If something of this sort could happen to me three times, how much of this behavior probably is occurring on our planet? I believe that this is a major problem and that university/college students need to be warned about it.

An example of this problem regarding access to an extremely important medical research article. Walsh and Pignone (2004) had an extremely important article concerning cardiovascular health published in the *Journal of the American Medical Association* in 2004. In recent years I have had substantial difficulty obtaining information about that article through use of Google Scholar. I will state emphatically that it is obvious that the drug industry is strongly influencing results of Internet searches, including Google Scholar searches, relating to statin drugs.

Factors and circumstances which tend to either degrade quality of information or reduce access to high quality information. Below is a list of problematic factors and circumstances which I think contribute to these difficulties. These sentences or paragraphs are not numbered or arranged according to subject.

I'll clarify that "misinformation" is giving incorrect information but not doing so intentionally. "Disinformation" is intentionally giving incorrect information.

Elsewhere in this book, I have expressed the opinion that, if a person is persistent and knowledgeable in conducting Internet computer searches, it is likely that the person will be able to obtain high quality information. Since the passage of the 2017 Republican tax cut, I have numerous times been unable to obtain through repeated Internet searches information which I wanted and knew was available. I do not have expertise about computers or the Internet. I am currently very pessimistic about feasibility of getting needed information before a relevant excellent Wikipedia article appears.

As indicated by chapter 31 and 32, I have put significant intellectual energy into studying hunter-gatherer society of humans during the 200,000 bp-70,000bp period. I believe that in that context there was opinion leadership. So, less intelligent and knowledgeable persons tended to respect and possibly adopt opinions of more intelligent and knowledgeable person. I believe, in fact, that some of that effect probably occurred as late as the early 1800s in rural and small town America. It's, of course, obvious that that type of "grassroots" opinion leadership does not occur in the U.S. of Donald Trump.

For many Americans, purposeful lying by President Trump is a giant obstacle to becoming and being well informed.

The phenomenon of "fake news" obviously is importantly connected with many aspects of this subject.

Unfortunately, many people who write materials that come up in Internet searches are not qualified or competent to write high quality verbiage.

Over my long life, I have observed that it is not uncommon for an "expert" to be profoundly wrong about something in his or her area of expertise. Obviously, error of the experts reduces the likelihood that ordinary people will be able to obtain correct information on a given subject.

Belief in magic and the supernatural diminishes how well the public is informed. As you know, this includes belief in several visits of aliens to Earth. (There are programs about ancient aliens on the History Channel.)

Some types of religious beliefs conflict with apparently correct information.

Some religious activities discourage obtaining access to high quality information.

When research questions the quality of a product, the company that produces the product may vigorously attack the credibility of that research. This can diminish the quality of public information.

Companies often "stretch the truth" in marketing products. Though I am a strong believer in the efficacy of many alternative-health measures and products, I believe that their promoters sometimes make exaggerated claims.

Totally uninterpretable claims are made in advertising. I recently saw a sunglasses ad on TV. The announcer said, "Our sunglasses are ten times more accurate than our competitors'."

A political party and allied groups can engage in sustained attacks on the reputation of a public figure. I believe that occurred regarding Hillary Clinton.

The extreme political polarization in the U.S. now results in a lot of incorrect beliefs. If two people disagree about something, at least one of them is wrong.

In some respects, religious people and non-religious people disagree about important things. Again, when two people disagree about something, at least one of them is wrong.

Unfortunately, there are people who broadly doubt the efficacy of science. These people are likely to doubt information derived through use of the scientific method.

This distrust of science is expressed in arguments that global warming is not occurring and that, if it is occurring, it has not been caused by human activity. Of course, the expression of this sentiment often is funded by corporate interests, such as coal, oil, and gas industries, who believe they can benefit by diminishing belief in global warming.

There are many millions of Americans who are anti-intellectual. Genuine intellectual activity should utilize proven methods, such as the scientific method, to generate correct information. Anti-intellectual persons may publicly attack information legitimately generated by intellectuals. Many professors are intellectuals with command of a vast amount of high quality information. Some people doubt the believability of professors.

I believe that a high percentage of Americans treat physicians as though they are nearly gods. It follows that these people think that physicians are in-errant, which means they are never wrong and never make a mistake. Unfortunately, physicians are sometimes wrong about important things. For example, physicians tend to have strong knowledge about extremely expensive procedures utilized in their specialty to overcome dangerous illness, injury, or other abnormal conditions. They know much less about activities, such as prevention of heart and brain disease, that can produce extremely little income. Many physicians know extremely little about nutrition and nutritional supplements. As a result, physicians are often wrong about the prevention of disease, especially when it concerns nutrition.

Adults who have been paying attention in recent years know that experts have changed their recommendations several times regarding many important subjects, especially subjects relating to health. Much of the discredited information remains available and misleads people.

Unfortunately, many students attend poor schools and are taught by poor teachers. How can they overcome these disadvantages later in life?

In Africa 100,000 years ago, parents and other members of their hunter-gatherer band had strong grasps of thousands of items of information that children would need to use later in life. Gradually, the information was taught to the children. Unfortunately, it is obvious that now many parents do not do a good job of teaching important correct information to their children.

While I am not "into" social media, I have the impression that social media often disseminates incorrect information. My impression is that "fake news" has often been disseminated through social media, such as Facebook.

I believe that the 36 chapters of this book together suggest that even universities and colleges are failing in significant instances to disseminate important information.

I think that this book documents successes of advocates of political correctness in preventing generation and dissemination of important correct information.

Television channels at one time frequently aired excellent documentaries that were extremely well developed, written, and filmed. (I will admit that I watch more TV than a supposedly intelligent and well informed person should watch.) Now, the frequency of airing of excellent documentaries is very much lower. They are replaced by interesting series about things such as people living near and inside the Arctic Circle, nude men and women trying to survive in challenging natural settings, people who are reunited with lost relatives, etc. I can go on and on. Watching these series is like eating food without nutrition. They do not provide valuable information. On History Channel you get programs about Big Foot, unidentified flying objects, ghosts, and ice-road trucking. While it would obviously be possible for TV to provide a giant amount of high quality information, people apparently sometimes won't watch that stuff, and advertising corporations wouldn't sponsor it.

I believe from personal observation that some activists intentionally disseminate incorrect information to their movement's followers to increase the followers' feelings of outrage regarding how members of their group are treated. This can be a type of "brain-washing." I think that young Black male authors of recent books, especially Coates (2015), Watson (2015), and Butler (2017), were trying to do that in their books. Lowery (2016) describes how this was done relating to events in Ferguson, MO, by Black Lives Matter.

Ethnocentrism and xenophobia hinder good-faith attempts to discern and disseminate truth. For example, if a very different group maintains a particular belief, xenophobia may inhibit ascription to that belief by members of other groups.

As a student, professor, bridge player, and bridge teacher, I have developed a strong belief that a high percentage of teachers and "learners" dramatically underestimate the importance of repetition in learning usable knowledge. If sufficient repetition does not occur, usable information may not be gained by a significant percentage of people. I believe that, because of this, some university and college students gain very much less usable knowledge in higher education studies than the public assumes they gain.

President Trump recently said, "Journalists are sick people who don't like our country." (August 27, 2017) The giant amount of this Trump rhetoric will reduce the ability of many people to gain valuable information from journalists.

From the start of the 2015 Presidential primaries to the present, Americans have confronted very serious challenges regarding information quality. The hacking and cyber-war tactics by Russians tended to produce intentionally incorrect information.

My experience regarding Google Scholar's treatment of information in my two most important published articles suggests that there probably is a giant amount of that type of disinformation and misinformation going on.

A related type of misinformation. During the 1990s, I found a published article about the consideration of race in criminal justice decision making. It was written by a team composed of graduate students and one professor. They used bivariate and logistic regression, which are, I believe, very esoteric forms of regression. In my opinion, the researchers failed to configure the variables so as to be able to carry out meaningful statistical procedures. I contacted the journal and was told that it would be politically incorrect to publish a retraction of the article.

My guess is that mistakes of that type are much less common in "elite" disciplines, such as economics and psychology, than in lower-tier disciplines. If a psychologist has bad data, has the wrong type of data, uses the wrong statistical procedures, uses the right statistical procedures incorrectly, engages in unjustifiable inference, etc., it is very likely that his or her article will not be published in a refereed journal or even a non-refereed journal.

Ways to obtain high quality information and remain well informed. As mentioned above, I am currently disenchanted with doing Internet searches for something important, especially before a Wikipedia article on the subject is available.

Excellent magazines. Generally, we probably can to a significant degree trust excellent magazines. Here are search engines for magazines: MagPortal, 4magazines, Isleypubliclibrary.org. I encourage you to try each of them.

Scholarly journals. The traditional way to search scholarly journals on the Internet is Google Scholar.

Wikipedia articles. My impression is that Wikipedia articles tend to provide high quality information. There are about 5,543,954 Wikipedia articles on the Internet. Only 26,962 of those articles have been designated as "good" by that organization. If a particular article has been designated as "good", there will be a small circle with a plus symbol inside in the top-right corner of the first page of that article. About 5,219 articles have been designated "featured articles." I do not know how that designation is indicated.

Known credible authors/experts. Obviously, a person may attempt to find an article or book on a particular subject by a known credible author. In chapter 25 about erosion of much that is valued in the U.S., I mention "five of the many people who can talk about this much more intelligently than I can: Fareed Zakaria, Rachel Maddow, Pete Peterson, Nicholas Burns, and Thomas Friedman." Two of those people are Republicans. I will add William Cohen, another Republican, to my list of extremely capable and credible persons relating to government and foreign relations. You can search on MagPortal for "articles by Pete Peterson about the national debt."

Use of high quality search engines. Students and others should attempt to use excellent search engines. In the Criminal Justice field, helpful searches can be done on the National Criminal Justice Reference Service website.

Excellent television and radio programs. I believe that Charlie Rose made a giant volume of high quality information available to the public in his *The Charlie Rose Show* on public television from 1991 until late in 2017. I have the impression that the excellent *Rachel Maddow Show* has the highest ratings of programs in that category. I'll recommend two additional TV shows that help a person to be informed and, I believe, think intelligently: *Fareed Zakaria GPS* on CNN and *Nova* on PBS. While discussions on Fox and MSNBC strongly tend to be driven by ideology, that is not the case on Zakaria's show.

REFERENCES

Butler, P. (2017). *Chokehold*. NY, NY: The New Press.

Coates, Ta-Nehisi. (2015). *Between the world and me*. NY, NY: Spiegel & Grau.

Flaherty, Michael (1983). The national incidence of juvenile suicide in adult jails and juvenile detention centers. *Suicide and Life-Threatening Behavior*, Vol. 13, No. 2, pp. 85–94.

Lowery, W. (2016). *They can't kill us all*. NY, NY: Little, Brown and Company.

Memory, J.M. (1989). Juvenile suicide in secure detention facilities: correction of published rates. *Death Studies*, Vol. 13, pp. 455–63.

Memory, J.M., Guo, G., Parker, K., & Sutton, T. (1999). Comparing disciplinary infraction rates of North Carolina Fair Sentencing and Structured Sentencing inmates. *The Prison Journal*, Vol. 79, pp. 45–71.

Walsh, Judith M.E. & Pignone, Michael (2004). Drug treatment of hyperlipidemia in women. *Journal of the American Medical Association*, Vol. 291, pp. 2243–2252.

Watson, B. with Petersen, K. (2015). *Under our skin: getting real about race*. Carol Stream, IL: Tyndale Momentum.

──── CHAPTER 35 ────
Thinking and Writing Well in the Professions

Elaboration. The main goal of this chapter is to give information to high school and college/university students who like to write and want to use that skill in a working career. I hope this information will help readers to make good decisions about choosing an academic major. Also, some suggestions are given about "writing in the professions." **This chapter concerns nearly entirely non-fiction writing**.

The most important ideas in this chapter. To write well, you must think well. To think well, nearly everyone needs to exercise. In several chapters, I have given full information about the startlingly great benefits of physical exercise.

Here's strong supporting information. I knew well my first cousin, Jasper D. Memory, who had a PhD in physics and was a finalist for president of WFU and chancellor of NCSU; of course, I know very well my son Alex, who is a "star" in computer science and will soon receive a PhD; I know of a friend's son, who is a "super-star" at a Big10 university. What have those three had in common? Each one either got or gets very meaningful physical exercise during every work day.

Thinking well is hard work. As I am writing this, I am thinking about playing tomorrow in two 3½ hour duplicate bridge sessions in which I will need to make my old brain work really well for nearly the whole time. Sometimes, it helps to consciously decide to think as well as you can. Lazy

thinking tends to fail horribly in strong bridge games. Obviously, lazy thinking will tend to fail in writing.

Relevance of "critical thinking." An important source about
"critical thinking" is an article on the website of the Foundation for Critical
Thinking with the title of "Defining critical thinking." While I support what
appear to be the goals of proponents of "critical thinking," my guess is that
many people are confused by their exposure to that movement because of
the inclusion of the word "critical", which suggests that intelligent thinking
should contradict previous thinking.

Excellent writers to learn from. I would be remiss if I failed to mention the importance of learning from the examples of excellent non-fiction
thinkers/writers, such as Malcolm Gladwell and Thomas Friedman.

Increase in importance of writing skills. On the study.com website (2011), Sarah Wright argues that writing skills are now more important
than ever.

Author's relevant expertise and experience. I was an associate editor of
the *Wake Forest Law Review* (1967–68), a consulting editor of *Suicide and
Life-Threatening Behavior* (1987–89), and the developer and senior editor of
a 500-page reader (Memory & Aragon, 2001).

Early in the 1980s, I, with only one publication, felt very confident about
being an excellent writer. Not long after that, I somehow acknowledged the
truth: **I actually was not even a good writer**. I was writing documents that
combined elements of several types of bad writing—legal, military, social scientific, and bureaucratic writing. So, I bought the excellent Strunk and White
(1962) book about writing, read it carefully, and started working hard on
improving my writing. Managing to become a fairly good writer significantly
increased my ability to achieve enough success in my working career. To see a
list of my publications of various types, you can look at the references section
at the end of this chapter. Quite improbably, my one foray into "creative"
writing, *Some Relationships* (1997), resulted in excellent newspaper reviews.
Here is a verse from that book.

Some relationships involve trying to get nattily dressed.
Some relationships involve trying to get Natalie undressed.

The group who liked that book the most was composed of three men with doctoral degrees from Harvard. Twenty years after self-publication, I have many unopened boxes of that book.

Since the 1980s, I have had the ability to sense how well my brain is working. Now, at 74, I have to work to get my brain to work well. Unfortunately, ho-hum functioning of my brain does not reliably produce even fair ideas or writing. On a recent Sunday, I took heart- and brain-healthy supplements, walked nine holes of golf in the morning, ate a good lunch, took a short nap, and drank a cup of caffeinated coffee. Then, I started developing ideas for this book, as I watched golf on TV. I gradually realized that, fortunately, my brain was working very well.

As a professor, I wrote and distributed a sheet for a high percentage of classes. This facilitated class discussion and gave the students something to study before exams. When I lead a discussion these days, I always hand out copies of a sheet I have written.

Importance of this subject. In many professions, writing is an important activity. It is worthwhile to address this subject because, in my opinion, writing is a skill that can be improved through hard work. Over the last 40 years, I have heard progressively more grammatical and word-usage mistakes on radio and television.

Relevance for young adults. Nearly all professional fields require one or more types of fairly distinctive writing. I suspect that a high percentage of high school and college students who like to write and are good at it assume—incorrectly—that they should major in English in college.

An undergraduate course about this could cover examples of very high quality writing from a wide variety of professional and vocational fields. Obviously, many undergraduate majors can provide substantive information needed while working in a particular field. I believe that a student who has majored, for example, in environmental science will succeed more in getting a job in that field and while working in the field than an English major.

Ways of "pursuing truth" in various professions and other activities. In earlier drafts I referred to "discerning truth." Intellectual purists (if any read this) will like "pursuing truth" better. (I understand that there is a school of thought according to which there is no "truth.")

In academic disciplines, professions, and vocations in the U.S., you find many widely differing methods for "pursuing truth" Below, there is a list and brief discussion of some of those methods.

In about 2007, I heard a Unitarian-Universalist minister say, in effect, "Everything we really know we learned through personal experience." Partly because I often taught research methods as a Criminal Justice professor, I knew that he was wrong. So, I wrote the first version of this list.

The scientific method. The scientific method is the most robust approach for generating important information, such as knowledge about causation. That information is of such high quality that scientists can, as an example, confidently predict that an atomic bomb will explode with a certain level of force. The scientific method is used in the social sciences. For example, survey results can be interpreted using aspects of the scientific method.

Testing solutions and methods suggested by well-supported scientific theory, which is supported by scientific research. Engineering utilizes this information derived through use of the scientific method in development of problem solutions and other methods that can be used with a high level of confidence, which is required in engineering.

Other mathematical analysis. This includes solution of mathematical equations.

Qualitative research methods. Most research uses the scientific method and statistical methods. There is a second strong research method, qualitative research, which often involves getting immersed in the thing you are studying and developing "empathic understanding" of it. This method requires extensive and careful note taking. Participant observation is a special type of qualitative research favored by anthropologists and some sociologists. A good example is *Street Corner Society* by W.F. Whyte (1943). He lived with a street gang for several years and wrote a book about his experiences.

Behavioral archeology. This method is used by archeologists who utilize archeological artifacts and other information in attempting to determine how humans or pre-human hominids behaved even millions of years ago.

Personal experience. All of us have many types of personal experiences. Based on these experiences, we may reach conclusions regarding facts, reality, and causes. Unfortunately, our experiences sometimes mislead us into reaching incorrect conclusions. (Unfortunately, having one excellent golf score does not prove that you are an excellent golfer.)

Personal observation. This category overlaps with personal experience. Unfortunately, even personal observation may fail to provide "correct answers" about facts, reality, causes, and events. When a social worker goes to a home to collect information about whether a couple meet the criteria to become adoptive or foster parents, the social worker observes very carefully, asks questions, and takes notes carefully. This information is used in writing a report.

Opinion surveys. Unfortunately, because many people refuse to respond to opinion surveys, confidence in the validity of opinion surveys is declining in the U.S.

Market analyses. Businesses pay for studies to determine how much demand there is for particular products.

Intuition. It is assumed that women have strong intuitive ability to reach good conclusions about facts, reality, and causes.

Reading facial expressions and body language. Police patrol officers and investigators and lawyers often try to read a person's facial expressions and/or body language to acquire important information about that person. High-stakes poker players try to do this.

Stories about past events, facts, and reality told to younger persons by parents and other older persons. In primitive cultures, these stories are extremely important.

Participating in education. Of course, the "information" offered in education can have many types of sources and delivery. Most professors in colleges and universities claim to be experts in at least one of their teaching areas.

Logic. The early Greek philosophers did not have advanced methods for measuring things or the scientific method and statistical procedures to test hypotheses. So, they used logic to discern "truth." Logic helps one to make good decisions in everyday life and is central to the scientific method.

"Intelligence" collection and analysis. This refers to military and national security intelligence. Of course, this can involve observation by an individual or through use of "high tech."

Print and non-print journalistic "reporting." This can include investigative reporting. Wasn't it Will Rogers who said, "The only things I believe are what I read in the newspaper?" We all know that a high percentage of Americans have become skeptical about the believability of journalists. Ordinarily, a newspaper's editors write many editorials on a wide variety of challenging and important subjects.

Religious teachings. Of course, religious leaders often attempt to teach people about facts, reality, causes, and past events, such as the resurrection of Jesus. Very often, they base this teaching on a religious text. Many Christians unhesitatingly say, "It's in the Bible. I believe the Bible. That's the end of the story." The high status of some religious leaders, including ministers and priests, can contribute to the credibility of their pronouncements with believers.

Prayer. Many people use prayer in attempts to determine facts, reality, and causes. I believe that people who carefully pray about something as they are going to sleep probably may, during the following day and later, receive benefits from meaningful brain activity during sleep.

Trials. Courts attempt to determine "truth" through trials. In criminal cases, conviction requires "proof beyond a reasonable doubt." (The proof beyond a reasonable doubt standard is very high. As a result, even though in some cases "everyone" knows the defendant was guilty, the jury verdict may be "not guilty." In such a case, truth discernment has failed. A smarter person than me might say that the system has performed as intended.) In civil cases, the standard is "proof by the preponderance of the evidence."

Internet searches. While the quality of information available on the Internet is wildly varied, I believe that, if you are careful and determined, you can often eventually obtain valuable information. Of course, this "information" varies greatly regarding methods by which it was originally derived.

Investigations. Police, commissions of various sorts, and legislative committees often try to determine truth through investigation. When I was a military prosecutor, I did my own investigations of cases assigned to me.

Crime-scene analysis. Criminal investigators (probably detectives) in law enforcement agencies go as soon as possible to important crime scenes, take photographs, take measurements used in drawing diagrams, collect important physical evidence, and do other things, as required. As a very experienced expert about criminal justice, I will share my belief that this is the most interesting and sometimes the most important thing done by people working in the criminal justice and juvenile justice systems relating to a particular case.

Allowing yourself to be subjected to verbal arguments and attempts to persuade. This includes advertisements and other marketing of products. (Does watching a statin ad on TV help you in discerning truth concerning effectiveness and effects of statins?)

Coercion, such as torture

Interviewing persons under the influence of "truth serum"

Interviewing persons attached to a polygraph (lie detector)

Chemical analysis

Precise measurement of many types of things

If a particular method for "pursuing, determining, discerning truth" appeals to you, you can identify professions and jobs in which that method is used.

Pre-work exercise routine. I don't know anyone who thinks and writes better in a challenging profession than my son Alex. So, I'm giving below his description of his pre-work exercise routine.

> "Five-to-seven days a week I do 30 minutes of cardio on a stationary bike or stairmaster. Then, I do one or two strength exercises. I've been doing that for about 18 years. For fun while exercising, I've always done something I like, like reading a novel, watching a movie, or playing a video game."

Doing physical exercise is the best way to build your brain power. I don't have the slightest doubt that, in 19 years of doing his routine, Alex has built his brain power significantly.

Partly because of my excellent heart health outcomes in spite of very severe heart disease risk factors, I recommend that you consider doing what I have done about 8,000 times since 1982. Take carefully selected heart- and brain-healthy supplements, wait 20 to 30 minutes, and then get at least 20 minutes of exercise that is at least as strenuous as brisk walking (I call this my "vascular cleansing routine" (VCR)). Through recent personal experimentation, I have concluded that I need at least 17 minutes of very brisk walking to get my body to use the alpha-lipoic acid I have taken and produce glutathione, which is an important antioxidant with a wide variety of benefits, including help with cognitive functioning. All thinking improvement formulas I have seen include folic acid, vitamin B6, and vitamin B12. You can find detailed information about this in the first 15 chapters of this book.

Ideas about preparing to write your first draft.

Try to be realistic about types and levels of writing in which you might succeed. At any time in the U.S., many tens of thousands of people, many of them very intelligent, talented, knowledgeable, and determined, are at some stage in writing of "the great American novel." (Though I tend to be somewhat grandiose, I don't think I could write even a good novel.)

Select your subject. Selecting a good and important subject may allow you to write something that is worth reading.

Timing can be important. It would have been silly for me to have written about my heart and brain health routine (VCR) ten years after I started performing it. It is not silly 36 years after I started, when I am 74 years old and have excellent heart and brain health.

If needed, develop preliminary familiarity with your subject. Chapter 34 is mainly about problems people encounter in trying to be well informed.

Decide regarding having one or more co-authors. In recent decades, the average number of authors of articles in scholarly journals has increased. Co-authoring works.

Decide on questions you want to answer. I'll provide some words and phrases that suggest questions you might want to answer through something you will write. A writer can plan to answer many of these questions.

Who, what, when, where, why, how
Efficacy/effectiveness of an innovation or invention
Description of past events
Are certain criteria met? (I wrote an unpublished paper on whether George W. Bush meets the criteria for having an anti-social personality. No, I'm not giving my conclusion.)
Identification of causes and their effects
Provision of solution(s) of one or more problems
Evaluation and, possibly, comparison of quality of applicants, ideas, plans, etc. This can involve comparison of options.
Provision of a plan for accomplishing something
Determination of relevant facts; determination of the nature of relevant reality

Prediction of future events and/or developments

Measurement of something

Identification of risks and, possibly, development of ways to minimize risks and protect against undesirable occurrences

Identification of important opportunities and development of plans to capitalize on identified opportunities

Decision regarding action to be taken

Determination of things such as ownership, legality, feasibility, value, cost

Approval or disapproval of something

Is punishment authorized? If so, is it justifiable?

Measurement of opinions, attitudes, values

Statistical results (e.g., incidence, correlation)

If required, do a literature review. In several types of writing, it is very important to do an excellent review of the published literature relating to the subject. This can be true in historical analysis and is true in scientific, social scientific, and behavioral scientific writing relating to research. (Social sciences include sociology, anthropology, political science, criminology, and economics. Behavioral sciences include psychology and social-psychology.) Because I am a slow reader, I have emphasized reading of excellent articles instead of books. Good writers tend to cram their best thinking on a subject into a published article.

In much legal writing, the writer must review the relevant case law and statutory law. This type of legal research sometimes is done by a paralegal (non-lawyer employee of a lawyer).

Work hard collecting needed information. In many types of writing, you must do a good job collecting high quality information/data. I defended a court-martial case against a JAG captain who had graduated from Harvard Law School. He failed to get the facts by going to an enlisted men's club at Fort Bragg, NC, late on a Saturday night. As a result, he failed to get a conviction. He could not have written a factually correct pre-trial brief.

Try to "think outside the box" and be ready to realize that a previous writer has been seriously wrong. Nearly 30 years ago, I (Memory,

1989) was prepared to discern that an actual suicide rate was 165 times as high as a published suicide rate (Flaherty, 1983).

Execute well the relevant method(s) for determining "truth." This can involve informally "making sense" of available and collected information.

If needed, improve the quality of important ideas and develop additional ideas. Good writing requires good ideas, which may need to be novel/creative. I have tried to include in every chapter of this book at least two or three items of important information most people don't have. Here is an idea with which some readers will disagree. In a time in which everyone with a computer can do computer searches on a wide variety of subjects, giving in your writing cites to supporting studies/articles/books has become less important, and genuinely novel ideas, conclusions, insights, hypotheses, strategies, and problem solutions have become more important.

Write with integrity and decency. What you have written is probably of limited or no value if you haven't worked and written with integrity and decency. In many types of writing, it is clearly inappropriate for the writer to allow religious or political beliefs to influence conclusions. It is clearly inappropriate for a scientist, social scientist, or behavioral scientist to attempt, in research, to achieve a desired result (e.g., the result desired by the funding entity). Vast legions of writers are smarter and more talented, skilled, informed, and productive than me. I don't think many have more integrity than I do.

Write with courage. Chapter 24 is about exhibiting moral courage in the workplace and in government, including situations which require whistle-blowing. Engaging in those behaviors may take courage. An unfortunate reality in the U.S. is that people who write with courage often pay a significant price for doing so.

An approach to the document-organization process that has worked for me. Especially if I am writing a long and complex document on a subject that is fairly new to me, I use the following approach. (There is an accepted format for research reports in the sciences, social sciences, and behavioral sciences.)

(1) *Take notes from reading and information collection and from your "brainstorming."* During nearly all of the steps above, a writer takes notes and does some preliminary writing. I try to continue brainstorming through the entire writing process. Take your notes on sheets that can be cut into slips.

(2) *When you believe you have enough important information and ideas, cut your sheets into slips with one main point on each slip.* References and footnote information should be on the front of the slip.

(3) *Sit down on the floor, and put the slips of paper (possibly hundreds of them) in front of you.*

(4) *Start organizing the slips into sections. It's fairly easy to change the position of one slip or an entire section of slips.* Allow this process to nearly have a life of its own. This will help you to develop over-all sequencing and organization and see connections of different slips and sections.

(5) *When you are happy with the organization that has emerged, tape the slips onto blank sheets of paper, being careful to put the sheets in order.*

(6) *After going through what you have, maybe inserting some notes, word process your first draft from the slip-covered sheets.*

Once you have a first draft, work on relentlessly improving it. Going through several stages of developing ideas, writing/revising, setting the project aside, and then developing ideas, writing/revising some more can produce major improvements. More talented and capable writers than I probably don't do this as much as I do. On very difficult and important writing projects, I generally do full proofreading and correction, with improvement of organization and phrasing, several times. With word processing, you can do significant improvements of a document in much less than one tenth of the time required 50 years ago.

Get feedback on what you've written. In nearly all types of writing, getting feedback concerning the written product from qualified and trusted others can be helpful. It has nearly always been a mistake when I have asked a person to read and give me feedback about a very early draft of a document.

Articles about careers in which writing is an important activity. Here are the titles of two excellent articles on the Internet that are specifically about careers in which writing is an important activity.

"What kind of writer do you want to be?" Writing-World.com

"There's more to a career in writing than being a journalist." The Guardian website

Two models of professionalization. During my working career mainly as a Criminal Justice professor, I obtained interesting information about two types of professionalization. So, I wrote the document below. The traditional model on the left is exhibited in traditional professionals, such as medicine, law, and architecture. The model on the right is exhibited by professional persons who are employed in governmental agencies and, to some extent, in businesses. Thinking and writing well are important aspects of work in both models of professionalization.

TWO MODELS OF PROFESSIONALIZATION

Traditional (Medical-Legal)	**Bureaucratic (based on Weber ideas)**
Work is a high-skill activity.	Work is a high-skill activity.
University education beyond the bachelor's degree level is required.	Bachelor's degree with technical training in agency or business is likely.
Large body of cognitively demanding knowledge	Smaller body of more technical information
Many scholarly journals	Some more technical journals

Qualification as a generalist (high probability of eventual work as a specialist)	High level of specialization in training and work
Code of ethics developed by profession	No meaningful code of ethics. Behavior is governed by agency rules and regulations and policies and procedures.
Substantially autonomous work is likely. Work should conform to legally-established standards of the profession.	Work within a hierarchically organized agency or organization. Work is supervised.
Professional exercises relatively wide discretion applying relevant legally established standard of care in deciding how to serve client.	Any discretion is guided by policies and procedures, and exercise is probably supervised and may need to be approved.
Power can be based on knowledge, reputation, position in association of practicing professionals.	Most important power is exercised by head of hierarchical agency, organization, or business.
Autonomy in work selection and scheduling	Work is assigned by agency/organization but may be scheduled by professional.
Clients are accepted; there is a confidential relationship with client, and a high duty of care and performance is owed to client.	There may be no clients. If there are clients, they are assigned. There is no general guarantee of confidentiality owed to client. High duty owed to organization and possibly the public in handling of persons.
No requirement of merit hiring and promotion	Usually hiring and promotion are expected to be based on merit.
No guaranteed career	Tenure and guarantee of employment can be gained.
Compensation is variable and often is high.	Fixed compensation and pension; compensation is usually modest.

Will English departments offer this type of course? That would require that a faculty member in English have sufficient expertise relating to "writing in the professions" and willingness to teach the course. Partly because taking the course might convince some students to choose a major other than English, English departments may be slow to offer this course.

I recently heard a community college English professor on the radio talking about a course she often teaches in which she compares sonnets of obscure European poets with hip-hop lyrics. How can such a course help a student to prepare to be a competent, productive, self-reliant, healthy, and successful young professional?

REFERENCES AND CITATIONS TO MOST OF
THE AUTHOR'S PUBLICATIONS

Houston, M., & Memory, J.M. (2001). Problem solutions in culture and society. In J.M. Memory & R. Aragon (Eds.), *Patrol officer problem solving and solutions*. Durham, NC: Carolina Academic Press.

Memory, J.M. (1967). N.C.G.S. 15-4.1: "due process of law" under *Gideon v. Wainwright? Wake Forest Law Review*, Vol. 3, pp. 1–32.

Memory, J.M. (1981). *Work-related stress of state criminal trial court judges*. Unpublished doctoral dissertation, Florida State University, Tallahassee.

Memory, J.M. (1989). Juvenile suicide in secure detention facilities: correction of published rates. *Death Studies*, Vol. 13, pp. 455–63.

Memory, J.M. (1990). "Miss Dessa and Mr. James." *The State Magazine*. (September issue)

Memory, J.M. (1991). What is Riverton? in Wright, Marilyn (1991). *A sense of place*. Laurinburg, NC: Scotland County Historical Association.

Memory, J.M. (1997). *Some relationships*. (self-published)

Memory, J.M. (1999). Some impressions from a qualitative study of implementation of community policing in North Carolina. In M. L. Dantzker (Ed.) (1999). *Readings for research methods in criminology and criminal justice.* Woburn, MA: Butterworth.

Memory, J.M. (2001). Teaching patrol officer problem solutions to university students. *The Journal of Criminal Justice Education*, Vol. 12, pp. 213–28.

Memory, J.M. (2017). *Low-complexity, high-power duplicate bridge methods.* Unpublished. Available without charge in pdf.

Memory, J.M. (2017). *Lessons from the life of Jasper Memory.* Near completion.

Memory, J.M. Sentences and sentencing law: types. *Encyclopedia of Criminology.*

Memory, J.M., & Aragon, R. (Eds.). (2001). *Patrol officer problem solving and solutions.* Durham, NC: Carolina Academic Press.

Memory, J.M., & Aragon, R. (2001). Importance of proven problem solutions in policing. In J. M. Memory & R. Aragon (Eds.), *Patrol officer problem solving and solutions.* Durham, NC: Carolina Academic Press.

Memory, J.M., & Aragon, R. (2001). Patrol officer problem solving techniques. In J. M. Memory & R. Aragon (Eds.), *Patrol officer problem solving and solutions.* Durham, NC: Carolina Academic Press.

Memory, J.M., & Aragon, R. (2001). Selective nonenforcement and selective enforcement solutions. In J. M. Memory & R. Aragon (Eds.), *Patrol officer problem solving and solutions.* Durham, NC: Carolina Academic Press.

Memory, J.M., & Aragon, R. (2001). Conflict management and crisis intervention. In J. M. Memory & R. Aragon (Eds.), *Patrol officer problem solving and solutions.* Durham, NC: Carolina Academic Press.

Memory, J.M., & Aragon, R. (2001). Making patrol policing professional. In J. M. Memory & R. Aragon (Eds.), *Patrol officer problem solving and solutions*. Durham, NC: Carolina Academic Press.

Memory, J.M. & Evatt, Lynn (2012). *Vascular cleansing routines: safe and effective heart health programs for women (and men)*. Released by digital publishing at Wake Forest University.

Memory, J.M., Guo, G., Parker, K., & Sutton, T. (1999). Comparing disciplinary infraction rates of North Carolina Fair Sentencing and Structured Sentencing inmates. *The Prison Journal*, Vol. 79, pp. 45–71.

Memory, J.M., & Morris, B. (2001). Illegal, unethical, and discriminatory purported problem solutions. In J. M. Memory & R. Aragon (Eds.), *Patrol officer problem solving and solutions*. Durham, NC: Carolina Academic Press.

Memory, J.M., & Rose, C. (2002). The attorney as moral agent: a critique of Cohen. *Criminal Justice Ethics*, Vol. 21, pp. 28–39.

Memory, J.M., & Rose, C. (2002). A surrebuttal *Criminal Justice Ethics*, Vol. 21, pp. 55–57.

Memory, J.M., & Smith, B. (1988). *Line police officer knowledge of search and seizure law: results of an exploratory multi-city test*. National Institute of Justice: Washington, DC. (Data have been available from the Inter-University Consortium for Political and Social Research, Ann Arbor, MI.)

Rohe, W., Memory, J.M., et al. (1996). *Community oriented policing: the North Carolina experience*. Chapel Hill, NC: Center for Urban and Regional Studies, University of North Carolina at Chapel Hill.

Sroka, J. C., & Memory, J.M. (2001). Ordinances and police practice. In J. M. Memory & R. Aragon (Eds.), *Patrol officer problem solving and solutions*. Durham, NC: Carolina Academic Press.

(In addition, I have presented nine scholarly papers at conferences and have had about 15 newspaper op-eds published.)

Flaherty, Michael (1983). The national incidence of juvenile suicide in adult jails and juvenile detention centers. *Suicide and Life-Threatening Behavior*, Vol. 13, No. 2, pp. 85–94.

Strunk, W. & White, E.B. (1962). *The elements of style*. NY, NY. McMillan Publishing.

Whyte, W.F. (1943). *Street corner society: the social structure of an Italian slum*. Chicago, IL: University of Chicago Press.

Wright, Sarah (2011). Why writing skills are more important than ever. Study.com website. October 5, 2011.

—— CHAPTER 36 ——
High-Risk Activities and Decision Making

Elaboration. This chapter includes a description and discussion of many types of high-risk professional/vocational and recreational activities. It covers also behavior that is limited to high-risk decision making, such as high-risk investing. All of these activities require high skill to achieve success.

In many sectors of life activity, individuals want to get the best available things and outcomes, and many people are willing to take significant risks while attempting to get the best payoffs. "Nothing ventured, nothing gained." This partially explains why this is a very broad and important subject. (Amazon has a separate section for books about this: "Amazon high risk books.")

Definition of high-risk activity. High-risk activities present the possibility of a very negative outcome and, usually, also the possibility of a positive outcome, possibly an extremely positive outcome. Generally, which outcome is achieved is determined by the skill and judgment of the participants.

Level of risk sometimes accepted. Three "recreational" activities help us to understand how great risks can be even in recreational high-risk activities. Apparently, between 6 and 9% of persons who attempt to climb Mount Everest die in the attempt. Americans are becoming more aware of the risks of injury football players confront. Studies have shown that a high percentage of long-term professional football players suffer serious brain injury. Some very determined competitors in gymnastics experience serious injuries resulting from the strenuous exercise that is necessary.

War as a high-risk activity. Military action is often started when a country believes it can achieve a substantial benefit by using military force against another country or countries. The risks of military action are so numerous and great that able and responsible thinkers believe that a country should exhaust every other option that has potential to produce an acceptable outcome, prior to using military force.

George W. Bush did not exhaust all feasible options, such as extensive weapons inspections, before starting the second Iraq War in 2003. The adverse financial and human consequences of that war for the U.S. and for the Iraqi people have been extremely great and, regarding treatment of seriously injured combatants, will continue for many more years.

Author's relevant expertise and experience. Because I have had professional and recreational experiences in or related to several high-risk activities, I have written this chapter utilizing primarily knowledge and insights I have independently acquired or developed. I want to emphasize that professors who might teach a course on this subject would very likely have sufficient written materials from experts.

Similarity of my life to a high-risk activity. If you have read this book to this point, you may have concluded that I have several talents and capabilities that might have helped me to achieve fairly high quality of life. (Of course, I know there are much more talented people than me in all of my activity areas.) Unfortunately, I also have several very significant weaknesses and vulnerabilities. So, I have had to try to capitalize on my talents and capabilities, while trying also to prevent adverse consequences of my weaknesses and vulnerabilities. As I discuss in the "About the Author" section at the end of this book, very adverse outcomes were entirely possible, if not likely.

Author exposure to and experiences in high-risk activities. During my career as a Criminal Justice professor, my main specialty area was patrol police officer problem solving and decision making. I developed, edited, and was the main contributor to a commercially published reader on patrol police officer problem solving (Memory & Aragon, 2001). I, however, have not been an expert on high-risk, dangerous police operations. In a recreational high-risk activity, duplicate bridge, I have reached the rank, Gold Life Master, that is four levels above ordinary Life Master. I wrote and presented at a conference of criminal justice professors a paper (Memory, 2003) discussing the similarity of two-officer patrol policing and duplicate bridge regarding attempting to capitalize on positive opportunities, while minimizing risks.

In 2003, I engaged in a recreational high-risk activity—canoeing alone for 220 miles in 6.5 days on a severely flooded meandering river—without adverse events. If you're experienced in canoeing, you may be thinking that I couldn't possibly have averaged 33 miles per day. Take a canoe to the Lumber River near Wagram, NC, and see how long it takes you to canoe to within sight of Georgetown, SC.

Since 1967, I have consistently played golf as frequently as I could manage. Though I have an extremely ugly golf swing, during my 15 years of best play, my average score was in the 70s. As all golfers and many spectators know, golf is a high-risk, high-reward activity.

Importance of this subject. If you try to list professions and vocations that involve pursuit of very positive outcomes, while trying to avoid serious adverse occurrences (e.g., the military, national-security activities, law, medicine, architecture, law enforcement, structural engineering, many other engineering specialties, etc.), you will get a sense for how important this category is. All of those activities present very great risks and rewards.

A fraternity brother of mine heads a large law firm that handles only big-money law suits. He has vastly better talent and tolerance for stressful, high-risk activity than I would ever have had.

Relevance for young adults. I think it is natural for young adults to be drawn to high-risk activities. The earlier you start learning how to perform a high-risk activity well, the better will be the chances that you will be able to succeed in it and enjoy it.

Proposal of a college course on this subject. Later in this chapter, there is extensive discussion of "risk management," which entails identification and minimization of adverse risks and identification and capitalization on positive opportunities in the industrial context. I strongly believe that departments and colleges of business can justify offering a course on "risk management." There is a substantial body of literature on that subject. Such a course could devote a few classes to the study of high-risk activities in recreation, investing, and non-business employment. I believe there could be an excellent course on high-risk activities that would have much broader content.

The connection of "critical thinking" with high-risk decision making. Critical thinking has been defined as "the objective analysis of facts to form a judgment." Before you can make a good decision, you have to collect the relevant facts and consider them while deciding. If a lawyer, doctor, investor, or high-risk skier doesn't "get the facts right," he cannot decide and act intelligently and safely.

As mentioned earlier, one of my important interests has been problem solving. I believe that the varied steps involved in solving a problem are critical thinking activities.

The relevance of good judgment in high-risk activities. When a person makes a significant decision, the person is exercising judgment. While, as discussed earlier in this book, I think problem solving and hope are extremely important for humans, I believe that judgment is even more important. If you fail to exercise good judgment, you may fail and suffer adverse consequences. This can diminish your prospects and hope for the future.

I first studied this subject when I wrote my FSU criminology master's area paper (Memory, 1977), which was about police exercise of enforcement discretion. For example, a campus security officer stops a student for drunk driving (which makes this high-risk decision making) on campus three hours after the graduation ceremony in late May. The student is in his ROTC (Reserve Officer Training Corps) uniform with a shiny second lieutenant bar on each shoulder. The officer decides that arresting and charging the student might very adversely affect the just-graduated student's future. So, she decides not to do the following: arrest the student, take the student to jail, issue a ticket for drunk driving, and impound the student's car. Instead, the officer has the student call a friend to drive him home, leaving his car to be picked up later. You can decide whether that would be exercise of good judgment by the officer. (Of course, we know it couldn't be good judgment if the officer considered the race or gender of the student.)

All types of professionals, even professional artists and musicians, make important decisions. An excellent prosecutor has superb judgement about how to handle criminal cases, including offering of plea bargains. I'm sure that the best surgeons do an excellent job of making decisions that arise during surgery.

A type of my own judgment that I am trying to improve concerns decisions I make while playing duplicate bridge. Bridge is a carefully simulated high-risk activity. Though I have a fairly high level of achievement in bridge, I am still trying to improve. This is not simple or easy. The American Contract Bridge League (ACBL) has a magazine, *The Bridge Bulletin*. For three years, I have been carefully reading and rereading old issues of that magazine, trying to use this repetition to help me to learn advanced methods that are hard to understand, learn, and use. Recently, I have decided to stop competing primarily as an aggressive bidder, in favor of carefully considering the circumstances in deciding how to act. I assume that millions of Americans who make their own investment decisions go through similar thinking about their decision style and strategy.

During the middle 1980s, I directed a major research project concerning police officer knowledge of search and seizure law (Memory & Smith, 1988). In a secondary study of judge knowledge of search and seizure law, I found that the only activity that increased judge knowledge was regular self-study of the subject. So, that is what I am doing concerning bridge—regular self-study.

Quality of judgment can vary substantially in a given activity. I know that, though I am a very good bridge player, I can't exercise judgement in bridge as well as "top" players. Though I am a good writer (or probably was when I had a younger brain), I know that many, many writers in many different types of writing have exhibited substantially better judgment and creativity in writing than I have.

High-stakes poker is a high-risk activity. If you watch poker on TV, you hear very detailed analyses of the strategies of the players. Because luck is a major factor in poker, the players who exercise the best judgment don't necessarily win the most money. Recently, I watched the final table of a very lucrative poker tournament. The player who won the tournament had previously never had any significant success in tournament poker. A similar outcome would never occur in duplicate bridge.

We can use behavioral archeology to conclude that small groups of hunter-gatherer men in Africa 100,000 years ago who hunted together virtually always exercised superb judgment in dealing with the many types of serious danger they encountered. So, how can we justifiably conclude that? If they had not exercised superb judgment in dealing with many great dangers, some number of them could have been killed. For a hunter-gather band, having several men killed and several gravely wounded probably would have resulted in failure of the group to survive.

I strongly believe that in every difficult field the top practitioners have an uncanny ability to optimize good results and minimize bad results, to a large extent through excellent judgment in decision making. (Of course, other things, such as access to high-tech, creativity, and leadership, influence effectiveness and success.)

It is important to understand that some people who engage in high-risk activities do not have sufficiently good judgment. I recently played bridge against a masters-level engineer who presents himself as an excellent player. When he made a particular bid, I realized that it is impossible for him to ever become a competent bridge player.

So, how do I think people can improve their judgment in their chosen field? After excellent education, I think they can (1) do regular self-study of their field; (2) learn from the achievements of top people in their field; and (3) continue to learn emerging problem solutions and methods in their field. (You can search on the Internet for "10 ways to improve your decision-making skills" on the WISEBREAD website.)

A medium-risk activity gone bad. In the early 1990s, I was scheduled to lead about 25 Boy Scouts and their leaders on a four-mile float on the severely flooded Lumber River in south-central NC. After they arrived at the put-in place, I tried to convince them that it was too risky to have the float. The Scouts insisted on floating. (Novices often don't understand how great the risks in an activity are.) About five canoes capsized very soon after embarking. If we had continued, probably all of the canoes but mine might have been capsized, with some of the canoeists struggling to swim from under giant growths of poison ivy. I informed the leaders that I was stopping the float. It took two hours to get everyone back to the put-in place. I believe it is clear that I showed bad judgment in allowing the float to start. In more dangerous activities, a similar incident could result in deaths and/or serious injuries.

The best and worst high-risk judgment from members of the same family. In the Cuban missile crisis in 1962, President Kennedy took the U.S. and USSR to the brink of nuclear holocaust to force USSR leader Khrushchev to remove Soviet missiles from Cuba. Khrushchev backed down, and the missiles were removed. JFK exhibited remarkably fine judgment.

In 1999 JFK, Jr., demonstrated the worst possible judgment when he flew a plane in weather conditions he was not trained to cope with. Tragically, the plane crashed, causing the deaths of his two passengers—his wife and her sister—and JFK, Jr.

"Everybody makes mistakes." This is a well-accepted saying in the U.S. that has been used in the titles of songs and books. While I think that saying is true, I believe it is very important for us to try extremely hard to avoid making very bad, very harmful mistakes. JFK, Jr., made an extremely bad, extremely harmful mistake.

Risk management. Risk management is an important function in many industries. It involves attempting to capitalize on positive opportunities, while identifying and reducing risks. This short sentence fails to communicate the great importance of risk and opportunity management in many corporations. I have a friend who was a high-level executive in an aircraft manufacturing corporation, with functions relating to risk and opportunity management. She reports that executives vary greatly regarding skills in risk management.

Clint VanZndt is a retired FBI agent who heads VanZandt Associates, Inc., which is described on the Internet as "an international threat and risk assessment group, specializing in behavioral and forensic analysis." Since VanZandt is not concerned with positive opportunities and does not actually manage risks, I think "risk assessment" does describe his function.

The main relevant issues. In trying to think systematically about this subject, I think we should consider the following issues.

What are and how great are the potential gains?

How great are the risks? It is important to know that in some high-risk activities, there are more than one significant risk. There can be problems regarding being able to know how great the risks are. For example, in white-water kayaking, the participants may not be able to know for sure how dangerous some stretches of white-water will be. During the summer of 2018, a couple took their three daughters kayaking. All three daughters and their father drowned. I suspect that they didn't have life jackets on.

In duplicate bridge against even good opponents, I take risks that I would not even consider taking against genuinely superb players, such as the Joyces in Chapel Hill, NC. They have caught me doing something that was unreasonably risky several times.

How great is the skill of the individual(s)? Developing participants in a high-risk activity need to be informed and realistic about how well their skills are developing.

Is this level of skill sufficient for the present activity? At the first tee of the Beth Page Black golf course, there is a sign warning that the course is intended to be played by strong players.

How great a risk of serious injury or death or other very adverse outcome will be tolerated? Mount Everest climbers are willing to accept between a 1-in-11 risk and 1-in-16 risk that they will die in the attempt.

The importance of avoiding or dealing well with anxiety and stress (the physiological stress reaction), which can occur during a high-risk activity or decision making. Anxiety and the physiological stress reaction can adversely affect a person's performance in a high-risk activity or high-risk decision making. We can describe countless activities and situations in which troublesome anxiety or experiencing of the physiological stress reaction would make the person unable to perform adequately well or make decisions competently.

A person can be unaware that major anxiety and the stress reaction can arise during a high-risk activity or decision making. Obviously, it is important to deal with that possibility well ahead of time. Having been a very low-level professional musician, I will assure you that you cannot whistle well in front of an audience if you get nervous.

Risks presented by particular activities. An article ("Charted: the 20 deadliest jobs in America") on the Washington Post website reports that the most dangerous occupation in 2013 in the U.S. was logging, followed by commercial fishing and aircraft piloting. The information was from the U.S. Bureau of Labor Statistics. Below is a list of additional at least fairly high-risk work activities.

Military leadership at all ranks, either in combat or otherwise physically
   dangerous activities. All military service members may encounter
   great risks.
Spying, espionage
Many types of investing (Some investing is designed to be very low-risk.)
Policing (Types of policing vary greatly in risks involved.)
Handling dangerous animals
Many types and aspects of practice of law, including trials
Some aspects of politics (e.g., spending much of your net worth in a run
   for office)
Very competitive industries involving substantial monetary investment
Many types and aspects of medical practice
EMT
Producing plays
Entering a costly and competitive field of education and employment
Working on a bomb squad
Bail bondsmen trying to apprehend bail-bond jumpers
Some types and aspects of engineering
Aspects of construction (Fifty thousand Chinese Nationalists died
   building a highway across Taiwan.)
Building demolition
Airplane piloting
Lending to risky startup-up businesses

Recreational activities which are sometimes genuinely risky activities
Risky snow skiing with risks of avalanches, dangerous falls, and collisions

Rock climbing
Bicycling in difficult mountainous terrain while performing difficult
    dangerous tricks
Risky white-water canoeing
Some other types of boating and sailing
Sports betting and other types of betting
Casino gambling
High-stakes poker
Some types of hunting
Many types of racing
Some types of animal training
Several sports, including football and golf, have high-risk aspects

Recreational activities which simulate a high-risk activity
Bridge
Chess
Low-stakes poker

Military parachuting. For nearly three years I was "on jump status" as an
Army parachutist in the 82nd Airborne Division. Risks confronted by parachutists in combat are limited in the following ways: (1) the planes fly low;
(2) the parachutes cause the soldiers to descend quickly, which limits the time
enemy soldiers can shoot at the parachuting soldiers; (3) the parachutes are
not "guidable", because that type of chute increases collisions of parachutists
in the air; (4) landing on the ground using an ordinary Army parachute is as
severe as jumping off of a 16-foot building; therefore, parachutists are trained
in making a PLF (parachute landing fall) to reduce injuries.

High-risk decision making. Driving is a high-risk activity in which we
engage in important decision making. A college student decides to attend a
university or college that will require incurring substantial higher education
debt. The student is accepting the risk that, after graduation, he or she will
not be able to obtain high paying work that would make prompt payment of
the debt possible. Similarly, when a student selects a college major and then
continues that education on the graduate level, the student is taking the risk
that she or he will not be able to obtain reasonably high paying work in that

field. In 1981, eight history doctoral students at Florida State University were awarded a PhD. I was told that only one of them got work related to history during a reasonable job-search period. That person became the curator of a museum.

I recently learned that the music department at a campus of the University of North Carolina does not allow any students to major in music performance. Though thousands of music-performance majors graduate from college in the U.S. every year, only about 175 music-performance jobs become available every year. The writer of the foreword of this book, Dr. Barbara Memory, graduated with high honors with a major in music performance (violin) from Michigan State University. Though she has had many successes as a professional violinist, she pursued music therapy as her career. She earned a PhD in music education from MSU and had a very successful career as a professor teaching music therapy.

In important ways, parenting can be a high-risk activity. Barbara Bush was a highly successful first lady. I believe that you cannot convincingly argue that she succeeded in mothering in ways that would help her son to be an excellent president. (I assumed that GWB would be the worst president from FDR to the present. Unfortunately, it appears that I was wrong.)

Marriage can be a high-risk decision. A pre-nuptial agreement minimizes the risk for the one with a lot of money, high earning ability, and/or likelihood of significant inheritance.

Risk in investing. We all understand that investing can involve assumption of significant risks and that investment advisers can offer a variety of investment plans, from a low-risk, relatively low-return plan to medium-risk and medium-return plans to high-risk and high-return plans.

I know a man who in 2007 had accumulated an excellent investment portfolio that would easily have supported him and his wife in comfortable retirement for decades. During 2007, he talked with his investment adviser about "cashing in his chips" and putting his money in no-risk funds. He decided to leave his money in the risky funds. When the 2007 economic crash occurred, he lost a very high percentage of his money and lost his ability to ever retire.

Another man I know stayed for many years with a broker who was a friend. If this stock investor had gotten a better broker in a better company, he nearly surely would have come out at least $100,000 better off.

Many years ago I decided not to invest in stocks, making my own decisions, because I do not have (1) required knowledge and experience; (2) access to important information; (3) ability to absorb a significant loss; and (4) emotional makeup needed for high-risk investing.

Decisions about forces that influence world climate. Once scientists warned about the dangers of climate change, governments and industries around the planet have been making high-risk decisions relating to the future habitability of our planet. As of early 2018, experts apparently believe that it is too late to prevent extensive global warming and the resulting adverse effects.

A classic example of bad high-risk decision making in sports. In the Master's golf tournament in 1985, Curtis Strange was leading as the last nine holes started. In that nine, there were two moderately long par-five holes. Strange attempted to hit his second shot on to the green on each of those holes. Both times, he failed, and he scored a bogey 6, which was one over par. If he had "laid up" by hitting his second shot on each hole so that he would have had a short and comfortable third shot to the green, he probably would have scored a 4 on one hole and a 5 on the other, resulting in a victory in the Masters.

The opposite decision making was done by Zack Johnson in a recent Master's tournament. He never tried to hit his second shot onto the green of a par-five hole. He knew that he was extremely good in short wedge shots. Zack won the Master's.

Improving your thinking and memory to improve your decision making and judgment. I always take heart- and brain-healthy supplements and do a brisk walk before playing duplicate bridge. Similarly, top international poker player Chris Mortensen exercises before playing poker. For me to play golf well, I have to prepare my brain to perform well. That helps me to make good decisions and, I think, actually improves my ability to execute a good swing.

Taking a nap can have cognitive-functioning benefits. During WWII, U.S. military pilots were allowed to take a nap during long flights, with the co-pilot at the plane controls.

<u>Decision making in potentially self-destructive activities</u>. Chapter 16 is about self-destructive behavior. Potentially self-destructive activities often involve individuals taking risks that rational and responsible persons would not take.

REFERENCES

Memory, John (2003). "Application of the theory of Chicago-scoring partnership bridge to two-officer patrol policing." Presented at annual meeting of the Academy of Criminal Justice Sciences in Boston, MA.

Memory, J.M. (1977). PEND: police exercise of non-enforcement discretion. Unpublished master's area paper. Florida State University: Tallahassee, FL.

Memory, J.M. & Smith, B. (1988). *Line police officer knowledge of search and seizure law: results of an exploratory multi-city test*. National Institute of Justice: Washington, DC. (Data have been available from the Inter-University Consortium for Political and Social Research, Ann Arbor, MI.)

CONCLUSIONS AND IMPLICATIONS

<u>Several over-arching conclusions.</u>

(1) I strongly believe that the medical establishment and the pharmacological establishment in the U.S. engage in measures to keep ordinary Americans from independently obtaining and acting on non-medical, non-drug information relating to health, some of which I have included in the first 15 chapters. Fortunately for me, I have discovered much of that information over the last 36 years and have acted on it, resulting in great benefits and favorable outcomes for me.

(2) Working hard on your physical health, physical strength, mental health, heart health, and brain health for decades before becoming a "senior citizen" will strongly tend to "pay off" during old age. Even working hard on strength needed for golf can have great payoffs later in life.

(3) The industrial and financial complex in the U.S. operates to achieve maximum spending and borrowing by Americans. Unfortunately, spending and/or borrowing too much results in major financial problems for many millions of Americans.

(4) Political correctness seriously decreases ability in our society to get certain types of information needed in solution of problems and in other important actions.

(5) As discussed in several chapters, a rapid deterioration of race relations is occurring in the U.S. Both Black-on-White homicide and

White-on-Black homicide have increased significantly in recent years. Also, Americans believe that incivility has become a very serious problem in American society.

Though I am an agnostic, I believe that an important remedy for these very serious problems can be significant increase in behavior by individuals according to some religion's Golden Rule, "Do unto others as you would have them do unto you." (PfLaum Publishing Co. markets an excellent poster providing information about versions of the Golden Rule of many religious groups. If I had one or more young children, I would put one of those posters on a wall or bulletin board in our house.)

I have a fine Republican, agnostic friend who says, "I just try to live by the Golden Rule," and he clearly succeeds in doing that. I think that many billions of small acts of courtesy, kindness, helpfulness, and caring can make a big positive difference. For example, when I go to a nearby mall to walk briskly before duplicate bridge games, I go out of my way (without acting strangely) to open a mall door for one or more African-Americans. For another example, since I was in my late teens, I have enjoyed joking around with African-Americans, who generally have excellent senses of humor. I recently saw an African-American man, who is probably retired from Army active duty, at my golf course standing by his beautiful, shiny car. As I walked by, I asked, "Sir, do you ever do anything other than polishing that car?" He and I both laughed. If he had said the same thing to me, if roles had been reversed, I would have known he was joking and would have appreciated that friendly interaction. I understand that joking with a stranger can be risky and fear that ability to joke with strangers is becoming less common in the U.S.

If a White friend and I were scheduled to have a golf match for a few dollars against two Black male friends, I would consider it very friendly and fun for one of them to say, "Are you guys ready to get your butts kicked?" I would try to come up with a witty return. If roles were reversed, I, for sure, wouldn't ask, "Are you **boys** ready to get your butts kicked?"

Implications. I, a retired professor, listed 36 different clusters of information regarding a very high percentage of which I believe coverage in university and college courses is nearly certainly nonexistent or woefully deficient. My guess is that there are many retirees (including my twin brother David, who is a retired full professor of education) who have as much, or more, of this type of information as I have. If this is true, there is a very vast amount of important information which college students are generally not able to study in undergraduate courses.

If one assumes that nearly all of the information in this book is very seldom, if ever, covered in undergraduate university and college courses, an important and fascinating question arises: "Why isn't it often covered?" While there could be major research on that subject, I will offer some answers to that question in a long sentence. I think that some of the reasons that information covered in the chapters of this book is not often covered in college courses are political correctness, trepidation of professors regarding criticizing widely prescribed drugs (mainly statins), desire to avoid offending powerful industrial and financial groups, desire to avoid offending people working in the professor's field outside of academia, desire to avoid providing health information that might result in civil liability, desire to avoid communicating information and ideas that will be likely to prompt strong criticism by groups outside the university, hesitance to cover content that presumably is mainly of interest to "senior citizens," desire to avoid jeopardizing the professor's chance to gain academic tenure, lack of a professor who is competent to teach a course, lack of interest of professors in some possible courses, and lack of sufficient relevant literature.

As this book was being completed, I became aware of an important book by Ludianoff and Haidt (2018), *The Coddling of the American Mind,* which is cited in the preface. The authors argue that especially in recent years college and university students have been stridently, and effectively, protesting professor teaching of certain ideas and even using particular words. In this book, I have not adequately discussed possible influence of students regarding courses offered and course content. In chapter 25 I provide extensive and strident criticism of President Trump. If a college or university professor made such statements in class, it is likely that they would provoke strong objections by students who support Trump. This may give us hints about evolution of political correctness in the higher education context. It also suggests that, when a professor has correct, valuable, potentially important information that would be strongly resisted by a substantial percentage of students, it may not be feasible to teach that information. We can hope that professors in that situation will find other ways to disseminate that information.

A significant percentage of professors have numerous publications concerned with their primary area of specialization. While this is admirable, many professors may, as a result, have little information outside of their areas of specialization. Of course, there no doubt are additional explanations for absence of important information from college and university courses.

Ways to identify and collect "missing" important information. It seems to me that it would make sense for universities and colleges to attempt to "mine" the knowledge of their graduates for valuable ideas about important information to include in courses. Of course, independent scholars might undertake a project to identify and collect this information. This probably would require participation of a very large number of subject experts.

ABOUT THE AUTHOR

Now 74 years old, John Madison Memory grew up (1949–61) from age five in Riverton, a rural community in Scotland County in south-central North Carolina. He was an Eagle Scout and received the Vigil Honor in scouting. John is a 1965 Wake Forest College graduate (BA, History), holds the JD degree (WFU, 1968) and a PhD in criminology (FSU, 1981), and is a retired Army Reserve JAG LTC. He has one child, Alex, who is working in the computer field and will soon be awarded a PhD in computer science.

John's working career primarily involved teaching Criminal Justice at the college/ university level. He was an associate professor in his last position. Information about John's publications is given in the references section of chapter 35.

John's five years of Army active duty service (1969–74) included one year as the commander of a military police company in Korea (when he won the 7th Division handball tournament) and two years as a JAG in the 82nd Airborne Division. He was an active Army Reserve JAG lawyer for 17 years. All of his Army Reserve assignments involved giving legal advice and support to a commander (a colonel or general) and his widely diverse staff.

Since his last university teaching job ended in 2004, he has lived in Columbia, SC, for five years and in Hendersonville, NC, for nine years.

As he discussed in the chapter about recreation, John has put more time and energy into recreation, hobbies, and avocations than most people. Though he lettered in tennis in his last two years at WFC, his main sport in later life has been golf. In duplicate bridge, he achieved Gold Life Master in 2016, which is four levels above Life Master. As did his **very** distant cousin George Washington, John enjoys dancing. Since his early teens, John has enjoyed composing and performing music. In college and law school, he was in two excellent professional folk singing groups. He and several excellent female singing partners have performed "the old songs" (1999–2012) about 250 times, mainly for groups of senior citizens. To hear some or all of John's 2016 CD of his whistling to his guitar accompaniment of 17 of his tune compositions, search for "Whistlin' Memory's favorite tunes on Bandcamp." John recommends his favorite, #14.

In addition to his scholarly publications, John has, over the years, had dozens of unpaid non-professional writing projects, several non-scholarly publications, and more than 15 published newspaper op-eds.

Author's statement about his values and ideology. As I mention several times in this book, I have never voted for a Republican; Bernie Sanders has been my favorite U.S. Senator for many years; and I worked very hard (no pay) and, I think, constructively for the Obama campaign in 2008 and Secretary Clinton in 2016. I strongly believe in "progressive" approaches for dealing with a wide variety of problems in the U.S. As elaborated in chapter 23, I support many "core" conservative values. I grew up in a fine Southern Baptist church and feel fortunate that exposure to Christian morality, such as the Golden Rule, was an important part of my upbringing.

Extraordinary challenges encountered by the author. I will sadly note that my actual childhood trauma and health challenges have been significantly greater than described by me immediately below. I decided it was better not to provide some details. A list of trauma and challenges follows.

Several types of severe childhood trauma, including the tragic death of my father when I was five years old. As a result of childhood trauma, I experienced severe post-traumatic stress disorder (PTSD).

Grew up without a father. My oldest brother is a deeply disturbed and disabled paranoid-schizophrenic. Because of these things, I failed to learn much important information during my childhood. (Fortunately, I had an excellent mother.)

Amblyopia ("lazy eye") of left eye, with some double vision, resulting in lifelong extremely slow reading.

Sexually abused by much older male when I was 11. Sexual abuse of children is very likely to be traumatic.

In one of his excellent books, Malcolm Gladwell discusses research showing that older students in a school class tend to have better life outcomes than younger students. Because I started the first grade four months early, the oldest students in my school and college class were 16 months older than me.

Lifelong sleep disorder(s), preventing long healthful stretches of sleep. On an average night, I awaken and urinate between six and eight times.

Low thyroid function, which causes tendency to gain weight. I obtained remedial medication in about 2008. I learned early in 2018 that this medication has not been overcoming my low thyroid function. My integrative physician has prescribed medication that should be effective.

Some physicians believe that having very acid urine nearly all of the time indicates a dangerous tendency of the body to have pH that is too low (acid). My urine is always between acid and very acid.

Low dissolved oxygen, resulting in use of insurance-paid oxygen machine at night since about 2008.

Possibly as a result of low dissolved oxygen, I have had four types of cancer. In addition to non-metastasizing basal cell cancer (many times), I have had potentially metastasizing squamous skin cancer (many times), melanoma, and prostate cancer.

Extremely severe risk factors for heart disease, brain disease, metabolic syndrome, and type 2 diabetes ((e.g., high LDL, very high triglycerides, very low HDL, very small LDL and HDL particles (which increase health risks), high inflammation, high insulin resistance, high homocysteine)).

Tests in 2018 indicated that I am in the second from the most severe category regarding risk of developing Alzheimer's.

Since briefly taking Lipitor in 2001, I have occasionally had tachycardia (pulse 180 bpm), which for many people is life threatening. If my arteries had not been very strong and clear of occlusion, the first instance of tachycardia might have been fatal (heart attack or stroke).

I have had one deep-vein thrombosis (left leg) after a long occurrence of tachycardia and a pulmonary embolism after another long occurrence of tachycardia. DVT and PE, which are caused by blood clots, can be very dangerous.

Vulnerability to becoming depressed, inherited from my father and increased by low thyroid function.

Vulnerability to experiencing anxiety and the physiological stress reaction. Confirmed while practicing law in 1968–69.

My tendency to "do the right thing," probably resulting from an "over-active conscience." This resulted in bad outcomes for me about six times during my working career. If you have an "over-active conscience," you nearly certainly have also in that situation under-active rational capacity, of which I am not proud.

<u>Adverse outcomes that could have resulted from these things</u>

Becoming a non-surviving or surviving casualty of mental health problems (especially depression)

Emphatic professional/vocational failure

Financial failure, from which I would not have been able to recover

Death or severe reduction in quality of life resulting from heart attack or other aspect of cardiovascular disease

Early development of symptoms of Alzheimer's or other dementia

Death from metastasized cancer

<u>My actual outcomes at age 74.</u> None of these adverse outcomes have materialized. Because **I have worked very hard on mental health, physical health, heart health, and brain health for many decades,** I now have a very good life situation and quality of life and have an excellent relationship with my fine and capable son. I am pleased with my present capabilities in my important activities (e.g., bridge, golf, composing and performing music, dancing, writing). Recent cardiovascular health screenings indicate that I have excellent heart health. As discussed in this book, I am optimistic about beating prostate cancer. Recent in-depth brain function evaluation indicated that I have very good brain health and function. An Internet website produced a prediction that I will live until my early 90s.

CPSIA information can be obtained
at www.ICGtesting.com
Printed in the USA
BVHW081359031218
534638BV00001B/43/P

9 781480 865655